The American
Cardiovascular Pandemic

T0197882

McFarland Health Topics

The American Cardiovascular Pandemic

A 100-Year History

DAVID GORDON

MCFARLAND HEALTH TOPICS

McFarland & Company, Inc., Publishers

Jefferson, North Carolina

ISBN (print) 978-1-4766-8512-0
ISBN (ebook) 978-1-4766-4415-8

LIBRARY OF CONGRESS AND BRITISH LIBRARY
CATALOGUING DATA ARE AVAILABLE

Library of Congress Control Number 2021047582

Front cover image © 2021 pickingpok/Shutterstock

Printed in the United States of America

*McFarland & Company, Inc., Publishers
Box 611, Jefferson, North Carolina 28640
www.mcfarlandpub.com*

TABLE OF CONTENTS

Acknowledgments

I dedicate this book to my wife Susan, who has not only encouraged and supported me at every step, but who has also shared the insights she gained during her years at the Chicago chapter of the American Heart Association in the late 1970s, where she helped coordinate public smoking, blood pressure, and diet education campaigns. Her stories about their successful efforts to persuade city restaurants to ban cigarettes helped put a human face on the vital impact of local volunteer organization in the battle against cardiovascular disease. She has patiently listened to me try out my ideas on her. No one could wish for a better partner in life.

I also want to express special thanks to my dear friend Debra Roney for her wonderful illustrations of atherosclerotic plaques (Figure 5.2), the coronary arteries (Figure 10.1), and the cardiac conduction system (Figure 12.1).

I am also deeply indebted to the NIH—and specifically the NHLBI—where I am fortunate to have spent most of my career. I could not have hoped to find a more supportive professional environment or one that better embodies the values of scientific rigor and integrity. Working at the NHLBI has enabled me to join a community of talented and dedicated professionals at NIH and at the institutions it serves in an extraordinary enterprise far larger than ourselves, guided by the twin goals of advancing human knowledge and ameliorating human disease. I have had the good fortune to work with many brilliant and dedicated colleagues on the studies described in this book over the course of my long career—too many to acknowledge individually here. However, I want to specifically thank George Mensah who invited me in 2016 to collaborate with him on an article for *Circulation Research* about the decline in cardiovascular mortality, which was the starting point for the present book. I also want to acknowledge another co-author of that article, Michael

Mussolino, who provided the health statistics for that article, which I have also used liberally in this book. Additionally, I want to thank Jeff Cutler for his constructive feedback on the first draft of this book and Jacques Rossouw for his historical perspective on the Women's Health Initiative.

I also want to express my deep gratitude and affection to my early mentors, who introduced me to cardiovascular epidemiology and clinical trials and without whom I might never have found my calling: Basil Rifkind (who gave me my first opportunity in this field and supported me at every turn), Al Tyroler and Gerardo Heiss (who supervised my Masters research), and Dale Williams and Ed Davis (who welcomed me to their Lipid Research Clinics Data Coordinating Center in Chapel Hill in 1979–84).

I also want to acknowledge the many other collaborators and friends—too numerous to name here—that I have made in my 42 years at NIH. These include my former NHLBI colleagues, many of whom worked on projects cited in this book: Robin Boineau, Bryan Brewer, Denis Buxton, James Cleeman, Patrice Desvigne-Dickens, Ray Ebert, Debra Egan, Lawrence Fine, Jerome Fleg, William Friedewald, Larry Friedman, Nancy Geller, Suzanne Goldberg, Ronald Goor, Max Halperin, Ahmed Hasan, Tracy Hoke, Erin Iturriaga, Ruth Kirby, Michael Lauer, Eric Leifer, Alice Mascette, Marissa Miller, Stephen Mockrin, Chuke Nwachuku, Gerald Payne, Gail Pearson, Michael Proschan, Diane Reid, Yves Rosenberg, Beth Schucker, Monica Shah, Susan Shurin, Sonya Skarlatos, Joni Snyder, George Sopko, Paul Sorlie, Wendy Taddei-Peters, Momtaz Wassef, and Gina Wei. They also include my many collaborators and friends outside the walls of NIH: Colin Baigent, Noel Bairey Merz, Elizabeth Barrett Connor, Reagan Bradford, Maria Brooks, Barry Davis, Katherine Detre, Robert Frye, Curt Furberg, Saul Genuth, Scott Grundy, David Herrington, Judith Hochman, Howard Hodis, Donald Hunninghake, Anthony Keach, James Knoke, Lewis Kuller, Gervasio Lamas, John LaRosa, Jay Mason, Lemuel Moyé, Pamela Ouyang, Marc Pfeffer, Bertram Pitt, Stuart Pocock, Jeff Probstfield, Paul Ridker, Robert Simari, Neil Stone, Jonathan Tolbert, Joel Verter, David Waters, Paul Whelton, Janet Wittes, Jackson Wright, and Faiez Zannad. Thanks also to those who have shared their ideas or listened to or critiqued my ideas at a scientific symposium or in a casual conversation, and those whose journal articles I have read or who have read mine. To the many who have influenced my thinking and understanding in unknowable ways, I hope this book reflects well on what you have taught me.

Finally, I want to gratefully acknowledge the thousands of volunteers who have selflessly participated in the many cardiovascular clinical trials chronicled in this book. If it takes a village to raise a child, it takes a good-sized city to achieve the successes our community has realized together.

PREFACE

On a brisk October day in 1978, barely a year after I came to work as a medical officer for a major National Institutes of Health (NIH)-sponsored cholesterol trial, I took my seat in the back row of a conference room in Bethesda, Maryland, as an international group of experts convened to review the evidence of a promising recent trend in mortality from heart attack and stroke in the U.S. and abroad.[1] Speakers included such major luminaries in the relatively new field of cardiovascular epidemiology as Nemat Borhani, Fred Epstein, Lew Kuller, Framingham leader Bob Garrison, and NIH health statistics guru Thomas Thom. And, of course, prominently featured was the father of preventive cardiology, Jeremiah Stamler, then approaching age 60, who had famously faced down the House Un-American Activities Committee in 1965 and defeated them in the Supreme Court, and who remains a fierce and productive advocate of cardiovascular health 42 years later.[2] The speakers list and audience also included many of rising stars in the field. After two days, the conferees concluded that heart attacks and strokes had indeed declined by as much as 25% since 1968, although they could not pin down exactly why.

This seemingly modest decline in heart attacks and strokes was actually a very big deal. It may surprise you to know that the 1960s were not only an era of social turmoil and upheaval, but also a decade in which more than 6.3 million Americans died of heart disease (mainly heart attacks) and another 1.8 million died of strokes.[3] The per capita death toll from heart disease in the 1960s was higher than in any decade before or since and the total was 110 times the 58,220 U.S. fatalities recorded during the entire Vietnam War.[4] Yet as a medical student in the late 1960s and early 1970s, I had a blasé attitude toward heart attacks. Yes, heart attacks were the number one cause of death by far in the U.S. and other developed countries, causing twice as many deaths as cancer (which ranked second), but didn't they happen mainly to old people seemingly as the end result of a

1

degenerative process of aging, i.e., hardening and narrowing of the arteries which provide the heart with blood and oxygen? From the distant perspective of a 32-year-old man, I thought this was sad, but we are not meant to live forever.

Now, to be sure, heart attacks did not happen only to the elderly, but too often struck in middle age, especially in middle-aged men with a family history of high cholesterol and early heart disease. While most of the 8.2 million cardiac deaths in the 1960s occurred in older persons, approximately one-third of all cardiac deaths in 1968–77 occurred before age 65—about 20% before age 45 and another 20% between ages 45 and 54.[5] Thus, it was not unusual for seemingly healthy middle-aged men and even women to be stricken down at the peak of their productivity, leaving their dependent families bereft. I had witnessed this phenomenon first-hand in my own circle of acquaintances. Indeed, the cholesterol trial I was working on in 1978 specifically focused on otherwise healthy "middle-aged" men, aged 35–59, with high cholesterol, who were thought most susceptible to a "premature" heart attack and thus most likely to benefit from a cholesterol-lowering drug.

In 1978, no one really knew whether the recent 25% decline in mortality from heart attacks and strokes was just a chance fluctuation or the beginning of a trend, or (if the latter) what factors were responsible. The ensuing four decades have brought clarity. As of 2017, heart attack mortality rates had fallen by 81% since their peak in 1968.[6] Stroke mortality rates fell by 77% during this same period, continuing a trend that began 60 years earlier. This progress has been hard won by a combination of basic and applied laboratory research, broad and far-reaching epidemiological studies, and expensive multiyear clinical trials in human volunteers. Occasionally, the road to progress has been easy and direct; more often it has been marked by false starts, setbacks, detours, dead ends, and outright failures. But science thrives on the failure of its favored hypotheses to pan out. Human inquiry generally begins with an observation and a question—How? Why? What if?—and progresses to a theory. What distinguishes scientific from other kinds of inquiry is a compulsion to put our theories and explanations to a test, to disprove old truths, and replace them with new truths. In science, all truths are tentative. Science takes to heart Alexander Pope's dictum that "no one should be ashamed to admit they are wrong, which is but saying, in other words, that they are wiser today than they were yesterday."[7]

Today, our basic understanding of why people have heart attacks and strokes has been revolutionized, and effective treatment options have multiplied. Cardiovascular disease is no longer viewed as an inevitable feature of the natural course of aging, and complacency has given way to hope. In this book, I will offer my inside look as a 42-year NIH employee at how this remarkable success was achieved. It is a multifaceted story with many unexpected twists. Sometimes I can speak as an active player in this community enterprise, other times as a colleague or adviser, and occasionally as the proverbial fly on the wall. I hope to hit the highlights without overly dwelling on statistical detail, but some statistics are essential to the story. I will focus on developments that have demonstrably influenced the course of the rise and decline of cardiovascular mortality since 1900, but my story will also include a few notable dry wells. If this story is comparable to an Agatha Christie whodunit, it is *The Murder on the Orient Express*.[8] Multiple suspects had a hand in it.

1

A Gentle Pandemic?

Those of you who lived through the 1960s may be asking, "What coronary pandemic? Did I miss something?" The 1960s were known for the Beatles, Vietnam, the civil rights movement, hippies, Woodstock, and the moon landing—not a pandemic. Certainly, there was nothing like the current novel coronavirus pandemic, which threatens to rival the fierce and grisly 1918–19 influenza pandemic that killed 675,000 Americans and 40–50 million people worldwide in two years.[1] But not all pandemics are infectious, and not all pandemics are explosive and grisly. The 20th-century cardiovascular disease pandemic that peaked in the 1960s was an instance of a slow-moving non-infectious pandemic, which killed millions, but far more slowly and almost gently.

How is it possible to experience a pandemic without even realizing it? Let me begin with the story of A.L., a prosperous 53-year-old businessman I encountered as a medical student, who checked into a Chicago hospital in the early 1970s after experiencing crushing chest pain one spring night. His pain, which radiated down his left arm, and his electrocardiogram (ECG) were typical of an acute myocardial infarction (MI)—a "heart attack" in common parlance—which occurs when a fatty deposit (atherosclerotic plaque, in medical jargon) in the wall of one of the major coronary arteries, ruptures and forms a clot that suddenly and catastrophically obstructs the flow of oxygen-carrying blood to a portion of the heart muscle (myocardium). Confirmatory blood tests showed typically high levels of cardiac enzymes, normally found only inside cells, which had spilled into the bloodstream from oxygen-starved heart muscle cells.

Nothing about A.L.'s prior medical history was out of the ordinary. His blood pressure (BP)—160/90 mmHg—and cholesterol level—270 mg/dL—were elevated by today's standards but were then considered to be in the upper range of normal. He smoked a pack of cigarettes per day. He had a modest middle-aged paunch, but he was not obese and did not have diabetes. His father and an older brother had died of heart attacks in their late 50s, but three other siblings (a brother and two sisters) were fine and eventually lived past the age of 75. In some ways, A.L., who never lost consciousness, was fortunate in that many victims of a fatal heart attack simply collapsed and died on the spot or their bodies were discovered in their beds or chairs after being fine when last seen.[2] So A.L. was treated in the usual prescribed manner, spending 36 hours in intensive coronary care, where he was monitored closely and given oxygen, intravenous lidocaine (a chemical relative of cocaine and Novocain) to control his heart rhythm and suppress extra beats, and morphine (an opiate) as needed for sedation and pain control. No coronary angiogram was done (as it would be today) since no invasive procedures were contemplated. Coronary artery bypass surgery was still in its infancy at that time, and coronary angioplasty and stents were not yet in use. When his vital signs and heart rhythm were stable, A.L. was moved to a quiet private room to rest and recuperate. A few days later, during morning rounds, he was found dead on the floor of his private hospital room, having collapsed while shaving.

A.L. was not an unusual case. Indeed, he was one of approximately 2.15 million middle-aged American men, aged 45–64, who died of heart attacks during the peak of the pandemic in the U.S. in 1955 through 1974.[3] The pandemic did not spare women; almost 700,000 45- to 64-year-old women died of heart attacks during this period. Heart attacks also killed millions of older Americans, including 2.0 million men and 1.2 million women between the ages of 65 and 74 during these 20 years. Altogether, heart attacks accounted for 414–483 deaths per 100,000 Americans each year in 1955 through 1974.[4] In addition, the same pathological process (atherosclerosis) in the cerebral arteries, which supply oxygen-carrying blood to the brain, is a major contributing cause of stroke, which accounted for 136–183 deaths per 100,000 each year during this period.[5] Although perhaps one-third of strokes are due to bleeding rather than atherosclerosis, it is reasonable to assume that another 1.2 million Americans between ages 45 and 74 died of atherosclerotic strokes during these two decades. In 1968, the peak year of the pandemic in the U.S., 956,000 Americans died of heart disease or stroke— nearly half of the 1.93 million deaths recorded in the U.S. that year and about three times the death toll from cancer.[6] Atherosclerosis of the arteries of the heart and brain was likely the underlying cause for more than half a million of these deaths. Although this book will focus on trends in the United States, this surge in mortality was a worldwide phenomenon. Atherosclerotic heart disease was a true pandemic, similarly affecting industrialized countries throughout the world.

It had not always been this way. Let us flash back for a moment to 1900. The U.S. had only 45 states; Utah had just entered the union that year, and Oklahoma, New Mexico, Arizona, Alaska, and Hawaii had yet to be added. The U.S. population was roughly 76 million, of whom 30 million (39%) lived on farms.[7] The three leading causes of death—pneumonia and influenza, tuberculosis, and diarrheal and other gastrointestinal diseases— were all infectious.[8] Many of these deaths occurred in very young children, 10% of whom did not live to see their first birthday.[9] Thus, the average life expectancy was only 46.3 years for men and 48.3 years for women.[10] Heart disease was the fourth leading cause of death, but the age-adjusted heart disease mortality rate was only half of what it would become in 1968.[11] In other words, an American of any given age was twice as likely to die of heart disease in 1968 as in 1900.

Furthermore, many of these heart disease deaths were almost certainly unrelated to atherosclerosis, although it is impossible to say how many since separate mortality statistics were not recorded for heart attacks and other heart disease (rheumatic heart disease, congenital heart disease, cardiomyopathy, etc.) until 1950. However, Dr. William Osler, the preeminent turn-of-the-century Canadian American physician and medical scholar, observed that angina pectoris and its allied states (i.e., myocardial infarction) were relatively uncommon afflictions of men of high "station" over age 45. "It (angina) is an attendant rather of ease and luxury than of temperance and labor; on which account, though occurring among the poor, it is more frequently met with among the rich, or in persons of easy circumstances. It is remarkable how many prominent individuals have succumbed to the disease. We may say of it as Sydenham did of the gout, that more wise men than fools are its victims."[12] Putting aside Osler's conflation of wealth and wisdom in the last sentence and his conflation of lack of wealth with temperance and labor a few sentences earlier, Osler was quite correct in pointing to the remarkable frequency of prominent men (versus ordinary citizens) dying of heart attacks. According to their Wikipedia biographies, five of the nine presidents who served between 1876 and 1928 and escaped assassination (Hays, Cleveland, Taft, Harding, and Coolidge) died at ages 57–72 under circumstances suggesting coronary heart disease, and two others (Arthur and Wilson) died of strokes.[13] However, by mid-century, coronary heart disease flourished as Americans (and citizens of other industrialized countries) became plump and comfortable. Also, while angina pectoris may have been relatively uncommon in Osler's time, that is because many persons with coronary blockages died suddenly or in their sleep before ever seeing a doctor.

I have plotted the arc of the pandemic in Figure 1.1 for annual mortality from heart attack, all heart disease, stroke, and all cardiovascular disease in the U.S., expressed as deaths per 100,000 people and adjusted to the age distribution of the U.S. in 2000, covering more than a century from 1900 to 2017.[14] (Note also that reporting requirements were not uniform in all states and territories before 1932.) The "all cardiovascular disease classification" includes all heart disease, strokes, and other vascular diseases (like aortic aneurysms, venous thromboembolic disease, and peripheral artery disease).

It is clear in Figure 1.1 that heart diseases are the predominant component of cardiovascular death and that (at least after 1950) heart attacks are the predominant component of heart disease death. One sees that heart disease mortality more than doubled over the first half of the 20th century from only 265.4 per 100,000 in 1900 to 588.8 per 100,000 in 1950.

Age-Adjusted Mortality Rates

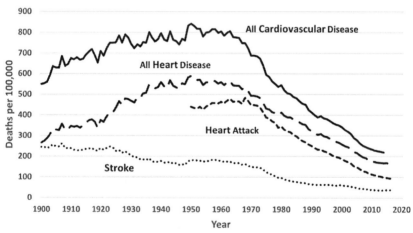

U.S. trends in age-adjusted mortality rates for Heart Attack (CHD), All Heart Disease, All Cardiovascular Disease, and Stroke, 1900–2017. Data were obtained from CDC Vital Statistics compilations.

Clearly, a significant pandemic had hit America. Total cardiovascular mortality increased less steeply because of the partially offsetting decline in stroke mortality during this period. While total cardiovascular and heart disease mortality leveled off in the 1950s, heart attack mortality continued to climb, peaking at 482.6 deaths per 100,000 in 1968. Since 1968, there have been sharp declines in all four of these categories over the ensuing five decades—81% in heart attack mortality, 69% in heart disease mortality, 77% in stroke mortality, and 71% in cardiovascular mortality. Translating these percentages into American lives, if conditions in 1968 had remained unchanged in 2017, an additional 1.13 million Americans (out of a population of 325 million) would have died of heart attacks and an additional 406,00 would have died of strokes.[15]

So why hasn't this pandemic been obvious all along? Outbreaks of infectious diseases have plagued mankind throughout history, going back to Biblical times and including the bubonic plague outbreaks of the middle ages and the introduction of smallpox and syphilis to the New World by European settlers. Indeed, the Book of Revelations names Plague as one of the four Horsemen of the Apocalypse. Even in the early 20th century, local outbreaks of cholera and yellow fever killed thousands, and millions died in the 1918–19 influenza pandemic, which attained global scope thanks to World War I. But the 20th-century heart disease pandemic was quite different. First, it was not contagious. Since most of its victims died quickly, quietly, and without much fuss, it did not incite panic or xenophobia. Second, unlike most infectious disease outbreaks, which thrive among poor people living in close quarters and with limited access to clean food and water, coronary heart disease epidemic began as a disease of affluence, promulgated by plentiful rich food and relative freedom from hard manual labor. Furthermore, the coronary heart disease pandemic happened over decades rather than months. By 1960, people suddenly collapsing and dying of heart attacks in their 50s and 60s became—not exactly normal—but part of the natural way of things. When then 25-year-old Paul McCartney and the Beatles poked gentle fun at the elderly in their 1967 song "When I'm 64," there is no doubt that people of that age were considered near the end of life, and that a quick and relatively painless cardiac collapse was sad but hardly shocking.[16] President Eisenhower, for example, was 64 years old when he had his first heart attack in 1955.[17] It is safe to say that Americans of that period would have been far more shocked at the idea that two men in their middle to late 70s would run for president in

2020 than by Eisenhower's condition in 1955.

Finally, although the heart attack rate at any given age has declined by more than 80% since 1968, this decline has served to put off coronary heart disease deaths to a later age, rather than prevent them entirely. Thus, if A.L. had been born 40 years later, he might still have died of a heart attack, but perhaps at age 73 instead of age 53, or perhaps he might have died of something else before his heart condition overtook him. So despite the steep fall in age-adjusted mortality rates over the past 50 years, heart disease has remained our leading cause of death, killing 655,000 Americans in 2017 and accounting for nearly one of every four deaths.[18] More than half of those deaths (365,914) were due to coronary heart disease.

Let us pause for a moment to consider the trajectory of the decline in heart attack mortality since it peaked in 1968. The decline is not linear. It can't be; otherwise the 50% decline in heart attack deaths per 100,000 over 23 years from 482.6 in 1968 to 240.6 in 1991 would have had to be followed by another 242 line deaths per 100,000 decline in the 23 years between 1991 and 2014, which would now leave us with a heart attack death rate below zero—an impossibility. So, when I tell you that heart attack mortality declined by 25% between 1990 and 2000, I mean that the heart attack

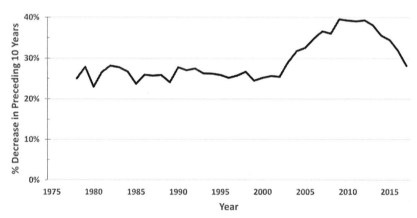

U.S. trend in rate of decline in heart attack mortality, 1978–2017. Each data point represents the 10-year decline in heart attack mortality rate over the preceding 10 years as a percent of the heart attack mortality rate 10 years earlier. Data were obtained from CDC Vital Statistics compilations.

mortality rate in 2000 had declined in the preceding decade by 25% of its 1990 rate—not by 25% of its 1968 rate. The percent decline per 10 years is plotted from 1978 to 2017 in Figure 1.2.

The percent decline per 10 years held steady between 23 and 28% before 2000. Mathematically, this is called a log-linear decline; that is, the *logarithm* of the death rate—not the death rate itself—declines linearly with the passage of time. The pace of decline then accelerated in the first decade of the new millennium, climbing to nearly 40% per 10 years in 2009–12, before falling back to 28% in 2017. I will return to this figure repeatedly in the coming chapters as I try to dissect the factors contributing to this pattern of decline.

The decline in heart disease rates since 1968 is clearly manifested in a gradual increase in life expectancy (Figure 1.3).[19]

As stated earlier, the average American born in 1900 could expect to live fewer than 50 years, largely due to the ravages of infectious respiratory and gastrointestinal diseases, which had a high death toll in children as well as adults. Heart disease (137 deaths per 100,000) ranked only fourth, while cerebrovascular disease (107) and cancer (64) were fifth and eighth, respectively.[20] Thanks to the profound decline in deaths from infectious diseases due to improved sanitation and the development of vaccines and antibiotics, life expectancy increased by 20 years (to 68.1 years in 1950) over the

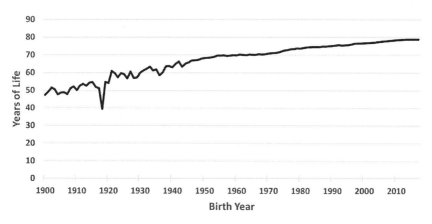

U.S. trend in life expectancy at birth, 1900–2017. Data were obtained from Berkeley and Macrotrends websites.

next five decades, despite the rise in vascular diseases and cancer, which displaced infectious diseases as the leading causes of death. (The transient 12-year life expectancy drop in 1918 reflects the profound impact of the 1918–19 influenza pandemic.) The rate of improvement slowed slightly in 1950–68, but then accelerated dramatically from 70.4 years 1968 to 78.9 years in 2013, until the recent rise of opioid deaths flattened the curve. The current coronavirus pandemic another—hopefully transient—1.5 year dip in 2020 (https://www.cdc.gov/nchs/pressroom/nchs_press_releases/2021/202107.htm). In the coming chapters, we will explore how this much overlooked 8.5-year gain in life expectancy over the past 50 years, largely reflecting the 81% declines in age-adjusted heart attack and 77% decline in stroke rates during this period, came about. It is a story of the success of scientists, physicians, health professionals, and public officials working tirelessly and collaboratively to understand atherosclerosis and to develop ways to prevent or treat its dire consequences on an individual and population level.

2

FRAMINGHAM,
MASSACHUSETTS

On April 12, 1945, as cardiovascular mortality was nearing its peak in the U.S., President Franklin Delano Roosevelt succumbed to a massive cerebrovascular hemorrhage (stroke) at age 63. Although his death shocked the American public, which had just elected him to his fourth term as president five months earlier, we know that FDR was suffering from malignant hypertension (his last blood pressure was a sky-high 300/190 mmHg) and advanced heart failure.[1] Indeed, one had only to look at the gaunt figure sitting between Churchill and Stalin at Yalta in February 1945, cigarette in hand, two months before his death, to realize that death was imminent.[2]

From 1935 to 1937 to 1941, FDR's blood pressure rose from 136/78 to 162/98 to 188/105—a level that would now be considered alarming. But at that time, although his 105 diastolic pressure (the blood pressure while the heart was between beats) was considered moderately elevated, his 188 systolic pressure (the blood pressure while the heart muscle is contracted) was considered a clinically inconsequential result of the normal arterial stiffening accompanying aging. No treatment was prescribed. No one advised him to stop smoking. It was not until 1944 when his chest X-ray showed an enlarged and failing heart, that the clinical significance of his high blood pressure was appreciated, and treatment—with digitalis and salt restriction—was initiated. It was perhaps the best that medicine could offer at that time, but it was too little, too late.

The profound ignorance and impotence of the most eminent medical specialists of the age to deal with the advancing cardiovascular pandemic, as illustrated by the fate of FDR, was the backdrop for the passage in Congress of the National Heart Act.[3] This act, which was signed into law by Harry Truman in October 1947, called for the establishment of the National Heart Institute as part of the National Institutes of Health (NIH) and for the

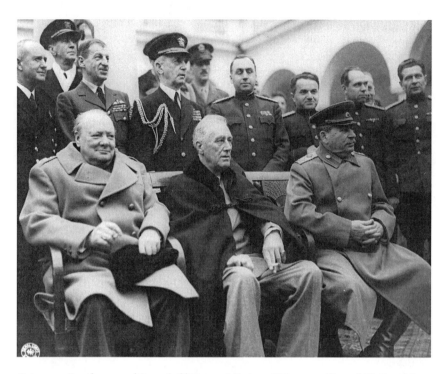

Crimean Conference. (From left) Prime Minister Winston Churchill, President Franklin D. Roosevelt, and Marshal Joseph Stalin at the palace in Yalta, where the Big Three met. National Archives, photo no. 111-SC-260486. http://loc. gov/pictures/resource/cph.3a10098/

design of an epidemiologic study of cardiovascular disease. Framingham, a middle-class (mostly white) Massachusetts factory town of 28,000 residents about 23 miles west of Boston was selected as the site of that study, because of its geographic proximity to Harvard and Boston University and because of its enthusiastic participation in the Framingham Tuberculosis Demonstration Study two decades earlier. Framingham's town hall style of government and its low rates of inward and outward migration also made it ideal for a long-term epidemiologic study. The Framingham study's first medical director, Dr. Gilcin Meadors, examined its first study participant on October 11, 1948. In April 1950, the directorship passed to Dr. Thomas Dawber, who along with Patricia McNamara and Dr. William Kannel, were responsible for its major early publications starting in 1957.[4]

So what is epidemiology? It is a science, dating back to the mid–19th century, in which investigators attempt to understand and control the outbreak of a disease in a population by learning as much as possible about the characteristics, habits, and environmental exposures of the persons in that population who got the disease did versus those who did not. It is essentially detective work, in which all the evidence is circumstantial. One does not need prior knowledge or even a prior working hypothesis as to the biological cause or pathology of the disease, although analysis of epidemiologic data may yield important biological clues. The prototypical epidemiologic success story was that of John Snow who used epidemiologic methods to trace the source of a severe outbreak of cholera in London's Soho district 1854 to contaminated water from the Broad Street pump.[5] Snow did not know or need to know that cholera was caused by a specific microbe (*Vibrio cholerae*); Pasteur, Koch and others did not establish the germ theory of infectious disease until almost 30 years later. Snow did not even know that the contamination came from diapers washed in a nearby leaky cesspool. All he knew was that all the cholera cases occurred in people who drank water drawn from the Broad Street pump; Soho residents who got their water from other sources—even those living in close proximity to affected households—did not contract cholera.

Cardiologists of the 1940s had better working hypotheses on the causes of heart disease than John Snow had to work with on cholera, but not enough to formulate coherent strategies on how to stem the pandemic. So, taking a page from the book of their predecessors in infectious disease, they turned to epidemiology. In 1948, the Framingham Heart Study (FHS) was the first major epidemiologic study of cardiovascular disease undertaken in the U.S. and the centerpiece of the research portfolio of the newly established National Heart Institute.[6] The study was quite simple in concept. Just over half (5209) of the town's 10,000 adult residents (ages 28–62) were recruited and enrolled over a four-year period. Each volunteer completed a detailed history and physical exam at their initial visit, and appropriate blood and urine samples were collected. Some samples were analyzed immediately for cholesterol, glucose, and other putative cardiovascular risk factors, while others were frozen and stored for future analysis. Then, participants were brought back at two-year intervals to assess their overall well-being and to perform additional examinations. Hospital records were collected for participants who had suffered a cardiovascular "event" (heart attack, stroke, cardiac procedure, etc.), and death certificates were collected for persons who died. Then at periodic intervals, the data were analyzed to relate the likelihood of a cardiovascular event in a particular person over a defined interval to that person's characteristics when they first entered the study. In this way, the study investigators could identify the "risk factors" that best predict a future heart attack, stroke, etc. Three major modifiable risk factors were identified—high systolic blood pressure, cigarette smoking, and high serum cholesterol level.[7] Older age and male sex were the two major non-modifiable risk factors. Somewhere between modifiable and non-modifiable, diabetes was also associated with a three-fold elevation of cardiovascular risk.

In the seven decades since its founding, the National Heart Institute has grown to become the National Heart, Lung, and Blood Institute (NHLBI), and the town of Framingham has grown to an incorporated city of 72,000 residents.[8] The NIH has funded a number of other epidemiologic studies in diverse populations—including Stamler's early studies in Chicago's Peoples Gas and Western Electric employees, the Jackson Heart Study in African Americans, the Hispanic Community Heart Study, the Strong Heart Study in Native Americans, the Honolulu Heart Study in Asian-Americans, the Cardiovascular Health Study in the elderly, the Coronary Artery Risk Development in Young Adults study, and the Women's Health Initiative, among others too numerous to list here.[9] Furthermore, although all of the original 5209 FHS participants have either died or have passed the age of 95, the study itself is alive and thriving, having spawned cohort studies of its second, third, and fourth generations, which have continued to contribute greatly to our modern understanding of genetic and familial patterns of cardiovascular diseases as well as expanding our understanding of patterns of cardiovascular risk. These studies have generated thousands of scientific research papers and have provided complex risk models. The newest models incorporate race, diastolic (as well as systolic) blood pressure, and high-density lipoprotein (HDL) (as well as total) cholesterol, as well as age, sex, diabetes, and cigarette smoking. Each of these risk factors is related in log-linear fashion to risk of adverse cardiovascular outcomes; that is, there is an approximate straight-line relationship between each risk factor and the log of the cardiovascular event rate. But there is no need to unearth your old Algebra 2 textbook! Instead, I have prepared a table of selected values of the 10-year risk of a heart attack or stroke in the model adopted by the American Heart Association (AHA) and American College of Cardiology (ACC) for defining risk categories in their current clinical treatment guidelines for high cholesterol and high blood pressure (Table 2.1).[10] You can go to this website to calculate your own 10-year cardiovascular risk.

Without getting bogged down in the details of epidemiologic models, three "big picture" features emerge.

- Risk factors have a cumulative impact. For example, in 40-year-old White men, each single risk factor increases 10-year risk by only 2.0–3.5-fold, but in combination they increase risk 50-fold from 0.6% to 30.5%.
- Age is an extremely potent risk factor—i.e., cardiovascular diseases affect the elderly more than the middle aged. However, the incremental impact of most other risk factors tends to decrease with increasing age. High blood pressure is an exception, because of its strong relation to stroke, which most affects the elderly.
- The most obvious lifestyle trends correlated temporally with the rise of heart disease in the first half of the 20th century—the availability among the affluent of a rich and abundant diet and the replacement of hard physical labor with more sedentary occupations—are conspicuously absent from the list of risk factors.

Table 2.1. Ten-Year Risk of Heart Attack or Stroke

Risk Factors	White Males				White Females			
	40	*50*	*60*	*70*	*40*	*50*	*60*	*70*
Low-Risk Index Subject*	0.6%	2.2%	6.2%	14.3%	0.3%	0.8%	2.5%	7.9%
Diabetes	1.2%	4.2%	11.5%	25.8%	0.7%	1.6%	4.7%	14.8%
Smoker	2.1%	4.9%	9.8%	17.3%	1.4%	2.4%	5.3%	12.9%
BP =180/100 mmHg	1.3%	4.4%	12.2%	27.0%	0.8%	1.9%	5.5%	16.9%
Cholesterol = 280 mg/dL	1.5%	4.1%	9.2%	17.7%	0.9%	1.5%	3.6%	9.1%
HDL Cholesterol = 40 mg/dL	1.1%	3.4%	8.2%	17.1%	0.8%	1.4%	3.3%	8.7%
All of the Above	30.5%	43.8%	56.8%	68.5%	28.9%	27.4%	35.4%	52.0%
Risk Factors	African American Males				African American Females			
	40	*50*	*60*	*70*	*40*	*50*	*60*	*70*
Low-Risk Index Subject*	2.5%	4.4%	6.7%	9.7%	0.3%	1.2%	3.7%	9.5%
Diabetes	4.8%	8.1%	12.5%	17.7%	0.7%	2.8%	8.7%	21.3%
Smoker	4.3%	7.4%	11.4%	16.2%	0.6%	2.4%	7.3%	18.1%
BP =180/100 mmHg	5.2%	8.9%	13.5%	19.2%	2.6%	5.9%	11.5%	19.9%
Cholesterol = 280 mg/dL	2.9%	5.0%	7.7%	11.0%	0.4%	1.8%	5.6%	14.1%
HDL Cholesterol = 40 mg/dL	2.9%	4.9%	7.6%	10.9%	0.8%	2.1%	4.7%	9.2%
All of the Above	20.4%	32.7%	46.3%	59.7%	39.4%	54.4%	67.8%	78.7%

Non-diabetic, non-smoker, BP = 120/80 mmHg, cholesterol = 180 mg/dL, HDL cholesterol = 60 mg/dL

Before we go any further, we need to remind ourselves of what epidemiologic models can and cannot tell us. Observational epidemiologic studies like the FHS tell us only which factors best predict certain outcomes, not if and where those factors fit in the causal chain leading to those outcomes. In order to win the "competition" among the candidate variables that are tried in an epidemiologic model, a variable must be precisely and reproducibly measured, and the true differences in that variable among the participants being studied must well exceed the variability of the measurement. For example, in a population like ours, where everyone buys their food from similar grocery stores and people cannot accurately recount the exact foods and the precise amounts of each that they ate during a particular day or week, a measurement of serum cholesterol will "outcompete," say, dietary fat in any risk model, even if it is the fatty diet that raised the population cholesterol levels in the first place. Similarly, blood pressure is a far stronger risk factor than high salt intake, even though a high-salt diet is an important cause of high blood pressure and helps explain why high blood pressure was more prevalent in mid-century in Asian countries like Japan, which relied heavily on salt to preserve food, than in America, where refrigeration was more widely available. Even when a variable is readily and precisely measurable, it is often displaced from the model by risk factors that are more proximate to the outcome. For example, although obesity is a significant underlying cause of high blood pressure, high cholesterol, and type 2 diabetes in the U.S., these latter more proximate risk factors for heart attack and stroke drive obesity out of the Framingham and many other risk models.

On a more fundamental level, Framingham and other purely observational epidemiologic studies can demonstrate only the *association* of certain characteristics with certain subsequent disease outcomes, not whether those factors are contributing *causes* of the disease in question. Some risk factors—race for example—may be mere bystanders or "markers" for other biological characteristics or behaviors (diet, blood pressure, diabetes, etc.) that lie directly in the causal chain. Even more importantly, no purely observational study can tell us where to find treatments to ameliorate those risk factors or tell us whether any particular treatment will work. For example, if a study showed that 50% of bank robberies occurred on Fridays, it would be absurd to conclude that you could cut bank robberies in half by closing banks on Fridays. Thus, as useful and enlightening as epidemiologic models may be, they represented only a tentative first step in stemming the growing cardiovascular pandemic of the mid–20th century. By elucidating associations between certain characteristics and adverse cardiovascular outcomes like heart attack, stroke, and death, large cohort studies have been enormously valuable in pointing the way toward promising preventive and therapeutic approaches in at-risk persons. However, the heavy lifting of reliably identifying and proving which drugs or procedures will be beneficial in which patients requires something more definitive—clinical trials. Because cardiovascular disease is multifactorial and its clinical course may run years or even decades in a given patient, these trials may entail treating thousands of patients over nearly a decade. Clinical trials can be quite expensive and must be chosen with great patience and care. Sometimes their results are surprising—showing unexpected efficacy or, more often, lack of efficacy of seemingly promising treatments, as we shall see in the next chapter.

3

CLINICAL TRIALS

So how does the science of medicine bridge the gap between knowing the correlates and potential causes of a disease and finding treatments that work and are safe? Our most important tool is the clinical trial. Clinical trials are simple in concept. One defines a group of patients that will potentially benefit from a particular treatment of unknown value, give some of them the new treatment (added to the existing standard of care) and some of them only the existing standard of care (the "control" group), wait a predefined amount of time, and compare the response of the treatment versus the control group. There are many variations on this theme. The response may be death versus recovery, incidence versus prevention of a known complication, development of an antibody response to a vaccine, etc. One may have more than one active treatment groups using different drugs or different dosages of the same drug. The treatment may not be a drug at all, but rather a surgical procedure, a diet, a vaccine, or even a diagnostic testing strategy. Each study participant may have to be treated only one time or continually and may have to be followed for days, weeks, months, or even years to determine outcomes. The required number of participants in the trial may be 100 or 10,000. But it always boils down to comparing one or more predefined regimens to a predefined control group for a predefined outcome in a predefined target population.

As pointed out by my former division director Michael Lauer in a 2010 presentation, clinical trials have been around for a long time. In 17th-century London, a clinical trial of the ancient practice of bloodletting for treating fevers (an offshoot of the theory of "humors"—nothing to do with comedy) was announced in the following colorful language:

> Come down to the contest ye Humorists: Let us take out of the Hospitals or the camps or elsewhere, 200, or 500 poor People, that have Fevers etc. Let us divide them in Halfes, let us cast lots, that one half of them may fall to my share and the other to yours; I will cure them without bloodletting...; but do you do as ye know.

We shall see how many Funerals both of us shall have: But let the reward of the contention or wager, be 300 Florens, deposited on both sides: Here your business is decided.[1]

The outcome of that particular "contest" is lost to history, but in the 1740s, a Scottish émigré to Maryland, Dr. Alexander Hamilton (no relation to the founding father), published the following account of a similar trial in patients with febrile infections:

It had been so arranged, that this number was admitted, alternately, in such a manner that each of us had one third of the whole. The sick were indiscriminately received and were attended as nearly as possible with the same care and accommodated with the same comforts. Neither Mr. Anderson nor I ever once employed the lancet. He lost two, I four cases; whilst out of the other third [treated with bloodletting by the third surgeon] *thirty-five patients died.*[2]

Unfortunately, this resounding rejection of the efficacy of bloodletting, published while George Washington was a teenager, could not save the good general from the ministrations of his physicians in 1799, who treated him for a bacterial infection in which his breathing was obstructed by an inflamed and swollen epiglottis by performing bloodletting and a host of other noxious procedures (emetics, enemas, blistering his throat, forcing him to gargle molasses) instead of a administering a potentially life-saving tracheotomy (which was available in 1799).[3] Even in 1892, almost a century later and after the germ theory of infectious diseases had been firmly established, the eminent physician William Osler opined: "During the first five decades of this century the profession bled too much, but during the last decades, we have certainly bled too little."[4] So the problem was not only that few clinical trials were done, but that even the wisest and most respected physicians persisted in their mistaken beliefs and practices despite contrary evidence.

As simple as clinical trials are conceptually, they can be extraordinarily complex, resource-intensive, and expensive to operationalize. The fact that clinical trials entail experimental research in human volunteers imposes significant ethical and regulatory requirements. Moreover, clinical trials must be designed to address the following challenges:

1. How can one know that any observed differences between treatment and control groups can be attributed to the treatment itself and not due to extraneous differences between groups (i.e., "confounding" variables)?

2. How can one know that any observed differences between treatment and control groups signify a true treatment effect and not merely the play of chance?

3. How applicable (generalizable) are the results of a clinical trial in a selected group of volunteers to the broad population of patients affected by the condition being studied?

While the science of clinical trials is far too complex to cover here, I will provide a primer that will impart a basic understanding of the evidence behind (and perhaps even a critical eye toward) modern clinical recommendations flowing from the myriad of heart disease trials that have been conducted. I encourage readers who want to know more to check out the excellent textbook by Friedman et al.[5]

Controlling for Confounding Variables

When evaluating treatment X for a new or unstudied disease (COVID-19, for example), one starts with an accepted standard of care (e.g., bed rest, Tylenol for fever, hospitalization for those needing oxygen, intensive care for those requiring a ventilator). One knows that a fraction of patients will recover under standard care, and that this fraction may vary from more than 99% in young previously healthy patients with mild symptoms to less than 40% in older or sicker patients in the intensive care unit. Obviously, if we want to know whether treatment X works, we have to be certain that the patients receiving treatment X are comparable those in the control group when the trial begins. We clearly would not believe a study in which treatment X were given only to the sickest patients, while the control group included the full spectrum of disease—or vice versa. Variables that differ between the actively treated and control groups and could affect treatment outcomes are called "confounders." The surest way to know that our treatment and control groups are comparable when we begin is to assign eligible patients randomly to one group or the other. This process, called randomization, is considered a fundamental attribute of a well-designed clinical trial. While there are some circumstances where randomization to treatment versus control may be unfeasible or unethical (for example, when a disease is 100% fatal under standard care), you should generally look askance at any clinical trial that is not randomized.

But randomization is only the first step to control for confounding. Even if the treatment and control groups are similar when they start the trial, how can we ensure that they remain similar thereafter in all regards except for the one critical difference of whether they are assigned to the group receiving treatment X or to the control group? For example, what if a number of patients who are assigned to the control group start taking treatment Y while those assigned to treatment X do not? How can we be certain that any differences in recovery rate are due to treatment X and not treatment Y? Or what if the study investigators attribute some adverse outcome they observe in control patients to the disease under study, but fail to make the same attribution in patients assigned to treatment X? The surest remedy for this kind of confounding is "blinding"— or the more politically correct (until recently perhaps) "masking." In a single-blind study, the participants are kept ignorant of whether they are in the control group or the group receiving treatment X. This is generally accomplished by giving the control group a placebo pill that looks, feels, smells, and tastes just like treatment X but contains no active agent. In a double-blind study, which is even better, both the participants and the investigators are kept ignorant of whether a particular person has been assigned to the active treatment or control group. In order to carry out a double-blind study, clinical trial investigators generally outsource the necessary functions of randomization, provision of the assigned treatment (X or placebo) and compiling and analyzing unmasked data to a separate data coordinating center, which reports periodically to an external data and safety monitoring board (DSMB). The DSMB periodically evaluates how the data are trending and judges whether it is safe and necessary to continue the trial.

Confounding may also rear its ugly head in the analysis of a trial. For example, if one is conducting a trial in free-living volunteers, a number of them may move away or decide to withdraw from the study. It is not safe to assume that these "drop-outs" are random or will not create spurious differences between treatment groups. It is therefore incumbent upon investigators to make every effort to find these people and establish at least whether they are dead or alive. Investigators may also be tempted to exclude some participants *post hoc* because they have not complied with the treatment or because they have certain outcomes that do not fit the original design. One of the important tenets of the science of clinical trials is to analyze data by "intention to treat" rather than by whether participants actually complied with the treatment to which they were randomized. This seems counter-intuitive, but when you start excluding or reclassifying people you have randomized, you no longer have a randomized trial and you open the door for confounding. The better alternative is to build in a margin for non-compliance in the trial design by randomizing more participants than you think are needed and to do everything possible to maximize compliance during the trial, while still respecting the rights of the participants to autonomy in decision-making.

Ruling Out the Play of Chance

When one performs an experiment in the physical sciences, say on the force exerted by the earth's gravity on a 20-pound iron block, one may assume that one 20-pound iron block is very much like another and eschew the use of multiple blocks and complex statistical analysis to interpret the results. This is not true for clinical trials, which are conducted in human beings, whose characteristics and responses to treatment vary widely. Thus, clinical trial results must necessarily be judged by probabilistic criteria, in which one asks how likely is it that a result at least as good as the one observed could have happened by chance? Typically, a probability (often called the P-value) of 5% (or one in 20) is taken as the arbitrary threshold for statistical significance, that is for rejecting the possibility that the result happened by pure chance. To put this threshold in context, the chance of the number 22 coming up on an honest roulette wheel is one in 38, or roughly 2.6%. The probability of shooting a "natural" 7 or 11 at the crap table is 8/36 or roughly 22%. So clinical trials "pay off" on a probability that is roughly half as stringent as the probability of winning on a single number at roulette and 4.5 times as stringent as that of shooting a natural at the craps table.

Every good clinical trial is designed with the objective of having enough patients to yield a strong probability (or "power") of producing a "significant" ($P < 0.05$) result if the starting hypothesis is correct. The way to do this is by calculating in advance how many patients you need to enroll to detect the hypothesized effect. Typically, most cardiovascular trials have been designed with at least 80% power, although 85 or 90% is even better. The smaller the effect you wish to detect, the more patients you will need for your trial. If you are evaluating a new antibiotic in patients with a highly lethal infectious disease and you expect an 80–90% cure rate, as few as 50 participants may be sufficient to demonstrate a significant benefit in a matter of weeks or months. In a chronic condition like coronary heart disease, where the standard of care already includes many established effective drugs, establishing the modest incremental benefit of a new drug may require 10,000 patients followed for seven years or more.

The number of patients required for a well-powered cardiovascular trial—i.e., its sample size—depends on the nature and frequency of the primary outcome (or end point) and the nature and size of the treatment effect one is trying to confirm. In general:

- Trials in which the primary outcome is an infrequent discrete event like death or a heart attack require larger sample sizes than trials looking at a continuous outcome (like weight loss) or the incidence of a more frequent event.
- When the primary outcome is a cardiovascular event or death, primary prevention trials—i.e., those performed in participants with risk factors but without known cardiovascular disease—require larger sample sizes than secondary prevention trials—i.e., those performed in participants with known cardiovascular disease.
- Trials in which a new treatment is compared with a known effective standard treatment require larger sample sizes than trials in which the new treatment is compared with a placebo or no treatment.
- Effectiveness trials, which look at the "real world" impact of interventions, tend to require larger sample sizes than efficacy trials, which look at treatment effects under well-controlled conditions.

Most of the cardiovascular trials discussed in this book are in the moderately large (1000–9999 participants) range. The smaller trials tend mostly to be efficacy trials of secondary prevention. Most of the "megatrials"—i.e., those with 10,000 participants or more—are either primary prevention trials in healthy participants or effectiveness trials looking for modest outcome differences in real world settings. Many examples of each of these categories of trials will be discussed in the coming chapters.

Probabilities only make sense if all the relevant parameters—the treatment, the population and outcome of interest, the primary analytic method, and the criteria for stopping—are specified in advance, i.e., before the experiment has begun. No casino that wanted to stay in business would pay a customer who placed his bet after seeing where the ball landed. Likewise, a trial designed to test the effect of a new drug on all-cause mortality cannot claim a positive result if it shows a significant decrease in heart attacks but no change in mortality. A trial may specify more than one primary outcome or a subgroup of especial interest, just as a roulette player may gamble on a group of numbers (odd or even, red or black). But just as the payoff is less for the roulette player who hedges his bet, the statistical criteria for claiming a significant result become stricter when multiple primary outcomes are specified.

Generalizability

Every trial designer is faced at the outset with a decision on how to define the trial's target population. At one extreme, a trial may target a very specific group of patients—for example COVID-19 patients on a ventilator for at least 24 hours or 35- to 59-year-old men with no history of heart attack or diabetes and serum cholesterol > 265 mg/dL. This may give you a better chance (in theory at least) to get a positive result but will leave a lot of unanswered questions about whether your therapy works in other groups. At the opposite extreme, you may include all comers with the condition in question at the risk of getting a muddled result if the treatment works better in some groups than others. Sometimes one can strive for the best of both worlds by incorporating a broad population and including enough members of key subgroups to power at least exploratory analyses in those groups, but often this means making the studies prohibitively large and expensive. A good rule of thumb is to design the study with specificity when prior lab or animal studies provide ample grounds to predict that a treatment might work better in one group than another but not to make arbitrary exclusions when such grounds are lacking.

Factorial Designs

Factorial trials are a somewhat arcane wrinkle on clinical trials, which have grown more popular as cardiovascular trials have grown ever more complex and expensive. Readers who are in a hurry may skip over this section now and refer back to it when the subject comes up in later chapters.

Basically, the factorial design is a clever strategy to do two or more trials for the price of one. In the simplest version, the 2×2 factorial trial (Figure 3.1), there are two treatments (A and B), each with its own control, and participants are randomized independently to Active or Control for each treatment.

FIGURE 3.1. A Simple 2×2 Factorial Design

Treatment A	Treatment B	
	Active	Control
Active	A and B	A but not B
Control	B but not A	Neither A nor B

When the trial is analyzed, all participants randomized to Active A are compared to all participants randomized to Control A (irrespective of whether they were randomized to Active B or Control B). Similarly, all participants randomized to Active B are compared to all participants randomized to Control B (irrespective of whether they were randomized to Active A or Control A). This design requires a study population in whom it is appropriate to randomize every member to all four possible combinations of treatments A and B. An example of a simple 2×2 factorial trial is the Women's Health Study (WHS), in which almost 40,000 women with no prior history of a heart attack were randomized to receive low-dose-aspirin versus placebo and vitamin E versus placebo; neither reduced subsequent major cardiovascular events (the primary outcome) significantly.[6] The validity of this design rests on the assumption that the efficacy of treatment A is not influenced by treatment B and vice versa; i.e., the treatments do not interact. If this assumption were false, the trial would have to be analyzed as four separate groups and the efficiency of the factorial design would be lost.

More complicated versions of the factorial design exist. In a partial factorial design, not everyone is randomized to treatment B. The ACCORD diabetes trial (illustrated in Figure 3.2) is a variant of this partial factorial design, in which all participants who are not randomized to Treatment B versus control are randomized instead to Treatment C versus control.

FIGURE 3.2. A 2×2 Partial Factorial Design

Subset I	Treatment A	Treatment B Active	Control
	Active Control	A and B B but not A	A but not B Neither A nor B
Subset II	Treatment A	Treatment C Active	Control
	Active Control	A and C C but not A	A but not C Neither A nor C

This trial, in which the primary objective was to compare mortality rates in diabetic patients receiving intensive versus standard diabetes management in 10,251 diabetic patients will come up in Chapters 4, 7, and 9.[7] The ACCORD design required that every participant have either high blood pressure (BP) or a lipid disorder called metabolic syndrome in addition to diabetes. The subset of participants with high BP were randomized secondarily to receive intensive versus standard BP management, while the subset with metabolic syndrome was randomized secondarily to receive the drug fenofibrate or a placebo. So everyone was randomized twice, but only the first randomization was the same for every participant. Other variants of factorial designs include the 2×2×2 factorial, in which each participant is randomized independently with respect to three treatments, the 2×3 factorial design, in which there are two independent randomizations, but one of them involves comparing two dosage versus placebo, and many others. However, the more complicated the design, the harder it becomes to identify and recruit the appropriate population, and the more likely that the treatments will interact. So, mercifully, more complicated factorial trials are rare.

Negative Trials

It is safe to say that everyone who participates in a clinical trial is thrilled when their trial's result is positive and disappointed when it is negative. After all, who among us would not prefer to have their ideas proven right than proven wrong? However, one must not conflate a negative trial with a bad trial. There are many reasons a trial may be negative.

Some trials turn out to be negative because of flaws in their design—most often, overly optimistic assumptions about how many participants they will need, how many they can recruit, compliance, and the choice of primary endpoint. Even the best designed trial may fail if it is poorly executed. However, a well-designed and well-executed trial that obtains a robust negative result may be just as valuable as a positive trial by establishing unequivocally that the new treatment is not beneficial, or even harmful. Such a result may even produce a paradigm shift that leads to new ways of thinking about a disease and new avenues of research to explore. Disappointing as this may be to the investigators and sponsors of such a trial, these results may save millions of future patients from receiving an ineffective or harmful treatment and redirect societal resources to finding a treatment that works. The story of the Cardiac Arrhythmia Suppression Trial (CAST) illustrates this point.[8]

The normal heart has a network of specialized fibers that generates and conducts the electrical signals that initiate and regulate the heartbeat so that fresh oxygen-carrying blood is pumped into the arteries about once every second (see Figure 12.1). When a heart attack occurs, this specialized conducting system in the heart may get damaged and put out stray signals even after the heart recovers its pumping capacity. These stray signals may generate runs of irregular heartbeats (arrhythmias), which at best are upsetting and at worst may commandeer the heart to beat too rapidly (tachycardia) or even to beat chaotically (ventricular fibrillation) in a way that disables its function as a pump. When this happens, the heart must be quickly shocked to restore normal rhythm and prevent death.

Given these dire possibilities, the development of well-tolerated orally administered drugs that reduced the frequency of irregular heartbeats in heart attack survivors was welcomed in the 1980s as a potential game changer. Intravenously administered anti-arrhythmic drugs like lidocaine were widely used at that time in the intensive coronary care setting but were not suitable for outpatient use. So it was broadly assumed that anti-arrhythmic drugs that could be prescribed to outpatients would save lives—so much so that many physicians had ethical reservations about even doing a randomized trial with a placebo control group. Nevertheless, the NIH undertook the CAST trial in June 1987, and set out to randomize 4400 post-heart attack patients to receive one of three anti-arrhythmic drugs (encainide, flecainide, moricizine) or placebo. The fact that any given patient was roughly three times as likely to receive an active drug than a placebo helped ease some of the ethical reservations about including a placebo control group.

Well, it turned out that the patients who received the placebo were the lucky ones. In April 1989, less than two years into the trial, the study's DSMB stopped the trial because of a 3.6-fold *increase* in arrhythmic deaths in the patients randomized to the encainide and flecainide groups—a highly significant finding, which turned expectations on their head.[9] Indeed, the DSMB almost failed to act because they had elected to be blinded as to which group was which (a terrible idea) and had blithely assumed that it was the placebo group with the higher mortality until a junior statistician at the coordinating center alerted them to the truth. The findings were less stark in the patients assigned to moricizine, who were allowed to continue in the trial until August 1991, when it was learned that they too were experiencing more harm (excess deaths) than good from their anti-arrhythmic drug treatment.[10]

So was CAST a failure? It was certainly a harrowing experience, in which some trial participants died who might not have died if they had been left untreated. But would they have been left untreated if they had not been enrolled in CAST? Almost certainly not! The three drugs used in CAST were widely prescribed in clinical practice by physicians who thought they KNEW that suppressing arrhythmia saved lives. In clinical practice, where there would be no DSMB monitoring their experience and comparing them with a control group, far more undoubtedly would have died. And because of CAST, thousands of later patients did not receive these harmful drugs. Therefore, I would argue that CAST was just as important as the positive trials we will talk about later, which established the benefit of many of the drugs and medical procedures we use today.

What's in a Name?

Cardiovascular clinical trialists often express their latent creativity by giving their trials a descriptive name, that encapsulates what their trial is about and lends itself to a catchy acronym. In a few instances, like the MRFIT acronym (pronounced Mister Fit) for the Multiple Risk Factor Intervention Trial, the inconclusive non-blinded 1972–82 NHLBI trial of a multi-pronged special intervention strategy involving lifestyle changes and antihypertensive medication versus "usual care" in high-risk

35- to 57-year-old men, the marriage of trial and acronym is perfect.[11] More often, as in CAST, the acronym is serviceable if not particularly relatable to the nature of the trial. In some trials, like the Lipid Research Clinics Coronary Primary Prevention Trial (LRC-CPPT), the investigators didn't even try to come up with a creative acronym.[12] Other trialists have gone into great contortions to add extra words to the name of their trial or hop-scotch through its name, taking an initial here and three interior letters there, to create a catchy acronym. For example, a trial of the anti-diabetes drug pioglitazone was named the PROspective pioglitAzone Clinical Trial In macroVascular Events, which becomes "PROactive," when one selects the bolded letters.[13] Perhaps the most extreme example of runaway creativity is when the pharmaceutical company AstraZeneca gave names lending themselves to celestial acronyms to an entire constellation of rosuvastatin trials, under the umbrella name Galaxy.[14] I'm not a big fan, but acronyms like JUPITER, METEOR, and STELLAR are catchy and pronounceable, even if they tell you nothing of what the trials are about. In any case, you will come to know many cardiovascular trials by name in the course of reading this book.

Meta-Analysis

Cardiovascular trials that address major health outcomes like mortality, heart attack, stroke, etc., are dauntingly complex, lengthy, and expensive enterprises, which always leave some questions unanswered, even when they are successful overall. They may show a significant overall benefit but may lack sufficient power to address important subgroups of interest. Or they may be negative overall but show promising effects in some important subgroup. Or they may show benefit for some outcome not specified in the study design. Meta-analysis is a statistical technique for combining the results of multiple similar trials to tease out beneficial or adverse effects of treatment that no single trial is large enough to address.

Unfortunately, meta-analysis is easy to manipulate or misuse. Most meta-analyses are performed after the fact—sometimes by investigators with an axe to grind—leaving the meta-analyst free to cherry-pick results by including trials that fit his/her hypothesis while finding sensible sounding reasons to exclude trials with inconvenient results. Before the statin trials came along (Chapter 5), the cholesterol field was full of competing meta-analyses drawing diametrically opposite conclusions from the same body of evidence.[15] Indeed, one-time Framingham director William Castelli once threw up his hands in mock despair at a 1992 research conference and wittily proclaimed that "meta-analysis is to analysis as meta-physics is to physics." The problem with retrospective meta-analysis is similar to that of analyzing the results of a horse race the following day. With the benefit of hindsight, one can think of all sorts of rationalizations for why one horse exceeded expectations and another disappointed. But the only analysis that matters is the one you make *before* the race is run.

In the 1990s, researchers at Oxford have developed and refined a technique called "prospective meta-analysis," which enables us to combine the results of multiple similar clinical trials without falling prey to selection bias.[16] In a prospective meta-analysis, a written protocol explicitly laying out all rules about which trials to include, which subgroups to analyze, etc., is published *before* the results of any component trial are known. Ideally, patient-level data (not just the published group-level data) are provided by the investigators of each participating trial. Then, when the results of the meta-analysis are published, the scientific audience can see for themselves that the meta-analyst has adhered to the protocol and has not cherry-picked which trials to include after the fact. As we shall see later, prospective meta-analysis has played a major role in amplifying and extending the power of cardiovascular trials to address multiple subgroups and positive and adverse outcomes that no single trial can adequately address.

In the coming chapters, we will see how insights gained from the laboratory, population science, and targeted clinical trials, and meta-analysis have gone hand in hand to tame the many-headed monster of cardiovascular disease over the past 50 years.

4

LOWERING THE PRESSURE

While simple organisms can get what they need from the environment via simple or assisted diffusion, all higher animals have a circulatory system to deliver oxygen and nutrients to cells that are not in direct contact with the external environment. The circulatory system consists of a vehicle—the blood—to carry oxygen and nutrients to the various organs, a heart to pump the blood, and conduits—the arteries, capillaries, and veins—to carry blood to the organs, perfuse them, and return blood to the heart, respectively. Human beings and other mammals actually have two circulations connected in series—the low-pressure pulmonary circulation, which sends oxygen-depleted blood from the right side of the heart to the lungs and returns oxygenated blood to the left side of the heart, and the high-pressure corporal circulation which send oxygenated blood from the left side of the heart to the rest of the body and returns oxygen-depleted blood to the right side of the heart. The term blood pressure (BP) refers to the force generated by the heart that propels blood from the left ventricle through the arteries in the corporeal circulation. BP is traditionally measured with an inflatable cuff applied to the upper arm and connected to a column of mercury (sphygmomanometer) and a stethoscope to detect changes in the sound of blood flow through the brachial artery in the crook of the elbow. At any given sitting, two pressures are measured—the systolic, when the left ventricle is fully contracted and the pressure is at its peak, and the diastolic, when the left ventricle relaxes and the pressure is at its lowest. In a healthy 35-year-old adult, a pressure sufficient to support a 120-millimeter (mm) column of mercury (Hg) at systole and 80 mm at diastole is typical and is recorded as 120/80 mmHg. The absence of a blood pressure due to massive blood loss and/or a failing heart is incompatible with life.

Blood pressure is not static. It may vary with body position (lying, sitting, or standing), time of day, activity, or state of nervous excitement.

Blood pressure normally differs between the arms and legs and may differ between one arm and the other under pathologic conditions like thoracic outlet syndrome. High salt intake can raise blood pressure and may help explain the relatively high prevalence of high blood pressure in traditional Asian cultures. Blood pressure is also regulated by hormones like aldosterone, serotonin, angiotensin, epinephrine (adrenaline), and norepinephrine; derangements in their metabolism by neuroendocrine tumors or kidney failure may raise blood pressure. (The relation of blood pressure and kidney function actually goes both ways; high blood pressure may cause thickening of the kidney arteries and impaired kidney function, while impaired kidney function due to other causes may release angiotensin into the circulation and raise blood pressure.) However, most instances of high blood pressure have no discernable physiologic cause or explanation other than the commonly observed gradual stiffening of arteries with increasing age (arteriosclerosis). This form of hypertension used to be called "idiopathic" or "essential" (meaning that the underlying cause and biological pathways were not understood), but we now recognize that it is largely due to modifiable lifestyle factors, especially diet.

The recognition of high blood pressure (or hypertension) as a condition associated with adverse clinical conditions such as heart failure (subsumed under diseases of the heart), stroke (largely cerebral hemorrhage), and kidney failure—the three leading non-infectious causes of death in 1900—long pre-dates the invention of the sphygmomanometer in 1896.[1] Indeed, the recognition of "hard pulse disease" goes back to ancient times. However, the remedies applied over the ages—bloodletting, severe sodium restriction, cutting the sympathetic nerves, and administering pyrogens to cause fever—were neither safe nor effective. Although severe or "malignant" hypertension, defined as a lethal syndrome of extreme rises in BP (e.g., 300 mmHg systolic), retinopathy (arterial changes in the retina that may lead to loss of vision), and kidney failure, leading rapidly to heart failure and/or (usually fatal) bleeding in the brain, was recognized in 1928, the medical establishment remained skeptical about treating lesser elevations in blood pressure. By the 1930s, insurance companies were already well aware of the value of BP in their actuarial calculations.[2] Yet in 1937, while President Franklin Roosevelt was suffering from moderate hypertension, eminent American cardiologist Paul Dudley White opined that hypertension was "an important compensatory mechanism that should not be tampered with."[3] Six years earlier, British professor John Hay had

34

gone one step further by opining that "the greatest danger to a man with high blood pressure lies in its discovery, because then some fool is certain to try and reduce it."[4] The question was moot in any case. It was not until after World War II that effective blood pressure-lowering drugs—tetramethylammonium chloride, hydralazine, and reserpine—became available, and it was not until a decade later that the development of the thiazides, well-tolerated oral diuretics derived from the sulfa antibiotics, made the treatment of high blood pressure practical on a mass scale. Other safe and effective drugs—beta- and alpha-adrenergic blockers, calcium channel blockers, angiotensin converting enzyme (ACE) inhibitors, angiotensin receptor blockers (ARB)—would follow in the ensuing two decades.

Although, no systematic surveys of the prevalence of high blood pressure exist before 1950, one can infer from the decline in deaths from associated conditions like stroke (Figure 4.1) and kidney failure, that the prevalence of high blood pressure almost certainly declined between 1900 and 1950, while other cardiovascular risk factors were still on the rise.

Now, stroke is complicated, because it reflects a mixture of obstruction of the arteries by ruptured atherosclerotic plaques and thrombosis (clotting) and bleeding in the brain. Today, atherothrombotic strokes are more common, but cerebral bleeds are more lethal. In the early 20th

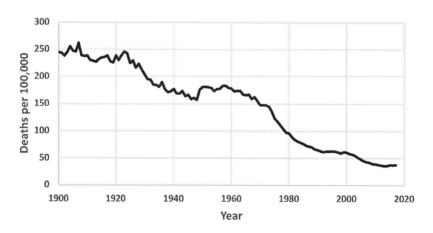

U.S. trend in age-adjusted stroke mortality, 1900–2017. Data were obtained from CDC Vital Statistics compilations.

century, cerebral bleeds were both more common and more lethal. The pre–1950 decline in strokes in the face of an increasing trend in atherosclerosis almost certainly reflects a decline in cerebral bleeds and, by inference, hypertension. Since no effective blood pressure treatments existed at that time, this decline may reflect declining salt intake as broad access to refrigeration decreased the reliance on salt to preserve meats. In any case, by the time the Framingham Heart Study began, mortality from strokes (including cerebral bleeds) had already declined by 40% since 1900 and mortality from nephropathy (kidney failure) had declined by 80% (from 88.6 to 17.4 per 100,000).[5]

When the Framingham Heart Study published its initial follow-up results in the early 1960s, moderate "essential" hypertension (that is moderately elevated BP with no known primary biological cause) was still considered a relatively benign condition.[6] According to a prominent 1965 review article, "It is common experience that many patients live medically uneventful lives in spite of prolonged and considerable blood pressure elevation."[7] Of course, a life ending in a sudden fatal heart attack at age 64 was probably considered "medically uneventful" at that time. A common clinical rule of thumb was that a systolic BP below 100 plus the person's age was considered normal.

Landmark Blood Pressure Trials

Spurred by the early Framingham results and the development of the thiazide diuretics, the U.S. Veterans Administration (VA), a nationwide network of hospitals established to treat military veterans, undertook a groundbreaking randomized clinical hypertension trial.[8] The VA Cooperative BP Trial, which began in 1964 under the leadership of Dr. Edward Freis, was the first of many major research trials conducted by the VA and was the among the first trials worldwide to address the treatment of hypertension.[9] It had two components:

1. a placebo-controlled trial in 143 male veterans with **severe** (but not malignant) **hypertension** (diastolic BP of 115 to 129 mmHg) in which the active treatment group received a combination of hydrochlorothiazide, reserpine, and hydralazine, which lowered their BP by 43/30 mmHg, for a period averaging 1.5 years, and
2. a placebo-controlled trial in 380 male veterans with **mild to**

moderate hypertension (diastolic BP of 90 to 114 mmHg) employing the same three drugs, which lowered their mean diastolic BP by 19 mmHg, for a period averaging 3.8 years.

Although both were very small trials by modern standards and were designed only to detect differences in composite outcomes, including stroke, retinal hemorrhage, heart attack, heart failure, and dissecting aortic aneurysm, as well as mortality, both studies showed that the veterans receiving active drug treatment to lower their blood pressure fared far better than those receiving placebo. In the **severe hypertension** trial (published in 1967), only one adverse cardiovascular events (no deaths) occurred in the drug-treated patients versus 27 events (including 4 deaths) in the placebo group.[10] In the (larger and longer) **mild to moderate hypertension** trial, which was published in 1970, 22 adverse cardiovascular events (including 8 deaths) occurred in the group receiving active drug treatment versus 56 events (including 19 deaths) in the placebo group.[11] Thus, by 1970, the earlier prevailing view that essential hypertension with diastolic BP < 130 mmHg was "benign" had become untenable. By the time I finished medical school in 1973, it was standard practice (at least in theory) to treat all patients with diastolic BP > 90 mmHg, but the goal of attaining diastolic BP below 90 mmHg was seldom attained. The rule of thumb at that time was that only half of all hypertensive patients were diagnosed, only half of those diagnosed were treated, and only half of those treated attained the therapeutic goal of < 90 mmHg diastolic.[12] Thus, overall, only one of every eight hypertensive patients was adequately treated.

The VA Cooperative Trial was only the first step. The study was relatively small and did not include women (who comprised only a small fraction of VA patients). Also, the VA trial used a fixed drug regimen, rather than targeting a blood pressure goal. So, in 1971, the NHLBI initiated the Hypertension Detection and Follow-Up Program (HDFP), a non-blinded community-based randomized trial, which used a stepped-care regimen of six blood pressure-lowering drugs in 10,940 men and women, aged 30–69, with diastolic BP > 90 mmHg (average BP = 158/101 mmHg).[13] This trial was initiated at NIH by William Friedewald and Gerald Payne, and Herbert Langford, Jeremiah Stamler, Nemat Borhani, and Coordinating Center Director Mort Hawkins were prominent in the study leadership. Patients in the active treatment arm began with a dose of the thiazide-like diuretic (chlorthalidone), and escalating doses of other drugs were added at prespecified intervals according to a standard protocol until the diastolic BP was brought below 90 mmHg. Patients in the control group were referred to outside physicians for standard care (which would presumably reflect the inadequate level of BP control in the community at large). As expected, BP control was significantly better in the stepped care group than in the control group. This difference was enough to bring about a statistically significant (P < 0.01) 17% reduction (6.4 versus 7.7%) reduction in mortality, including a 20% reduction in the milder cases (diastolic BP between 90 and 104 mmHg at baseline).[14] Mortality was reduced in both men and women and in both Black and White, and for ages 50–59 and 60–69 years.[15] Strokes were also significantly reduced by about one-third (1.9 versus 2.9%) in the stepped care group.[16]

While skeptics might have dismissed the VA trial results as those of a small trial in an unrepresentative patient population, they could not dismiss the power and generalizability of the HDFP results. Having established the unequivocal value of treating mild to moderate diastolic hypertension, medical scientists around the world began clinical trials to address unanswered questions about how broadly the lessons of these early trials ought to be applied and the role of the many new antihypertensive drugs entering the market as we entered the 1980s. I will focus on a few NHLBI-sponsored clinical trials which were at the center of the U.S. efforts in this arena.

The first question on the post–HDFP agenda was the treatment of systolic hypertension. In the early days, physicians focused on treating elevated diastolic BP, even though systolic BP was the stronger risk factor in the Framingham and other epidemiologic cohort studies. So, even after it was accepted that hypertension, defined by diastolic BP > 90 mmHg, was not a benign disease and that blood pressure lowering drugs could reduce mortality and strokes, questions remained about whether and how to treat the large number of older patients (projected at the time to affect eight million Americans by 2025) whose arteries lost elasticity as they aged and presented with elevated systolic BP (> 160 mmHg) and a normal diastolic BP.[17] After all, these were the very sort of patients in whom John Hay and Paul Dudley White had cautioned against medical interference a generation earlier, and their skeptical attitude still prevailed in many quarters. If one were to treat their "isolated systolic hypertension," would one not risk lowering their diastolic BP to troublesome levels that would produce dizziness, fainting, falls, and even broken bones in fragile seniors? Would lowering BP reduce cardiovascular complications enough to offset these potential risks?

After a successful pilot study led by Steve Hulley and McFate Smith, the NHLBI initiated the Systolic Hypertension in the Elderly Program (SHEP) in 1985 to address this important condition. SHEP was a double-blind placebo-controlled randomized trial in 4736 men and women aged 60 years and above with isolated systolic hypertension (systolic BP > 160 mmHg but diastolic BP < 90 mmHg). The active treatment group received chlorthalidone, supplemented with the beta-blocker atenolol and/or reserpine as needed to lower systolic BP by at least 20 mmHg and to a level below 160 mmHg. The primary outcome of interest was the combined incidence of fatal and nonfatal stroke. The trial was led by many of the same investigators who led the HDFP, but now with Curt Furberg, Jeff Cutler, and Jeff Probstfield leading the NHLBI project team. Once again, the results were resoundingly positive. After an average of 4.5 years of follow-up, a 12 mm Hg reduction the average systolic BP (143 versus 155) was accompanied by a 36% reduction in strokes in the chlortalidone versus the placebo group (5.2% versus 8.2%, P = 0.0003).[18] Chlorthalidone treatment also brought about substantial and statistically significant reductions in heart attacks, all major cardiovascular events, and mortality from all causes. The SHEP results confirmed that hypertension, even when confined to elevated systolic BP in older patients with stiff arteries, was a clinically significant condition whose treatment was demonstrably lifesaving.

The next critical question was brought to the fore by the many emerging antihypertensive drug options and the difficulty of attaining adequate BP control with any single drug. The Antihypertensive and Lipid Heart Attack Trial (ALLHAT) was undertaken in 1994 (with a substantial contribution from Pfizer, which provided two of the first-line drugs plus logistical support) to address the question of which drugs, singly or in combination, were best for controlling BP and preventing adverse cardiovascular outcomes.[19] ALLHAT was one of the most complex trials the NHLBI has ever undertaken. Not only was it huge—42,448 participants (of whom 47% were women and 53% were non–White)—it included randomization to one of four first-line drugs—lisinopril (an ACE inhibitor), amlodipine (a calcium channel blocker), doxazosin (an alpha-adrenergic blocker), and a low-dose (12.5–25 mg) chlorthalidone (diuretic) control arm.[20] Each of these drugs had up to three different prescribed dosage levels which somehow had to be titrated to attain a BP < 140/90 mmHg in each patient (in conformity with the expert guidelines at that time) while maintaining the double-blind design.[21] Participants who were unable to attain this goal on the maximum dosage of their first-line drug were also given atenolol (a beta-adrenergic blocker) as a second-line drug; hydralazine, reserpine, and clonidine were used as third-line drugs for patients not controlled on two drugs. Furthermore, to treat and track so many patients, ALLHAT's 625 clinical sites were distributed into nine administrative regions, each with its own separate leadership structure. And if all that wasn't enough, one-quarter of the study participants were simultaneously enrolled in a non-blinded pravastatin trial using a partial-factorial design (see Chapter 3). Much of the ALLHAT leadership—Study Chair Curt Furberg (now at Wake Forest Bowman Gray University), Program Director Jeff Cutler, Project Officer Gerald Payne—had been part of the NHLBI leadership team for SHEP, and many of the ALLHAT regional directors and deputy Study Chair Jackson Wright were also SHEP investigators. The Coordinating Center, now led by Barry Davis, remained at the University of Texas at Houston.

The final ALLHAT results showed no significant differences among the four treatment arms in the primary outcome—the combined incidence of fatal and non-fatal heart attacks—or in most of the secondary cardiovascular outcomes and total mortality.[22] The exception was a significantly lower rate of heart failure diagnoses and hospitalizations in the chlorthalidone control group and significantly higher rates of heart failure in the doxazosin group.[23] (The latter finding, along with its lower efficacy in achieving BP control, caused the doxazosin arm to be terminated early.) It should be noted that the clinical significance of the ALLHAT heart failure results is uncertain because diuretics tend to alleviate heart failure by decreasing fluid retention, while doxazosin tends to increase fluid retention. At the time, the ALLHAT results were touted because they showed that the least expensive drug (chlorthalidone) was as good or better than the newer more expensive drugs. But even now, almost two decades later, when inexpensive generic versions of all these drug classes are available, ALLHAT was useful in establishing the therapeutic equivalence of these drug classes, which are now often used in combination, since one drug is rarely sufficient to achieve optimal BP control.

The final major remaining question in treating hypertension was how low is low enough. Two non-blinded 21st-century randomized trials set out to determine whether cardiovascular outcomes might be further improved by lowering the goal for systolic BP from < 140 mmHg ("standard control") to < 120 mmHg ("intensive control"). The first trial, initiated by Peter Savage and Jeff Cutler, was conducted in 2001–09 in a 4733-participant subset of a type 2 diabetes trial called Action to Control Cardiovascular Risk in Diabetes (ACCORD), which employed a partial factorial design (see Chapter 3).[24] The second, the Systolic Blood Pressure Intervention Trial (SPRINT), was initiated by Jeff Cutler and project officer Larry Fine and conducted in 2010–15 in 9361 non-diabetic patients.[25] Both trials achieved substantially lower SBP in the intensive than in the standard control groups,. SPRINT found a statistically significant 25% reduction in the primary composite cardiovascular outcome and a significant 27% reduction in total mortality in non-diabetic patients randomized to intensive versus standard control.[26] However, the ACCORD trial found only a small (12%) non-significant reduction in cardiovascular events in diabetic patients randomized to the intensive versus standard treatment group.[27] At first glance, these two trials appeared to show better results for intensive BP control in non-diabetic than diabetic hypertensive patients. However, a subsequent analysis of the ACCORD BP trial showed that the benefit of intensive BP control in ACCORD participants who were randomized to standard glycemic control—a 23% reduction in cardiovascular events—was essentially identical to the 25% reduction in SPRINT.[28] This squares with a subgroup analysis of the SHEP trial, in which lowering systolic BP to 140 mmHg or less significantly reduced adverse cardiovascular outcomes in older diabetic, as well as non-diabetic participants.[29] It was only the ACCORD patients who were randomized to the failed intensive glycemic control strategy who did not benefit from the intensification of BP control. It should also be noted that the improved cardiovascular outcomes in the intensive BP treatment groups in both the SPRINT and ACCORD trials came at the cost of statistically significant increases in complications related to low BP—dizziness, fainting, injuries sustained in falls, etc., although the benefits clearly outweighed the risks. The 2017 ACC/AHA High Blood Pressure Clinical Practice Guidelines revised the threshold and treatment goal for hypertension to 130/70 mmHg, reflecting the SPRINT results.[30]

Quantitative Overview of BP Trials

The studies I have highlighted in this chapter represent only major landmark trials, which were sponsored mainly in the U.S. public sector, although sometimes (especially in ALLHAT) with significant participation from non–U.S. sites and in-kind contributions from pharmaceutical firms. The reason for the preeminence of NIH, the world's largest public funding source for biomedical research, in the blood pressure field is that trials of stepped care approaches to BP control using combinations of drug classes and trials of head-to-head drug comparisons are generally not in the wheelhouse of drug manufacturers, who as a rule are interested in proving the efficacy of their specific drug. (As we shall see in Chapter 5, the pharmaceutical industry has played a far more prominent role in cholesterol trials.) However, these large NIH trials are but the tip of the iceberg of BP trials conducted in the U.S. and throughout the world.[31] A 2016 retrospective meta-analysis, found 123 qualifying BP trials, including 613,815 participants.[32] Notwithstanding the many pitfalls of retrospective meta-analysis (see Chapter 3), these investigators were quite meticulous and transparent about their eligibility criteria. Also, by 2016, the overall benefit of the BP treatment was no longer controversial; the authors' intent was simply to quantify the relationship between BP lowering and various cardiovascular outcomes is specific subgroups. Their main findings were as follows:

1. The risk of major adverse cardiovascular outcomes fell by 20% (strongly significant) for every 10 mmHg reduction in systolic BP. This is actually larger than the 12% decrease in 10-year risk associated in observational studies with a 10 mmHg drop in systolic BP in a 60 year-old White male non-smoker without diabetes.[33]

2. Every 10 mmHg in systolic BP was also associated with a 17% decrease in risk of heart attack, a 27% decrease in risk of stroke, a 28% decrease in risk of heart failure, and a 13% decrease in mortality—all strongly significant.

3. Similar benefits of BP lowering at all baseline levels of BP.

4. Similar benefits of BP lowering in patients with and without cardiovascular disease at baseline.

5. Similar benefits of BP lowering for most classes of drugs, with the exception of beta-blockers (which were significantly less effective than other drug classes with respect to all outcomes except heart attack).

Impact of BP Control on Decline in Heart Attack Deaths

In a span of 60 years, the treatment of hypertension has traveled a long road from therapeutic nihilism, with no effective treatments available anyway, to a clear mandate for lowering BP below 130/80 mmHg, with a wide variety of safe and effective drugs to accomplish this goal in most patients. Indeed, four of these drugs—lisinopril, amlodipine, losartan, and hydrochlorothiazide are—ranked first, fifth, ninth, and twelfth among the most frequently prescribed drugs in the U.S. in 2017 with more than 270 million prescriptions among them.[34]

Clearly, our progress in developing blood pressure drugs and demonstrating their efficacy has profoundly affected clinical practice, expanding the definition of hypertension and increasing the proportion of hypertensives successfully treated. A recent analysis of data from the National Health and Nutrition Examination Survey (NHANES) documents this progress.[35] In the 1999–2000 survey, 31.8% of persons with hypertension were treated and controlled to BP <140/90 mmHg. By 2013–14 this percentage had climbed to 53.8%. However, this percentage has tailed off to 48.4% in 2015–16 and 43.7% in 2017–18. This unfortunate trend probably reflects the relaxation of the systolic BP treatment goal from < 140 to < 150 mmHg in the eighth Joint National Committee (JNC 8) treatment guidelines in 2014.[36] It remains to be seen whether the incorporation of the SPRINT results in the newest national guidelines, issued in 2018, will reverse that trend.[37]

To what extent do these trends explain the observed decline in mortality from heart attacks and strokes? Ford et al. have used a sophisticated model called IMPACT to address this question for coronary disease (heart attack) mortality in the U.S. for the 20-year period 1980–2000, during which heart attack mortality declined by 45.9% from 345.2 to 186.8 deaths per 100,000.[38] This model, which I will be citing throughout this book, analyzes prevalence and mortality rates, broken down into specific categories by age and gender, and applies regression coefficients estimated from the best available observational data for BP and other risk factors. It estimates that the change in mean systolic BP from 129.0 to 123.9 mmHg would be expected to have prevented 68,000 heart attack deaths in 2000—about 20.1% of the observed reduction in heart attack mortality.

The obvious problem with the IMPACT model is that it does not consider advances in BP treatment or declines in heart attack mortality after 2000, when heart attack mortality declined at its fastest pace (see Figure 1.2) and the proportion of hypertensive patients who attain a BP < 140/90 mmHg nearly doubled. Lacking access to the IMPACT software and the required input data, I have devised a method to update the published 1980–2000 result to 2014 using the NHANES reports cited above (see the appendix for details). Applying the fact that the improvement in BP control from essentially zero in 1968 to 53.8% in 2014 is 2.47 times the improvement from 10% in 1980 to 31.8% in 2000, we calculate that BP lowering accounted for 26.7% of the 79.5% decline in heart attack mortality during that period (see Table A.2).[39] This figure understates the total cardiovascular benefit of BP control, since it does not include the considerable impact of BP control on strokes and heart failure. However, this estimate would drop to 22% if we used the 2017–18 NHANES BP control figure. In either case, our advances in the treatment and control of high blood pressure since 1960 are a major success story and have taken a big bite out of the mid–20th-century cardiovascular pandemic.

FIGHTING CHOLESTEROL

Cholesterol ($C_{27}H_{46}O$) is a waxy organic fat-soluble substance (or lipid), which is an essential structural component of the membranes of all animal (but not plant) cells (Figure 5.11).

It is synthesized mainly in the liver and is abundant in diets containing meat, dairy, and other animal products. In addition to its structural role, cholesterol is also the common precursor of bile acids and all the steroid hormones, including cortisone and the sex hormones, which are synthesized in the adrenal glands, testes, and ovaries.

Because it is not soluble in water, cholesterol requires "carrier" proteins (apolipoproteins A, B, and others) to emulsify it so that it can travel through the blood in particles called lipoproteins. Lipoproteins were discovered in the 1920s and classified by their density, which is assessed by the degree to which they sink or float in an ultracentrifuge. In general,

The cholesterol molecule.

lipoproteins with high protein and low fat content sink and those with low protein and high fat content float. There are four broad classes of lipoproteins (going from heaviest to lightest): (a) high-density lipoprotein (HDL), which contains mainly apo-A and cholesterol, (b) low-density lipoprotein (LDL), which contains mainly apo-B and cholesterol, (c) very low-density lipoprotein (VLDL), which contains apo-B, C, and E and cholesterol and large amounts of triglyceride, and (d) triglyceride-rich chylomicrons, which transport dietary fats from the small intestine and are normally found in the blood only after meals. In the typical American or European, at least 65% of the circulating cholesterol is carried by LDL. In 1967, Fredrickson et al. classified the pathologic states associated with high lipoprotein levels.[1] Their second category (type II), in which LDL levels are elevated, will concern us most in this chapter.

Felix Marchand coined the term atherosclerosis in 1904, to describe the inflammatory changes that had been observed in the blood vessel walls of patients dying of cardiovascular causes fifty years earlier by the pathologists Karl von Rokitansky and Rudolf Virchow.[2] The term refers to the hardness of the artery ("sclerosis") and to the gruel-like consistency ("athero") of the substance (cholesterol, fats, and cellular debris) extruded when the lesion (or plaque) is cut. Figure 5.2 depicts an atherosclerotic plaque that partially obstructs an artery longitudinally and in cross section. From there, it was an easy leap to tie clinical cardiovascular events like heart attack and stroke, which involve the sudden and catastrophic obstruction of the blood supply. of vital organs like the heart and brain, to atherosclerosis.

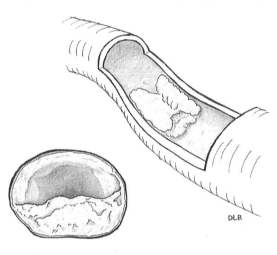

The "cholesterol hypothesis" placing cholesterol in the causal chain for atherosclerotic cardiovascular disease got

Longitudinal and cross-sectional drawings of an atherosclerotic plaque. Artwork by Debra L. Roney.

its start in 1913, when the Russian pathologist Nikolai Anichkov was able to reproduce atherosclerosis in rabbits by feeding them cholesterol that had been extracted and purified from egg yolks.[3] This is not easy to replicate experimentally in humans, in whom you can look at circulating cholesterol levels, but not—at least not easily—the lesions themselves. In the classical human feeding study by Ancel Keys, the short-term impact of dietary cholesterol intake on serum cholesterol was modest; the relative amounts of dietary saturated fats (hard fats typically found in meats, butter, and tropical plants) and unsaturated fats (soft fats and oils typically found in plants and fish) had a larger impact.[4] Other circumstantial evidence supported the cholesterol hypothesis:

1. The transitory 30% decline in cardiovascular mortality rates in Norway and other European countries occupied by Germany during World War II, when meat, dairy products, and eggs were in short supply.[5]

2. The Honolulu Heart Study of Japanese migrants, which showed a rise heart attack rates and fall in stroke rates as migrants adopted a western diet and lifestyle.[6]

3. The Seven Countries Study, which compared the populations of the U.S., Canada, Australia, England, Wales, Italy and Japan and found higher cardiovascular mortality rates in the countries consuming the most animal fat.[7]

However, none of this evidence came close to being dispositive. By the time Framingham and other prospective epidemiologic studies identified serum cholesterol as a major cardiovascular risk factor in the 1960s, medical science had little to offer for the treatment and control of high blood cholesterol and could offer no definitive proof that doing so would prevent heart attacks and other cardiovascular events. Until the development of the statins in the late 1980s the only approved cholesterol-lowering drugs were:

1. The bile acid sequestrant resins cholestyramine and colestipol, which inhibit the reabsorption of bile acids (a product of cholesterol) in the small intestine, thus forcing the liver to divert some cholesterol to the production of more bile acids. These drugs can theoretically lower LDL cholesterol by 25%, but they were administered as a gritty slurry (earning them the nickname "sand"), which must be drunk in large daily quantities and often cause constipation and abdominal discomfort. The

resins remain within the intestine and do not enter the body and are therefore quite safe; nevertheless, patient compliance is problematic.

2. Niacin, a vitamin which moderately (10%) lowers LDL and VLDL and raises HDL cholesterol, when given in high doses. Niacin also has significant vasomotor side effects (hot flushes), which limit patient compliance.

3. Clofibrate, which has a similar pharmacological effect to high-dose niacin but fewer side effects. Two newer fibrate drugs, gemfibrozil and fenofibrate, are in use today.

Until the mid–1970s, most of the trials using these drugs and/or cholesterol-lowering diets were secondary prevention trials in a few hundred patients. Blood cholesterol was typically lowered by 10% or less, and the results were mixed.[8] The largest trial was the Coronary Drug Project initiated by the NIH in 1966.[9] This double-blind placebo-controlled randomized trial in 8341 men with known heart disease had five active treatment arms (a) niacin, (b) clofibrate, (c) dextrothyroxine (a thyroid hormone analog), (d) low-dose estrogen, and (e) high-dose estrogen. None of the five drugs reduced mortality (the primary outcome). The men treated with niacin did show a significant favorable trend in recurrent coronary events.[10] But the dextrothyroxine and estrogen treatment arms had to be stopped early due to net *adverse* trends in cardiovascular outcomes.[11] (It should be noted that estrogen was used in this trial to mimic the relative "protection" of women from atherosclerotic cardiovascular disease, not to lower cholesterol levels.)

The World Health Organization (WHO) also initiated a large (15,763 participants) primary prevention trial using clofibrate in Edinburgh, Prague, and Budapest in 1962.[12] After five years of treatment, 25% more deaths were observed in the clofibrate than in the placebo group. However, after 13.5 years of extended follow up, mortality did not differ between groups.[13] Although the dismal results of the CDP and WHO clofibrate trials removed clofibrate as a viable cholesterol-lowering drug, two newer fibrate drugs, gemfibrozil and fenofibrate, have fared better in subsequent trials.[14]

The Lipid Research Clinics Coronary Primary Prevention Trial (LRC-CPPT)

In 1973, the NHLBI, after rejecting the concept of a large diet-heart trial as unfeasible, initiated the Lipid Research Clinics Coronary Primary

Prevention Trial (LRC-CPPT), a double-blind placebo-controlled primary prevention trial of cholestyramine in 3806 35- to 59-year-old men with type 2 hypercholesterolemia (LDL cholesterol > 175 mg/dL after three months of dietary treatment).[15] The study, which cost more than $150 million in *circa* 1980 dollars, was among the most expensive cardiovascular trials ever done. As a junior member of the NHLBI's LRC-CPPT management team, I can personally attest that no effort or expense were spared in the execution of this trial. Not one of the 3806 trial participants were lost to follow-up, and all cardiovascular hospitalizations and deaths were independently reviewed by a blinded panel of cardiologists to insure rigorous and objective classification of study endpoints. The trial had the strong backing of Donald Fredrickson and Bob Levy, two of the architects of the lipoprotein classification system, who had risen to the directorship of the NIH and NHLBI, respectively. Many of the twelve Lipid Research Clinics at which the trial was performed were alumni of Fredrickson's NIH laboratory, who had become eminent researchers in their own right. The data coordinating center was set up at the University of North Carolina, one of the country's leading schools of public health, and the Centers for Disease Control (CDC) standardized all cholesterol and lipoprotein measurements. The Lipid Metabolism Branch of the NHLBI, which was led by Dr. Basil Rifkind after Dr. Levy assumed the NHLBI directorship, was abundantly staffed with clinical trials experts, epidemiologists, nutritionists, and laboratory scientists who helped manage the trial.

However, when the much-anticipated trial results were announced in January 1984, they were underwhelming.[16] The difference in the primary outcome, the combined incidence of fatal and nonfatal heart attacks, was small—155 in the cholestyramine group versus 187 in the placebo group—and of marginal statistical significance. Although this 17% relative reduction in the primary endpoint was supported by similar reductions in secondary endpoints like stroke, other adverse cardiovascular outcomes, and the conversion of annual graded exercise tests from negative to positive, there was essentially no difference in total mortality—68 deaths in the cholestyramine group versus 71 deaths in the placebo group. The main problem was that cholestyramine, which lowered cholesterol by as much as 25% in small short-term trials, produced only a mean 8% cholesterol reduction in the LRC-CPPT due to deteriorating compliance over the trial's 7–10-year duration. The investigators pointed out that a 17% reduction in cardiac events was almost exactly what predictive models (like Framingham) would have anticipated for an 8% cholesterol reduction. A model based on internal analysis of the trial data showed o 49% reduction in heart attacks among LRC-CPPT participants who did maintain a 25% cholesterol reduction.[17] However, the LRC-CPPT certainly did not offer the clarity of the early hypertension trials and did not boost prescriptions of cholestyramine or other available cholesterol-lowering drugs. The cholesterol hypothesis seemed to be stuck and might have remained so but for two developments in the laboratory while the LRC-CPPT was underway—the identification and elucidation of the LDL receptor gene, for which Michael Brown and Joseph Goldstein won the 1985 Nobel Prize in Medicine, and the discovery in Japan of an antibiotic secreted by a penicillium fungus, which eventually became the prototype statin drug.

Familial Hypercholesterolemia and the LDL Receptor Gene

A Norwegian clinician, Carl Muller, first recognized familial hypercholesterolemia (FH) as an autosomal dominant inherited disorder characterized by high serum cholesterol and early severe cardiovascular disease in 1938.[18] Children who inherit copies of the mutated gene from both parents (homozygotes) have serum cholesterol levels approaching 1000 mg/dL, resulting in cholesterol deposits in their skin, tendons, and corneas, and severe atherosclerotic cardiovascular disease, manifesting in heart attacks and often death before they reach adulthood. Since these severely affected children respond poorly to cholesterol-lowering drugs, their treatment relies on plasma apheresis, a dialysis-like procedure in which the non-cellular (plasma) portion of the blood is cleansed of LDL perhaps twice a week. Persons who inherit a mutated gene from one parent and a normal gene from the other have milder manifestations with cholesterol levels in the 300–400 mg/dL range; these persons do respond to cholesterol-lowering drugs but still tend to have heart attacks in middle age and to die prematurely. The combined frequency of the many FH mutation variants is about one in 1000 in the U.S. This means that the prevalence of the severe homozygous form of the disease is about one in a million (the probability of inheriting a defective gene from both parents), while the milder heterozygotes comprise about 0.2% of the population, or more than 600,000 Americans. Brown and Goldstein demonstrated that the mutations that cause FH entail alterations in the structure of receptor molecules that enable LDL to move from the blood into the liver and other organs where the cholesterol it contains can be repurposed for the production of hormones and other essential molecules.[19] If these receptors are disabled, the liver and other organs must make their own cholesterol, while LDL levels in the bloodstream climb. According to the cholesterol hypothesis, these high circulating levels of LDL promote atherosclerosis. Thus, upregulating the production of LDL receptors in patients who have them would be an effective therapeutic strategy to reduce circulating LDL levels and inhibit atherosclerosis.

The Statins

In April 1971, Akira Endo, a Japanese pharmacologist employed by Sankyo, became interested in finding an antibiotic that would inhibit the synthesis of cholesterol and, inspired by the legendary discovery of penicillin by Alexander Fleming, began screening 3800 species of fungi for suitable compounds.[20] After about a year, his research produced citrinin, a potent inhibitor of 3-hydroxy-3-methylglutaryl coenzyme A (HMG CoA) reductase, the key rate-controlling enzyme in the synthetic pathway for cholesterol. Although animal experiments showing severe kidney toxicity quickly ruled out the use citrinin in humans, its discovery paved the way for the discovery of a second active compound called compactin several months later. For reasons never fully explicated, Sankyo abandoned compactin in 1980 after several years of animal studies and sold the rights to Merck, who developed a similar compound of its own called mevinolin (or lovastatin) with a superior safety profile. After years of testing, the U.S. FDA approved the clinical use of lovastatin for lowering LDL cholesterol in 1987, although randomized clinical trials were still needed to prove its efficacy in reducing rates of heart attack and other cardiovascular events. Still, because of its relative freedom from side effects and its ability to lower serum cholesterol by 20–30% under real-world conditions, prescriptions of lovastatin quickly surpassed the resins. Lovastatin was soon joined and surpassed by many other statin drugs—pravastatin (Pravachol), simvastatin (Zocor), fluvastatin (Leschol), atorvastatin (Lipitor), rosuvastatin (Crestor), pitavastatin (Livalo)—which offered advantages in potency and/or side effect profiles. According to ClinCalc, atorvastatin, simvastatin, pravastatin, and rosuvastatin were the second, eighth, 26th, and 39th most prescribed drugs in the U.S. in 2017, with more than 205 million prescriptions among them.[21]

The case for the cholesterol hypothesis was further bolstered in 1990 by the report of an unusual randomized trial in which partial ileal bypass surgery, in which the final segment of the small intestine (where bile acids are reabsorbed) is bypassed by joining the previous segment of the small intestine directly to the colon.[22] This procedure is tantamount to a more drastic and permanent version of cholestyramine resin. As one might imagine, recruitment was difficult and protracted; only 838 patients were randomized over nearly eight years. However, because the surgery produced a sustained 24% cholesterol reduction, there was a highly significant 35% reduction in the combined incidence of fatal and nonfatal MI, although the reductions in the two primary outcomes—mortality from coronary disease and from all causes—fell short of statistical significance. While the results of this trial provided proof of concept that a treatment that could actually produce a sustained cholesterol reduction of 20% or more could prevent heart attacks, the actual treatment used in this trial had little practical value.

So, returning to the mid–1980s, the NHLBI could have aptly portrayed LRC-CPPT results as hopeful but not definitive while awaiting results from the ongoing statin trials to perhaps provide the required proof. But they chose a riskier and more controversial route, promoting the LRC-CPPT results as having definitively provided the last missing piece to prove the cholesterol hypothesis. The NHLBI leadership argued that the LRC-CPPT findings should be viewed in the broader context of evidence from epidemiology and the laboratory (including the findings of Brown and Goldstein), and pointed to the development of new and more powerful cholesterol-lowering drugs (the statins) looming on the horizon. They established the National Cholesterol Education Program to promote public awareness of cholesterol and issued treatment guidelines (analogous to those for BP) which mostly emphasized diet and then stepped back to await the results of the pharmaceutical industry's ongoing statin trials.[23] While the NHLBI's promotional efforts laid the groundwork for the statins, they stirred up a firestorm of controversy.[24] Some of the objections were arcane (e.g., quibbles over the criteria for statistical significance), and others were silly (e.g., attributing biological importance to the flukish 11–4 excess of deaths by accident, suicide, or homicide in the cholestyramine group).

However, critics of the LRC-CPPT included many serious scientists who were justifiably skeptical of orchestrating an entire public health campaign based on the trial of a treatment that few patients would tolerate for a week (let alone a lifetime), which showed only a small, marginally significant benefit at best, and which was then extrapolated to cholesterol-lowering therapies that had not even been tested yet. This approach could easily have backfired if the statin drugs had not panned out.

But the statin drugs did pan out—and in a big way. In November 1993, Merck announced the results of its Scandinavian Simvastatin Survival Study (SSSS) in 4444 patients with prior heart attacks, in which simvastatin significantly reduced heart attacks, heart attack deaths, and total mortality by 34%, 42%, and 30% respectively.[25] A year later, Parke Davis announced similarly positive results of their West of Scotland Coronary Prevention Study (WOSCOPS) of pravastatin in 6595 hypercholesterolemic men without prior heart disease.[26] Twelve additional statin trials with acronyms like CARE (pravastatin) Post-CABG (lovastatin in patients with coronary bypass grafts), AFCAPS/TEXCAPS (lovastatin) LIPID (pravastatin), GISSI-P (pravastatin, not blinded), LIPS (fluvastatin), HPS (simvastatin), PROSPER (pravastatin), ALLHAT-LLT (pravastatin, not blinded), ASCOT-LLA (atorvastatin), ALERT (fluvastatin),and CARDS (atorvastatin) all reported results in the ensuing decade, and were included in the 2005 report of the Oxford Cholesterol Treatment Trialists prospective meta-analysis, which included 14 statin trials with 90,056 participants.[27] Except for the two non-blinded trials, where there were high rates of crossover to statin treatment in the control group, all reported statistically significant reductions in major vascular events. When the results were expressed in terms of risk reduction per 1.0 mMol/dL (38.6 mg/dL) lowering of LDL cholesterol, the results fit a straight line with a slope of 23% reduction in risk of major coronary events (mainly heart attacks) per mmol/dL decrease in LDL cholesterol. Similar reductions were observed for other cardiovascular events, including strokes and heart attack deaths. Statins had no adverse effect on cancer or other causes of death; mortality from all causes was significantly reduced by 12%. The percent reduction in major vascular diseases was similar and robust across patient subgroups— for example, 22% in patients with a prior heart attack versus 28% in patients with no prior heart disease, 26% in patients below age 65 versus 19% in seniors, 24% in men versus 18% in women, 21% in hypertensive patients versus 25% in others, 22% in diabetics versus 23% in others, etc.

In an updated 2010 analysis of 170,000 participants, which included twelve additional statin trials (five of which compared high- versus low-dose statins), the Cholesterol Treatment Trialists found more of the same.[28] In the 21 placebo-controlled trials, a mean 1.07 mmol/dL (41.3 mg/dL) mean reduction in LDL cholesterol, brought a highly significant 22% decrease in major vascular events (heart attacks, strokes, etc.). The results of these 21 trials are plotted against the LDL cholesterol reduction after one year is provided in Figure 5.3.

Although there is considerable variability around the regression line, the general trend comes through—the greater the reduction in LDL cholesterol, the greater the reduction in risk. In the five trials of intensive (high-dose and or high-potency) statin treatment, an additional 0.51 mmol/dL (20 mg/dL) mean reduction in LDL cholesterol brought an additional significant 15% reduction in major vascular events. In general, reductions of 22% in major vascular events and 10% in total mortality were observed for every 1 mmol/L (38.6 mg/dL) reduction in LDL cholesterol.

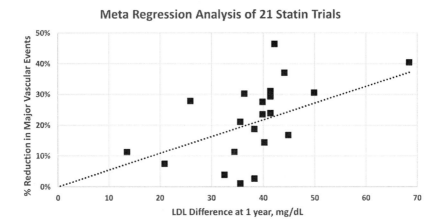

Meta Regression Analysis of 21 Statin Trials

Meta-regression analysis of 21 statin trials. Percent reduction in risk of major vascular events for 21 statin trials is plotted versus LAD cholesterol difference at one year. The trials are SSSS, WOSCOPS, CARE, Post-CABG, AFCAPS/TexCAPS, LIPID, GISSI-P, LIPS, HPS, PROSPER, ALLHAT-LLT, ASCOT-LLA, ALERT, CARDS, ALLIANCE, 4D, ASPEN, MEGA, JUPITER, GISSI-HF, and AURORA. Data were obtained from the Cholesterol Treatment Trialists (CTT) Collaboration, Lancet 2010; 376: 1670–1681. The dashed line represents a weighted linear regression in which each trial was weighted in inverse proportion to the standard error of its estimated risk reduction.

Thus, a patient receiving intensive statin therapy who attained the typical 1.58 mmol/L (61 mg/dL) decrease in LDL cholesterol (versus placebo) can expect to attain a net 32% reduction in the risk of major vascular events and a 15% reduction in risk of death. The risk reductions were again similar in all relevant subgroups—men and women, older and younger persons, persons with and without prior cardiovascular disease, persons with or without diabetes or hypertension, and persons starting from different baseline LDL cholesterol levels. There was no increase in cancer or other non-cardiovascular deaths in participants who received statins. Although statins still have their detractors and no drug is tolerated by everyone, no class of drug has been studied more thoroughly and rigorously than the statins regarding safety and efficacy in as many persons and has emerged with as clean a slate. The worst that can be said for the statins is that they can cause significant muscle inflammation (which can lead to kidney failure and death in extremely rare cases) in a small fraction of persons. Also, statins cause small increases in blood sugar that may complicate their use in diabetics; however, statins are the single best class of drugs for preventing major vascular events—the leading cause of death—in diabetics.[29]

Several non-statin cholesterol-lowering drugs have also emerged in the 21st century. Ezetimibe (Zetia), an oral agent approved in 2002, is often used in conjunction with a statin to add another 10–15% reduction in LDL cholesterol level. The most promising new drugs are the proprotein convertase subtilisin kexin 9 (PCSK9) blockers evolocumab (Repatha) and alirocumab (Praluent), which are monoclonal immunoglobulins that help the liver clear LDL cholesterol by blocking a protein called PCSK9, which interferes with LDL receptors.[30] These drugs, which can be given only by injection, mimic a naturally occurring human PCSK9 mutation which is characterized by very low levels of LDL cholesterol and correspondingly low rates of cardiovascular disease. PCSK9 blockers are especially useful in FH heterozygotes whose LDL cholesterol levels remain elevated even after taking statins; when they are used in combination with a statin, LDL cholesterol reductions of 65% or more may be achieved. However, since the efficacy of all these drugs requires LDL receptors, they are not very effective in FH homozygotes. The recent approval of lomitapide (Juxtapid), which partially blocks the production of LDL particles, may offer these patients some relief.

In summary, the treatment of high BP and high LDL cholesterol are the twin bulwarks of modern preventive cardiology. The BP and cholesterol stories have many parallels but also some important differences. The major randomized trials establishing the importance of BP lowering were completed by 1992, before the first major statin trial was published, while people were still arguing over whether the cholesterol hypothesis was a myth. While physicians had their choice of multiple classes of effective BP drugs that were generally used in combinations, physicians had no good options for lowering LDL cholesterol until the statins came along and even today rely primarily on the statins. The NHLBI has remained a central player in BP trials into the 21st century (SPRINT) but has played only a minor supporting role in cholesterol trials since 1984.

Impact of Cholesterol-Lowering on Heart Attack Deaths

Like hypertension, the treatment of high blood cholesterol has traveled a long road from acrimonious controversy to consensus, but within half the time. Unlike hypertension, the road was for cholesterol was tortuous and laden with potholes. As recently as 1990, the state of cholesterol lowering drugs was little better than that of antihypertensive drugs in 1960, and some dismissed the cholesterol hypothesis as myth. It was not until 1994 that the first clinical trial demonstrated that statin treatment could prevent cardiovascular events, and it was not until 2001 that the National Cholesterol Education Program Expert Panel was able to give a full-throated endorsement to statins as the first line of pharmacologic treatment of high blood cholesterol.[31] In 1988–94, just before the first statin trial was published, only 3.4% of U.S. adults reported taking a cholesterol-lowering drug of any kind; that percentage grew to 9.3% in 1999–2002 and 15.5% in 2007–2010.[32] The percentage of American adults using statins doubled between 1999–2002 and 2010–11, growing from 7.4% to 15.9% in men and from 9.6% to 18.9% in women.[33] If one just looks at Americans over age 40, the prevalence of cholesterol-lowering drugs grew from 19.9% in 2003–04 to 27.9% in 2011–12, while the prevalence of statin use grew from 16.3% to 23.2% over the same decade.[34]

In 2018, the ACC/AHA Guidelines for cholesterol treatment have established LDL cholesterol < 100 mg/dL as the ideal and recommend intensive statin treatment to achieve that goal for patients without cardiovascular disease whose 10-year cardiovascular risk exceeds 7.5%.[35] They further recommend intensive statin treatment for all patients with established cardiovascular disease, with a goal of reducing LDL cholesterol by 50%. A recent analysis of 2012–13 data showed that while statin use was 27.9% among all Americans over age 40, roughly 60% of those with high risk due to existing cardiovascular disease and 50% of those with diabetes were using a statin.[36] The use of statins in secondary prevention has grown from zero in 1980 to 45% in 2000 to 72% in 2011.[37]

The IMPACT model of Ford et al. attributes 24.2% of the observed decline in heart attack mortality between 1980 and 2000—to the reduction in the mean population LDL cholesterol level in the U.S. population from 5.67 mmol/L in 1980 to 5.33 mmol/L in 2000, which according to the Cholesterol Treatment Trialists meta-analysis would translate to a 32% reduction in heart attack deaths in men and a 31% reduction in women.[38] Most of this reduction was likely due to the introduction of statins in the late 1980s. The model also estimated that statin treatment in various secondary prevention settings (after a heart attack, heart failure, coronary bypass surgery, hypertension, etc.) accounted for an additional 8.5% of the observed reduction in heart attack mortality. Thus, the introduction of statins drugs accounted for roughly one-third of the 46% reduction in heart attack deaths (from 345.2 to 186.8 deaths per 100,000) between 1980 and 2000. But what about the contribution of statins to the accelerating decline in heart attack mortality after 2000, as shown in Figure 1.2?

I have applied the method described for hypertension in Chapter 4 (and explained in detail in the appendix) to extrapolate the published IMPACT findings for statins to cover the 77.4% decline in heart attack mortality in 1968–2011 (the most recent year for which I have national statin usage data for all adults). Based on the increase in statin usage by a factor of 2.05 between 2000 and 2011, I estimate that LDL cholesterol lowering—mainly statin usage—in the general population (i.e., primary prevention) has accounted for 27.7% of the 77.4% decline in heart attack deaths between 1968 and 2011 (see Table A.2). Similarly, I estimate the increase in statin usage in persons who have already had a heart attack (i.e., secondary prevention) by a factor of 1.71 between 2000 and 2011, has accounted for 8.2% of this mortality decline (see Table A.4). All told, 35.9% of the 1968–2011 decline in heart attack mortality can be attributed to statins and other cholesterol lowering interventions. These figures probably understate the total cardiovascular impact of statins since they do not include reduction of atherothrombotic strokes. (Cholesterol lowering does not reduce strokes caused by intracranial bleeding.) It also does not model the increasing use of more aggressive statin regimens in secondary prevention and high-risk primary prevention, as recommended in the newest cholesterol treatment guidelines. All in all, it is fair to state that the development and promulgation of statins during the past three decades is probably the single greatest factor in the decline in heart attack deaths since 1968.

6

THE TOBACCO BANE

The story of the third potentially reversible Framingham cardiovascular risk factor, cigarette smoking, differs importantly from that of hypertension and high cholesterol in that cigarette smoke was already a proven carcinogen by the time the first Framingham results were reported in 1961. Therefore, efforts to control this risk factor were always a matter of changing public opinion and behavior more than proving that smoking caused heart disease. Furthermore, cardiovascular public health scientists took a back seat to specialists in lung disease and cancer in these efforts. Although the public sector, specifically the Surgeon General's office and the Centers for Disease Control and Prevention (CDC), played an important coordinating role, these efforts were spearheaded in the U.S. by national and local chapters of volunteer organizations like the American Lung Association (ALA), the American Cancer Society (ACS), and the American Heart Association (AHA).

The major epidemiologic studies of smoking were done in the early 1950s by Richard Doll and Bradford Hill in the UK and by Cuyler Hammond and Daniel Horn in the U.S.[1] In their landmark 1952 retrospective case-control study, in which men comprised 93% of all cases, Doll and Hill found that only seven of 1357 men with lung cancer (0.5%) versus 61 male controls (4.5%) were non-smokers.[2] There was a strong graded dose-response relationship, with lung cancer rates at least 10 times higher in heavy smokers than in non-smokers. The strong relationship between smoking and lung cancer was confirmed prospectively in 1954 by Doll and Hill in male physicians and in a larger ACS-supported U.S. study by Hammond and Horn in 187,766 50- to 69-year-old men.[3] By 1964, when the U.S. Surgeon General issued the historic report of his advisory committee on smoking health, implicating smoking in chronic obstructive lung disease and cardiovascular disease, as well as lung cancer, randomized trials of smoking were no longer ethically viable.[4]

Although tobacco has been with us since colonial times, cigarettes are a relatively recent phenomenon. Before 1900, most tobacco was either chewed or smoked in pipes and cigars, which because they tend to be consumed in modest amounts and their smoke is not deeply inhaled, are less addictive and less damaging to the lungs.[5] Annual per capita cigarette consumption in 1900 was only 54 cigarettes.[6] Lung cancer was quite rare. The development of technology for the mass production of inexpensive cigarettes circa 1900 changed all this. Per capita cigarettes in the U.S. rose almost 100-fold to 4345 cigarettes per adult per year in 1965, when 42.4% of Americans smoked them. By 1950, consumption, which comprised less than 1% of American tobacco consumption in 1880, accounted for 80% of American tobacco consumption. Lung cancer had become the leading cause of cancer death in American men in 1954, and surpassed breast cancer as the leading cause of cancer death in American women in 1987.

The prevalence of cigarette smoking in U.S. adults has declined steadily from the early 1960s to the present (Figure 6.1A), reaching a new low of 13.7% in 2018 (Figure 6.1A).[7]

The prevalence of cigarette smoking among youths under age 18 surged briefly in the 1990s but is now less than that in adults, although this trend has been more than offset by the rising popularity of electronic cigarettes.[8] Cigarette smoking has always been more prevalent in men than women but has declined more rapidly in men, and the gender gap has steadily declined from almost 30% in the mid–1950s to 3.6% in 2018 (Figure 6.1B).

Lung cancer mortality (which reflects the long-term, largely irreversible ravages of smoking on lung tissue) has been falling since 1993, lagging almost 30 years behind the decline in cigarette smoking, with annual declines of 1.9% in men and 0.9% in women.[9] The rise and decline in cigarette smoking closely parallels the trend in heart attack mortality (Figure 1.1), covering the same period. In contrast to lung cancer, there is no perceptible lag time behind the trend in smoking, because the cardiovascular effects of smoking tend to be acute and mostly reversible—if a person stops smoking.

This chapter will address three questions:

1. How did cigarettes become so popular?
2. How was the post–1963 decline in cigarette smoking achieved?
3. To what extent do the rise and decline in smoking from 1900–2020 explain the trends in mortality from heart attacks, strokes, and other cardiovascular causes?

A. Trends in **Cigarette** Smoking by Age

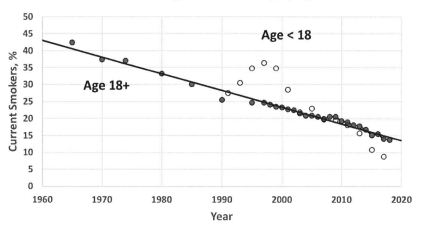

B. Trends in Cigarette Smoking by Sex

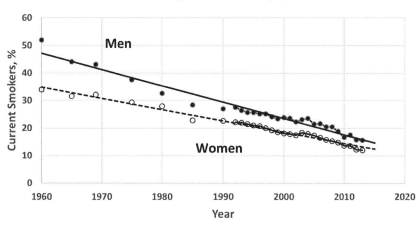

U.S. trends in cigarette smoking, 1960–2018, from the American Lung Association website. Trends are shown by age group (Figure 6.1A) and sex (Figure 6.1B).

The rise in the popularity of smoking in 1900–60 was fueled largely by changes in the tobacco curing process, producing a sweeter, milder blend, the portability and affordability of cigarettes, and the invention of safety matches. But cigarettes were also heavily marketed by direct advertising and by what would now be called "product placement" in movies and other popular entertainments. Cigarette smoking was popularly portrayed as relaxing and soothing, endorsed by doctors and celebrities; you can check out some of the more absurd examples on the internet.[10] They were endorsed by celebrities like Lucille Ball, Gary Cooper, Arthur Godfrey, and Steve McQueen. They were even marketed to women as a means of weight control, as in "Reach for a Lucky instead of a sweet" and (if you can believe it) as a remedy for the symptoms of asthma, bronchitis, and influenza. Although cigarette sales took a hit during the Great Depression and again in the early 1950s, following the studies linking smoking and lung cancer, tobacco companies countered by marketing filter cigarettes and other brands with reduced tar and nicotine content and/or menthol. Cigarette consumption quickly rebounded. By 1960, half of all cigarettes smoked in the U.S. had filters.[11] But new ads like those featuring a rugged cowboy called "the Marlboro Man" and an ad for a new cigarette brand for women called Virginia Slims ("You've come a long way, baby!") were still all over television in the 1960s. Pioneering newscaster John Cameron Swayze sat in front of a Camels logo on his daily newscasts, and the main characters in popular TV shows of the era (like Perry Mason) smoked cigarettes. In this environment, the 1964 Surgeon General's report exploded like a bombshell, creating a huge flurry of headlines and rating among the top news stories of 1964.[12] However, all this publicity made only a small dent in cigarette consumption.

Following the Surgeon General's report, the U.S. Congress passed two major pieces of anti-smoking legislation.[13] The Federal Cigarette Labeling and Advertising Act of 1965 required tobacco companies to put health warnings on all cigarette packaging and to air public service announcements publicizing the deleterious effects of smoking on health. The Public Health Cigarette Smoking Act of 1969 went a step further and banned all cigarette advertising in the broadcast media. However, these new laws did nothing to prevent tobacco companies from rechanneling their advertising budget into print advertising, billboards, etc. In 1975, five years after Richard Nixon signed the cigarette advertising ban into law, per capita cigarette consumption still hovered around 4000 per year, down only about 7% from its peak of 4300 in the early 1960s. Clearly, a broader grass-roots anti-smoking campaign was needed.

One offshoot of the 1964 Surgeon General's report was the establishment of the National Clearinghouse for Smoking and Health to track the progress of antismoking efforts. This organization soon evolved into the

CDC Office on Smoking and Health, which coordinates with national volunteer health organizations like the ALA, ACS, and AHA and their local chapters to support state and community anti-smoking programs, promote tobacco research, and ensure the public visibility of antismoking messaging. It is these grass-roots efforts, which focused on making cigarettes unappealing and curtailing and eventually banning smoking from public spaces, that finally sent per capita cigarette consumption plummeting by more than half during the last quarter of the 20th century. An important driver of these efforts was research on the adverse impact of secondhand smoke on non-smokers, especially children with asthma and other respiratory disorders.[14] Although secondhand smoke accounts for a relatively small number of lung cancers, the exacerbation of asthma and other lung conditions in children chronically exposed to tobacco smoke was for more pervasive and alarming. With this new evidence in hand, smoking cigarettes now could be said to involve more than a risky personal lifestyle choice; it also claimed the most innocent of victims.

In 1975, one could expect to be exposed to secondhand cigarette smoke at work, in bars and restaurants, on airplanes and trains, and in hotels. When I sat in a non-smoking section on a flight to Europe in 1973, the smoking section was right across the aisle, about two feet away. Efforts to change this culture began modestly with local campaigns—like a successful effort by the local chapter of the AHA in my hometown of Chicago in the late 1970s to persuade local restaurant associations to call for designated non-smoking sections in restaurants. Then, these efforts began gradually to pick up steam Some important landmarks in this battle are listed below:

Table 6.1 Anti-Smoking Landmarks, 1975–2000[15]

1975	Minnesota becomes the first state to require separate smoking areas in public places by passing the Minnesota Clean Indoor Air Act.
1984	The USFDA approves nicotine gum as the first drug designed to help people quit smoking.
1986	A new Surgeon General's report on the Health Consequences of Involuntary Smoking is issued, emphasizing the harmful effects of secondhand smoke.[16] A final definitive report was issued in 2006.
1987	Congress prohibits smoking on short domestic flights. Before this, smoking was allowed in the back rows of domestic flights.
1987	Aspen, Colorado, becomes the first city in the U.S. to require smoke-free restaurants.

1988	California voters approve Proposition 99, which imposed a 25% surtax on cigarettes and earmarked the additional revenue to create a statewide anti-tobacco control program.
1988	American Lung Association, American Heart Association and American Cancer Society establish Tobacco Free America to publish "State Legislated Actions on Tobacco Issues," which tracks relevant taxes, laws, and programmatic funding for every state.[17]
1989	Congress bans smoking on all domestic airlines.
1990	San Luis Obispo becomes the first city to ban smoking in all public buildings, including bars and restaurants.
1993	The U.S. Environmental Protection Agency published a report concluding that secondhand smoking is responsible for approximately 3000 lung cancer deaths annually in nonsmoking adults and respiratory impairment in hundreds of thousands of children.[18]
1998	California becomes the first state to issue a comprehensive ban of smoking in all bars and restaurants.
1998	Attorneys General from 46 states reach a multibillion dollar damages settlement with tobacco industry.
1999	The U.S. Department of Justice sues the tobacco industry under the RICO (racketeering) statute, claiming that they engaged in "a coordinated campaign of fraud and deceit." This lawsuit was decided in the government's favor in 2006.

Restrictions on smoking have continued to grow in the 21st century, and the prevalence of smoking has continued to fall, reaching a new low of 13.7% in 2018.[19]

The success of anti-smoking efforts has been predominantly in encouraging smokers to give up the habit, rather than preventing teenagers and young adults from acquiring it. The proportion of "ever-smokers" who have quit smoking has increased at a steady pace from 24.2% in 1965 to 61.7% in 2018.[20] By contrast, the proportion of 12- to 17-year-olds who start smoking rose from 12% in the mid–1960s to as high 16% a decade later, then fell back to 12% in the late 1980s and early 1990s, rose again to 14% in the late 1990, and fell to 11% in 2002–03.[21] The trend in 18- to 25-year-olds is somewhat more encouraging, falling from a high of 11% in 1968 to below 6% in the early 1980s and rebounding slightly to 7% in 2000–03.[22] However, more recently, starting in 2007, a new phenomenon—electronic cigarettes (e-cigarettes) or "vaping"—has taken hold among adults seeking a "safer" alternative to smoking and, more ominously, among teenagers, who are attracted to their candy-like flavors. While e-cigarette use has remained steady at roughly 3% in adults, there has been an alarming two-year increase in their use in high school-ers (11.7% in 2017 to 27.5% in 2019) and in middle schoolers (3.3% in 2017 to 10.5% in 2019).[23] Because of this sharp uptick in e-cigarette use, nearly one in three high-schoolers and one in eight middle-schoolers used some form of tobacco in 2019. While vaping may not deliver carcinogenic tars into the lungs, it does effectively deliver nicotine with its associated risk for cardiovascular disease and acute asthmatic attacks and is just as addic-tive as tobacco. In 2019, there were sporadic reports of unusual acute (and even fatal) respiratory distress syndrome in young consumers of flavored e-cigarettes and calls for banning these products.[24]

Cardiovascular Impact of Trends in Smoking

There is no doubt that the marked decline in cigarette consumption and in prevalence of smoking from 42% in 1965 to 14% in 2018 has saved millions of American lives and has extended life expectancy. Holford et al. calculated that the reduction in smoking between 1964 and 2012 increased life expectancy by 2.3 years in men and 1.6 years in women and has resulted in 157 million years of life saved.[25] These gains in life expectancy represent just under 30% of the observed 7.8- and 5.4-year overall gains during this 48-year period in men and women, respectively. Reducing cigarette smok-ing, which has reduced incidence of and mortality from lung and other cancers and chronic obstructive lung disease, as well as cardiovascular dis-ease, is probably the single most impactful public health accomplishment of the last half of the 20th century.

But in keeping with the object of this book, let us focus more nar-rowly on the role of the anti-smoking effort in quelling the cardiovascu-lar pandemic of the 20th century. The IMPACT model estimates that the decline in cigarette smoking was responsible for 11.7% of the 46% decline in heart attack mortality between 1980 and 2000.[26] Given the fact that the decline in cigarette smoking from 40% in 1968 to 14% in 2017 was 2.57 times as great as the decline from 33% in 1980 to 23% in 2000, this extrap-olates to smoking cessation accounting for 16.4% of the 81% decline in heart attack mortality since 1968 (see the appendix, Table A.2).

One can apply the same approach to extrapolate the published IMPACT results of 1980–2000 back in time to analyze the contribution of cigarettes to the onset of the cardiovascular pandemic. In contrast to BP and cholesterol, we have reliable cigarette consumption data going back to 1900, when cigarette smoking first became popular (Figure 6.1). We must make two modifications:

1. Lacking national heart attack mortality data before 1950, we must base the analysis on the decline in heart disease mortality, which includes cardiomyopathy, rheumatic, congenital, hypertensive and other heart conditions, as well as heart attacks.

2. Ford et al. relied on non-randomized studies of smoking cessation, in which heart attack risk was reduced by 36%, rather than the roughly 50% reduction one would expect if heart attack risk returned to its pre-smoking baseline.[27] While this assumption is defensible in analyzing the decline in smoking since 1968 (which was driven by smoking cessation rather than preventing new smokers), it is clearly not valid when analyzing the rise in smoking between 1900 and 1968, in which each new smoker can be more reasonably assumed to have doubled his/her heart attack risk.[28]

After making these adjustments, I have estimated that the rise in smoking prevalence from 0 in 1900 to nearly 40% in 1968, accounted for nearly 28% of the 100% increase in heart disease mortality from 265.4 to 531.0 deaths per 100,000 between 1900 and 1968 (see the appendix, Table A.3). The contribution might be even larger if one assumes that cigarette smoking more than doubles the risk of a heart attack. Efforts to discourage teenagers and young adults from smoking may hold the key to further progress, although their short-term cardiovascular risk is low.

THE RISE OF DIABETES

After reading the last three chapters, which attribute more than half of the decline in heart attack deaths since 1960 to improvements in just three risk factors—BP, LDL cholesterol, and smoking—a reader might form the mistaken impression that taming this great pandemic was a direct march from one success to the next. However, the next three chapters, in which promising beginnings have ended in disappointment, offer a sobering look at how difficult and frustrating this process has often been.

Diabetes mellitus (a composite of the Greek word *diabainein* meaning "to pass through," referring to excessive urination, and the Latin word *mellitus*, meaning "sweetened with honey," referring to the spillage of the sugar glucose into the urine) is a complex metabolic disorder characterized by the inability to regulate blood sugar levels. The underlying defect in this disease, which affects 34.2 million Americans (10.5% of the U.S. population), is a deficiency of or resistance to the hormone insulin, which is normally synthesized in the pancreas by the islets of Langerhans.[1] This hormone, which is a dipeptide (two linked chains of amino acids that are shorter than proteins), is integral to the conversion of fat to glucose and enables glucose to enter muscle and other cells to be utilized as an energy source. Diabetes mellitus is actually two distinct diseases—one in which insulin is not produced (type 1) and another in which insulin is produced normally but the target cells are resistant (type 2).

Type 1 diabetes, which typically strikes in children and young adults and is often called juvenile-onset diabetes, has been around for at least 3000 years, since the days of ancient Egypt.[2] It is now widely seen as an auto-immune disease, in which the insulin-producing cells of the pancreas are destroyed by the body's own immune cells, perhaps triggered by a viral infection.[3] Without insulin, the constant loss of glucose in the urine produces dehydration, emaciation, and eventually a lethal condition called diabetic ketoacidosis in which blood glucose levels skyrocket and form ketones, the blood becomes more acidic, and coma and death ensue. Until Frederick Banting, James MacLeod, Charles Best, and James Collip, of the University of Toronto isolated insulin in a stable injectable form in the early 1920s—a discovery that won Banting and MacLeod the 1923 Nobel Prize in Medicine—most diabetics succumbed to this fate.[4] When Ely Lilly and Company began to mass-produce insulin from the pancreases of pigs and cows in 1923, diabetics gained a new lease on life. However, as diabetics began to live longer, the long-term chronic inflammatory effects of this disease on blood vessels became manifest.[5] Two kinds of blood vessel changes occur:

- Changes in the small vessels (microvascular disease) of the heart, kidneys, retina (eyes), nervous system, etc., which may lead to heart failure, kidney failure, blindness, neuropathy, and poor wound healing.
- Accelerated atherosclerosis of large blood vessels (macrovascular disease) in the heart, brain, etc.

Today, the leading cause of death among diabetes is not diabetic ketoacidosis but heart attack, as illustrated by the death of baseball Hall of Famer Jackie Robinson.[6] The availability of insulin saved him from an early death by ketoacidosis and allowed him to finish his baseball career, but it did not save him from near-blindness and a fatal heart attack on October 24, 1972.

After World War II, accompanying the post-war boom in prosperity, a once uncommon variant of diabetes called type 2 (or sometimes adult-onset or non-insulin-dependent) diabetes has emerged and has far surpassed type 1 diabetes in prevalence, accounting for 90–95% of all cases.[7] In contrast to type 1 diabetes, the pancreas produces more than enough insulin, but the target muscle and fat cells become resistant to insulin and require ever-increasing insulin levels to properly metabolize glucose.[8] Unlike the type 1 variant, type 2 diabetes is associated with obesity and manifests as a continuum from "metabolic syndrome" to "pre-diabetes" to frank diabetes. It often evolves slowly over many years (hence, its relative rarity in children). Blood glucose levels rarely rise as high in type 2 as in type 1 diabetes, and ketoacidosis is rare, occurring only in late cases after the ability of the pancreas to meet the ever-increasing demand for insulin has been exhausted. Many type 2 diabetic patients do not require insulin injections and can be adequately controlled by diet, alone or in combination with the myriad available oral agents that stimulate pancreatic insulin production or decrease insulin resistance. However, notwithstanding all these differences, the impact of type 2 diabetes on small blood vessels in the heart, kidneys, eyes, and nervous system is similar to that seen in type 1 diabetes. Like Jackie Robinson and his fellow type 1 diabetics, most type 2 diabetics eventually die of heart attacks, at a rate three times higher than persons without diabetes.

With diabetic ketoacidosis becoming less of an issue following the introduction of insulin and the rise of the type 2 form of the disease, the attention of medical science has focused on how to prevent or ameliorate the cardiovascular consequences of diabetes that shorten the lives of those afflicted and impair the quality of their lives. Since the early 1970s, improving blood glucose control has seemed the most likely avenue to improve the longevity and quality of life in diabetes. Two developments made it possible to pursue this research.

1. Discovery of a superior marker of metabolic control in diabetes: Measuring blood glucose itself is an unsatisfactory marker of metabolic control, since its levels fluctuate widely over the course of each day, depending on how recently one has eaten and the content of the most recent meal. When I was in medical school, the cumbersome glucose tolerance test, which required a series of timed blood draws following ingestion of a measured glucose load, was typically used to diagnose diabetes. The discovery and development of glycated hemoglobin (HbA1c) in the early 1970s provided an easily measured blood marker of metabolic control for tracking the progress of diabetics without worrying about transitory fluctuations in blood glucose levels.[9] Selvyn et al. showed in 2010 that HbA1c was indeed a better predictor of future cardiovascular events in 11,092 nondiabetic adults than fasting blood glucose.[10] HbA1c levels below 5.7% are generally considered normal, levels between 5.7 and 6.4% indicate prediabetes, and confirmed levels of 6.5% or higher indicate diabetes.[11] In diabetics, where HbA1c levels may exceed 10% before treatment, the American Diabetes Association (ADA) considers HbA1c levels below 7% as the criterion for good metabolic control.[12]

2. Development of a wide variety of oral medications for treating type 2 diabetes.[13] Until the late 1990s, therapeutic options for diabetes beyond insulin injection were limited to the biguanides (mainly metformin), the sulfonylureas (glyburide, glipizide, glimepiride), and the meglitinides (repaglinide, nateglinide). Metformin, which improves

sensitivity to insulin, is generally considered the drug of choice.[14] It is currently the fourth most prescribed drug in the U.S., with 78,602,870 prescriptions written in 2017.[15] The less preferred sulfonylureas and meglitinides stimulate pancreatic insulin secretion and are often prescribed in combination with metformin. Many other options have become available during the past two decades, as you will see later in this chapter.

Numerous randomized trials using one or more oral drugs instead of or in addition to insulin have been performed to try to establish, analogous to the blood pressure trials described in Chapter 4, that achieving tighter glucose control in diabetic patients reduces their rate of heart attacks and other adverse cardiovascular events and to determine which if any regimens are most effective in this regard. The major diabetes trials are described below.

University Group Diabetes Program (UGDP)

Diabetes trials got off to a very inauspicious beginning when the UGDP trial was launched in 1960. The trial was originally designed with four treatment arms:

- Tolbutamide (an early sulfonylurea drug that is no longer used)
- Placebo for tolbutamide
- Insulin provided in a standard invariant dosage, set according to the patient's body weight
- Insulin provided in variable dosages designed to normalize fasting blood glucose levels

In 1961, two more treatment arms were added:

- Phenformin (which has been replaced by metformin in current practice)
- Placebo for phenformin

The study was partially blinded; patients knew whether they were receiving insulin or either of the two oral drugs but did not know whether they received the active or placebo versions of the two oral drugs. The tolbutamide arm was stopped in 1969 because of excess mortality in the group receiving active versus placebo tolbutamide, although the heart attack rates did not differ significantly. The phenformin arm was terminated for lack of efficacy two years later.[16] The insulin arms of the trial were allowed to run to completion, but at the end of the day, they were also no better than placebo in terms of preventing heart attacks or prolonging life. The decision by the investigators to abort the tolbutamide arm, which was leaked to the press three weeks before the results were presented at the annual ADA scientific meeting and caused stock prices to plunge, set off a firestorm of criticism, particularly in the pharmaceutical sector, which accused the investigators of bias.[17] However, subsequent laboratory studies have shown that tolbutamide (along with a related subset of sulfonylurea drugs) had specific toxic effects on heart muscle that may have accounted for the excess deaths. These drugs have given way to new safer sulfonylurea drugs. Phenformin has since been withdrawn because of its tendency to cause severe lactic acidosis, a metabolic complication that can cause kidney failure and sometimes death.[18] Metformin, which is far safer than phenformin, is currently the only approved biguanide drug, So the controversy about the two UGDP oral drugs has been rendered moot to some extent. Yet, the fact remains that it failed to offer "proof of concept" for the hypothesis that improved metabolic control prevents or ameliorates the cardiovascular consequences of diabetes. There things languished for more than a decade.

The Diabetes Control and Complications Trial (DCCT)

In 1983, the NIH's National Institute of Diabetes and Digestive and Kidney Diseases (NIDDK) launched a major randomized cardiovascular outcomes trial in 1441 patients, aged 13–39 years, with type 1 diabetes mellitus. Patients were stratified (as primary or secondary) based on the absence or presence of pre-existing diabetic complications in the small blood vessels of the eyes and/or kidneys and randomized to conventional or intensive therapy. Patients in the conventional therapy arm received one or two daily injections of a fixed insulin dosage, while patients in the intensive therapy arm received multiple daily doses of insulin with a goal of achieving normal HbA1c levels. The results were published in 1993.[19] Mean HbA1c levels of 7% were in fact sustained in the intensive group versus 8.5–9.2% in the conventional group. This difference in glycemic control brought about highly significant reductions in retinopathy (damage to the small blood vessels in the eyes) and other forms of diabetic damage to the microvasculature of the

71

nervous system from close to 60% in the conventional arm to 25% or less in the intensive arm. Reduced rates of other microvascular complications were also observed. However, the DCCT was unable to address the impact of the intensive treatment regimen on incidence of heart attack, stroke, and other macrovascular adverse outcomes, since participants were too young to be at high risk for these outcomes. Two small contemporaneous trials in Stockholm and Japan found similar results.[20]

UK Prospective Diabetes Study (UKPDS)

The UKPDS was a large complex non-blinded British multicenter randomized trial conducted in 4075 patients with newly diagnosed type 2 diabetes.[21] Its objective was to determine wither intensive diabetes control (target HbA1c < 7%) could reduce the incidence of microvascular and macrovascular complications of diabetes. The UKPDS stratified patients as overweight (N = 1704) or normal weight when they entered the study. Normal-weight patients were randomized to receive intensive care with either insulin or a selection of sulfonylurea drugs versus conventional care.[22] Overweight patients were randomized to intensive care with either insulin, a sulfonylurea, or metformin versus conventional care.[23] Thus, there were in effect seven treatment arms—5 receiving intensive treatment with either insulin, sulfonylureas, or metformin and two receiving conventional care. However, the metformin group was very small (N = 342). The results, published in 1998, were correspondingly complicated, but boiled down to the following:

- Intensive treatment in general significantly reduced microvascular complications.
- Heart attack rates were also reduced in the intensive care groups, but the reduction fell short of statistical significance.
- Intensive treatment had no impact on mortality.
- The intensive treatment metformin group appeared to fare slightly better than the other intensive treatment regimens in overweight patients, but the numbers were small, and the differences were not significant.

In general, the UKPDS results were far more encouraging than the UGDP. The good news is that they showed that intensive glycemic control mitigated the microvascular ravages of type 2 diabetes. The bad news is that they fell well short of proving that this treatment prevented heart attacks. The worse news is that they provided no evidence at all that intensive glycemic control prolonged life. However, the positive results for microvascular complications elevated the HbA1c < 7.0% treatment goal to standard practice and thereby made it mandatory that this treatment goal be incorporated in the control arm of any future diabetes treatment trial. Thus, as the new millennium dawned, it was no longer possible to design an ethically acceptable randomized trial to prove that attaining that goal reduced mortality.

Diabetes trials in the first decade of the 21st century focused chiefly on two research questions: (1) trials comparing a new class of drugs, the thiazolidinediones, to the older drugs (insulin, metformin, and the sulfonylureas) in type 2 diabetes and (2) trials designed to compare even more intensive regimens of glycemic control to the new standard of HbA1c < 7.0%.

The Thiazolidinediones

From the time of the UGDP through the completion of the UKPDS, the medical management of type 2 diabetes relied on same four drug classes—insulin, biguanidines, sulfonylureas, and meglinitides. While phenformin gave way to metformin, tolbutamide gave way to glyburide, glipizide, and glimepiride, and insulin became available in multiple long-acting and short acting variations, the approval of the first thiazolidinedione, troglitazone, in 1997 appeared to represent a breakthrough. Like metformin, troglitazone addressed the basic metabolic defect of type 2 diabetes, by decreasing resistance to insulin. Unfortunately, troglitazone was withdrawn in 2000 because of case reports of significant toxicity to the liver. However, two other drugs of the same class but without the liver toxicity—rosiglitazone and pioglitazone—quickly filled the breech.

Several major cardiovascular trials were soon implemented to test whether these new drugs offered any advantage over the established drugs in reducing cardiovascular complications in diabetes:

1. The Rosiglitazone Evaluated for Cardiac Outcomes and Regulation of Glycaemia in Diabetes (RECORD) trial was a multicenter, randomized, non-blinded study, sponsored by SmithKlineGlaxo, that evaluated the incremental effect of rosiglitazone

(Avandia) on cardiovascular outcomes in 4447 patients with type 2 diabetes treated with metformin or sulfonylurea.[24]

2. The NIH-sponsored Bypass Angioplasty Revascularization Investigation 2 Diabetes (BARI-2D) trial (for which I was the initial project officer) was a 2×2 factorial trial in type 2 diabetic patients with heart disease who were candidates for elective coronary bypass surgery or placement of coronary stents.[25] In the diabetes component of the trial, participants were randomized to an "insulin-sensitizing strategy" of glycemic management built around rosiglitazone and metformin versus an "insulin-providing" strategy built around sulfonylureas and insulin. The HbA1c target was < 7.0% in both groups.

3. The PROactive (PROspective pioglitzAzone Clinical Trial In macrovascular Events) study was a multicenter randomized placebo-controlled trial sponsored by Takeda to evaluate the incremental effect of piaglitazone (Actos) above metformin and sulfonylureas on cardiovascular outcomes in 5238 patients with type 2 diabetes and pre-existing cardiovascular disease.[26]

None of the three trials showed significant improvements in their primary outcomes, although PROactive came close and did achieve a significant reduction in its major secondary outcome, the composite of all-cause mortality, and nonfatal heart attack. However, both rosiglitazone and pioglitazone have since been shown to be associated with significant excess risk of heart failure. This side-effect has relegated these drugs to second-line status in treating diabetes; they are not recommended for patients with known heart failure or significant heart disease.[27]

Intensification of Diabetes Control

At the outset of the 21st century, four randomized trials were implemented to evaluate the effect of more ambitious HbA1c targets on cardiovascular outcomes:

- The Action to Control Cardiovascular Risk in Diabetes (ACCORD) trial (described in Chapter 3) was an NHLBI-sponsored 2×2 partial factorial trial comparing intensive (HbA1c < 6.0% target, 6.4% attained) to standard (HbA1c 7.0–7.9%

target, 7.5% attained) glycemic control in 10,251 patients with type 2 diabetes who also had either hypertension or metabolic syndrome.[28] The primary outcome was all-cause mortality.

- The Action in Diabetes and Vascular Disease: Preterax and Diamicron Modified Release Controlled Evaluation (ADVANCE) trial was an international investigator-initiated trial supported by Servier, the manufacturer of the two preferred drugs used in the trial (gliclazide and a fixed combination of perinodopril and indapamide), which compared intensive (HbA1c <6.5% target, 6.5% attained) versus standard (HbA1c target based on local guidelines, 7.3% attained) in 11,340 patients with type 2 diabetes.[29] The primary outcome was the combined incidence of adverse microvascular and macrovascular complications.

- The Veterans Administration Diabetes Trial (VADT) compared intensive versus standard glycemic control in 1791 military veterans (nearly all men) with poorly controlled diabetes and attained HBA1c levels of only 8.4% in the standard group versus 6.9% in the intensive group.[30] The primary outcome was a composite of macrovascular complications.

- The Look AHEAD (Action for Health in Diabetes) study was an NIDDK-sponsored multicenter randomized trial of weight loss in 5145 overweight adults with type 2 diabetes.[31] The primary outcome was death from cardiovascular causes. The intervention produced an 8.5 kg weight loss and a mean HbA1c of 6.6% (versus 7.2% in the control group) after one year, but neither was sustained.

None of these four studies supported the hypothesis that more intensive glycemic control reduced heart attack, stroke, or other macrovascular events in diabetes. ADVANCE was the only one of the trials that showed a significant reduction in its primary outcome (which included microvascular complications as well as macrovascular events), but this reduction was due entirely to a reduction in microvascular events. Heart attack and mortality rates were no lower in the intensive than the standard group. The results of the ACCORD trial were even worse; the study was stopped early due to excess mortality in the intensive glycemic control group. One problem with trying to lower blood sugar levels aggressively is the risk of overshooting the mark and inducing hypoglycemia (low blood sugar), which can cause fainting, bodily injury, and even death if glucose is not administered promptly. The VADT was badly underpowered and showed no difference in the composite outcome. In the Look AHEAD study, patients in the intervention group quickly regained the weight they lost in Year 1; by the end of the 10-year trial, mean HbA1c was a mere 0.1% lower in the intervention group than in the control group, and of course there was no difference in cardiovascular mortality. Thus, an additional decade of clinical trials had brought us no closer to proving that intensive glycemic control improved heart attack rates or longevity in diabetes than we were in 2000.

Dipeptidyl Peptidase-4 (DPP4) Inhibitors

As the 21st century entered its second decade, a promising new class of diabetes drugs, the DPP4 inhibitors, came on the scene. Like sulfonylureas, they stimulate insulin secretion, but without the undesirable side effect of weight gain.[32] Early animal studies showed inhibition of atherosclerosis in rabbits and rodents. However, three large, randomized trials in humans—using saxagliptin (SAVOR), alogliptin (ExAMINE), and sitagliptin (TECOS)—have shown only that these drugs are equivalent to sulfonylureas in reducing adverse cardiovascular events in type 2 diabetes.[33]

Newer Drugs

Two additional classes of drugs have now been approved for clinical use in type 2 diabetes. the Glucagon–like Peptide-1 (GLP-1) receptor agonists, which include exenatide (which was first identified in gila-monster saliva), liraglutide, and several newer variants, must be injected and are expensive and therefore not widely used.[34] The newest drugs, the sodium-glucose cotransporter (SGLT) inhibitors like empaglifozin, dapaglifozin, and canaglifozin, reduce glucose reabsorption by the kidneys and thus increase the level of glucose in the urine while decreasing it in the blood.[35] Clinical trial data on long-term cardiovascular effects of these drugs are lacking.

Impact of Advances in Treating Diabetes on the Decline in Cardiovascular Mortality

We have come a long way in improving the lives of persons with diabetes in the past century. The discovery and mass availability of insulin means that they no longer have to worry about having their lives cut short by diabetic ketoacidosis at an early age. The application of clinical trial results showing the benefits of tight glycemic control has meant that most diabetic patients today will not end up like Jackie Robinson—white-haired and nearly blind by age 50 and dead at age 53. However, we still do not have a diabetes drug or combination of drugs that will demonstrably reduce morbidity and mortality from heart attack and stroke. Fortunately, we do have drugs that reduce cardiovascular mortality in diabetics by lowering their blood pressure and their LDL cholesterol.[36]

However, the bad news is that the prevalence of type 2 diabetes has exploded, especially during the past two decades (Figure 7.1).[37]

As recently as 1999, the prevalence of diagnosed diabetes in the U.S. was 4.0%. In 2018 (the most recent available data) it was 8.2%. Type 2 diabetes accounts for 90–95% of the disease burden, which is fueled, no doubt, by the rising prevalence of obesity in the U.S. (see Chapter 14). The

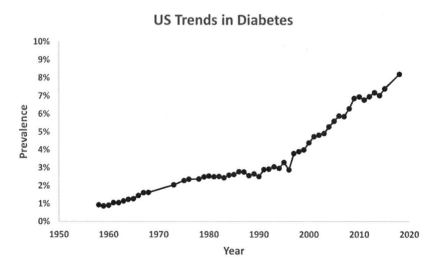

U.S. trends in diabetes, 1958–2015, from CDC data. https://www.cdc.gov/Diabetes/statistics/slides/long_term_trends.pdf

upward trend shows no signs of abating; if anything, it is growing steeper. And to make matters worse, despite the myriad available treatment options, only 20.9 % of diabetics in 2013–16 were treated and controlled.[38] By contrast, 45.2% of diabetics were treated but not controlled, 9.2% were diagnosed but not treated, and 24.7% were not even diagnosed.

Thus, it is evident that the decline in mortality from heart attack and stroke since 1960 has occurred *despite*, not because of, any progress we have made in controlling diabetes, where advances in treatment have been outstripped by its rising prevalence. Turning once again to the IMPACT model, its estimated 2.9% increase in the prevalence of diabetes between 1980 and 2000 *slowed* the decline in cardiovascular mortality in this period by 10%.[39] And, as we have seen, the prevalence of type 2 diabetes has risen to 8.2% since then.

However, while the rising prevalence of diabetes is a significant problem, its impact to date has not been quite as dire as this model portrays. The model estimates that the 2.9% rise in the prevalence of diabetes from 6.5% in 1980 to 9.5% in 2000 offset 10% of the decline in the annual heart attack mortality rate from 345 to 187 deaths per 100,000 during this period. In other words, were it not for the rise in diabetes, the heart attack mortality rate would have fallen by an additional 12 deaths to 175 deaths per 100,000. However, Ford's assumed diabetes prevalence rates are far higher the CDC prevalence rates—2.54 and 4.4%, respectively—plotted in Figure 7.1. Therefore, the model's estimate of the adverse impact of diabetes on heart attack mortality is almost certainly too high. Also, the IMPACT model does not consider any improvements in treatment that may have mitigated this impact either before or after 2000. Although treatments designed to lower HbA1c have not demonstrably altered the fact that diabetics have at three times the risk for heart attacks as non-diabetic, the IMPACT model doesn't consider the rapidly growing use of statins, which are now given to more than half of all type 2 diabetics and has reduced their heart attack mortality rate (as well as that of non-diabetics) by one-third.[40]

Therefore, rather than extrapolate the published IMPACT estimate to 2017, I have taken a different approach, which considers the other advances in treatment that have dramatically driven down CHD mortality rates in both diabetics and non-diabetics since 1968 (see the appendix, Table A.5). I have calculated that if the prevalence of diabetes had remained at its 1968 level (1.6%) rather than increasing to 8.2% in 2017, but we still had all the other modern treatments described in other chapters of this book, the CHD mortality rate in 2017 would have fallen by an additional 10.5 deaths to 82.4 deaths per 100,000. This represents an additional 11.3% drop relative to the actual 2017 mortality rate but only 2.2% of the 1968 CHD mortality rate. On the other hand, if the prevalence of diabetics were 8.2% in 1968, there would have been an additional 61.7 CHD deaths per 100,000 that year. Under either scenario, CHD mortality would have fallen by 82.9% rather than 80.7% if the prevalence of diabetes had been unchanged. So the big story is the 80.7% decline in CHD mortality due to treatments that reduced mortality in diabetics and non-diabetics alike, not the extra 2.2% decline we could have realized had the prevalence of diabetes not increased.

However, this is *not* a call for complacency about the long-term trend in diabetes. The trend line in Figure 7.1 is growing ever steeper and shows no sign of abating. In the meantime, the rate of decline in heart attack has fallen from 38% per 10 years in 2012 to 28% per 10 years in 2017. It is not unreasonable to attribute at least part of this deceleration to the rising tide of diabetes. If the prevalence of diabetes were to continue to climb apace and reaches 40% in the next twenty years or so, I have calculated that the CHD mortality could increase by 55% from 92.7 to 143.7 deaths per 100,000, unless we make major advances elsewhere (see Table A.5 in the appendix). Just as we were in the rising arm of an atherosclerosis pandemic in 1920, we may now be in the rising arm of a diabetes epidemic in the U.S. in 2020. And just as the 20th-century atherosclerosis pandemic rendered the great influenza pandemic of 1918–19 a historical footnote, the gathering 21st-century U.S. diabetes epidemic may be with us long after COVID-19 fades into history.

8

"Good" Cholesterol

Before 1977, high circulating levels of cholesterol and the lipoproteins that carry it were generally considered to be bad actors in the causal chain of atherosclerosis and its adverse cardiovascular consequences, even if this hadn't yet been proven in clinical trials. Thus, when the Framingham Heart Study published a report linking high levels of the previously overlooked small dense high-density lipoprotein (HDL) particles to *reduced* risk of heart attack, it created quite a stir.[1] Throughout the late 1970s, 1980s, and early 1990s, studies, perspectives, and editorials touted HDL cholesterol as a major cardiovascular risk factor, on a par with LDL cholesterol (but in the opposite direction), and dubbed it the "good cholesterol," although the cholesterol carried in HDL particles is of course the exact same molecule that is carried in LDL particles. HDL was thought to work by facilitating reverse cholesterol transport from the arterial wall to the liver, where it could be repurposed or cleared from the body, thereby undoing the mischief wrought by LDL.[2] The ratio of LDL to HDL cholesterol was promoted as a superior all-purpose risk factor and is included in lab panels even today; a ratio below 3.5 is good, and a ratio above 5.0 means trouble. I personally contributed to the HDL hype in a 1989 analysis of four published observational epidemiologic studies showing that levels of HDL and LDL were associated in an opposite and proportionate way to cardiovascular risk.[3] Thus arose the "HDL hypothesis" that raising HDL cholesterol levels would reduce the rate heart attack and other cardiovascular events.

However, as I also noted at the time, there were several major gaps in this tidy story.[4]

1. HDL is correlated with many other cardiovascular risk factors. Male sex (typically 40–50 mg/dL for men and 50–60 mg/dL for women), obesity, diabetes and pre-diabetes, and high triglyceride levels are associated with reduced levels of HDL cholesterol; exercise and alcohol intake are associated with increased levels of HDL cholesterol.

Although epidemiologic studies point to the independence of HDL cholesterol as a predictive factor, one could not rule out that HDL is merely a marker for poorly quantifiable healthy behaviors like physical activity and diet.

2. We lack a good genetic model (comparable to familial hypercholesterolemia for LDL cholesterol) for HDL "deficiency" in animals or humans.[5] For example, patients with Tangier disease (named for its discovery in Tangier Island in the Chesapeake Bay) have very low levels of HDL cholesterol, but their risk of heart attack is not elevated. Families with very high HDL cholesterol levels (> 100 mg/dL) and great longevity have been identified, but other families with high HDL cholesterol do not have increased longevity.

3. No practical pharmacological treatments to raise HDL cholesterol existed, with the possible exception of estrogen in post-menopausal women (we will see how that worked out in Chapter 9). The efficacy of weight loss and exercise to raise HDL are limited by compliance, and the pitfalls of prescribing alcohol are obvious.

4. Clinical trial evidence for the benefit of raising HDL cholesterol was completely lacking.

Fibrate and Niacin Trials

The lack of specific HDL-raising drugs did not stop investigators from trying to mount randomized clinical trials to establish the positive effects of raising HDL cholesterol in conjunction with lowering triglyceride levels, using two old classes of cholesterol-lowering drugs, the fibrates and niacin, in settings that minimized their impact on LDL cholesterol. Five such trials were conducted between 1980 and 2011:

- The Helsinki Heart Study (HHS) randomized 4081 asymptomatic 40- to 55-year-old men with non–HDL cholesterol > 220 mg/dL to receive either gemfibrozil or placebo.[6] Gemfibrozil raised mean HDL cholesterol by 11%, lowered mean LDL cholesterol by 11%, and lowered mean triglycerides by 35%. Incidence of the primary composite cardiovascular outcome was reduced by 34% (P = 0.02), but mortality was not reduced.
- The Veteran Affairs HDL Intervention Trial (VA-HIT) randomized 2531 men with pre-existing atherosclerotic heart

disease, HDL cholesterol < 40 mg/dL, LDL < 140 mg/dL, and triglyceride levels < 300 mg/dL to receive either gemfibrozil or a placebo.[7] Gemfibrozil raised mean HDL cholesterol by 6% and lowered triglyceride levels by 31%, with no change in LDL cholesterol. The incidence of the primary outcome (fatal and nonfatal heart attacks) was reduced by a statistically significant 22%.

- The Fenofibrate Intervention and Event Lowering Trial in Diabetes (FIELD) trial randomized 9795 50- to 75-year-old patients with type 2 diabetes. and triglyceride levels < 443 mg/dL in 63 centers in Australia, Finland and New Zealand to receive fenofibrate or a placebo.[8] Fenofibrate raised mean HDL cholesterol by 5%, lowered LDL cholesterol by 12%, and lowered triglycerides by 29%. The primary outcome (fatal and nonfatal heart attacks) was reduced by 11% in the fenofibrate group, but this reduction was not statistically significant. However, mortality was slightly (but not significantly) higher in the fenofibrate group.

- The Action to Control Cardiovascular Risk in Diabetes (ACCORD) trial, a 2×2 partial factorial NHLBI trial, randomized 5518 persons with type 2 diabetes, HDL cholesterol levels below 55 mg/dL for women and Blacks and below 50 mg/dL for everyone else, LDL cholesterol levels between 60 and 180 mg/dL, and serum triglyceride levels below 750 mg/dL to receive fenofibrate or a placebo.[9] Fenofibrate increased HDL cholesterol by about 1 mg/dL, decreased triglycerides by 25–30 mg/dL, and did not change mean LDL cholesterol levels. There was no significant difference in the primary outcome (major fatal or nonfatal cardiovascular events) or in any secondary outcome.

- The Atherothrombosis Intervention in Metabolic Syndrome with Low HDL/High Triglyceride and Impact on Global Health Outcomes (AIM-HIGH) trial[10]: This NHLBI trial randomized 3414 patients with metabolic syndrome and known cardiovascular disease, who were already taking high-dose simvastatin plus ezetimibe (as needed) to maintain LDL cholesterol levels between 80 and 100 mg/dL, to receive either slow-release niacin or a placebo. Metabolic syndrome was defined as HDL cholesterol below 40 mg/dl for men or below 50 mg/dl for women, triglyceride levels between 150 and 400 mg/dL, and LDL cholesterol below 180 mg/dL at entry. After two years, niacin produced a 4 mg/dL difference in mean HDL cholesterol, a -29 mg/dL difference in triglyceride, and a -4.5 difference in LDL cholesterol between the niacin and placebo group. However, there was no significant difference in the primary outcome (a composite of fatal and nonfatal major cardiovascular events) or any secondary cardiovascular outcome. There was a nonsignificant 2% increase in mortality in the niacin group.

The overall results of these studies were mixed at best. The two older gemfibrozil studies reported positive results, but the three later fenofibrate and niacin studies were all negative. None of the studies showed a beneficial effect on mortality. Only the HHS achieved more than a 6% increase in HDL cholesterol, but even in this best case, the reported improvement in cardiovascular outcomes could as easily have been attributed to the similar reduction in LDL cholesterol and/or the far larger reduction in triglyceride levels. Clearly, a drug that specifically produced substantially larger increases in HDL cholesterol was needed to truly test the HDL hypothesis.

Cholesteryl Ester Transfer Protein (CETP) Inhibitors

A new class of drugs, the CETP inhibitors, suddenly changed the landscape for the HDL hypothesis at the dawn of the new millennium. CETP is a protein that facilitates the movement of cholesteryl esters (cholesterol bound chemically to fatty acids) from HDL to LDL particles.[10] Inhibiting this protein raises HDL cholesterol and lowers LDL cholesterol, thereby (hypothetically) lowering cardiovascular risk. However, the evidence to support this hypothesis from naturally occurring mutations in CETP in animals and humans is mixed. Some families with defective CETP actually have increased cardiovascular risk despite high HDL cholesterol levels. In any case, by 2005, four such drugs were undergoing clinical evaluation—torcetrapib, dalcetrapib, evacetrapib, and anacetrapib—which could raise HDL cholesterol as much as twofold while lowering LDL cholesterol by as much as a statin. What was not to like?! Pfizer, the developer of torcetrapib, the first of these drugs, saw it as a blockbuster and eagerly awaited the results of its 15,067-patient ILLUMINATE trial, which they would use to market torcetrapib in combination with atorvastatin. Hoffman-LaRoche (dalcetrapib), Eli Lilly (evactrapib), and Merck (anacetrapib) were equally bullish about the three flagship trials of their drugs—dal-OUTCOMES (15871 patients), ACCELERATE (12,092 patients), and REVEAL (30,449 patients), respectively.[11]

The results were an unmitigated disaster—at least from the perspective of their sponsors, who had invested hundreds of millions of dollars in the development of these drugs. In the ILLUMINATE trial, published in 2007, the torcetrapib group experienced a 25% *increase* in cardiovascular events and a 58% *increase* in mortality—both statistically significant—despite a 74% increase in mean HDL cholesterol and a 25% decrease in LDL cholesterol.[12] Although the study investigators raised the possibility that the adverse result may have been due to "off-target" effects of torcetrapib on potassium and bicarbonate levels that were unrelated to CETP inhibition, all hopes that torcetrapib would be a breakthrough drug were dashed and hopes for CETP inhibition in general were cast into doubt. Five years later, the next domino to fall was dalcetrapib, a less potent CETP inhibitor without the off-target metabolic effects of torcetrapib. In the dal-OUTCOMES trial, adverse cardiovascular outcome rates did not differ between the dalcetrapib and placebo groups, despite a nearly 30% higher mean HDL cholesterol in the former group and no difference in LDL cholesterol.[13] Five years later, evacetrapib and anacetrapib completed the gloomy picture. In the ACCELERATE trial, there was no difference in cardiovascular event rates between the evacetrapib and placebo group, despite a whopping 133% increase in mean HDL cholesterol and 31% decrease in LDL cholesterol in the group receiving the active drug.[14] Finally, in the REVEAL trial, anacetrapib did modestly but significantly reduce the primary cardiovascular outcome (which included revascularizations as well as clinical events) by 9%, but this reduction was probably attributable more to the 17 mg/dL (18%) reduction in non–HDL cholesterol than the 43 mg/dL (104%) increase in HDL cholesterol,[15] Although the results suggested that anacetrapib was safe and also had a favorable effect on diabetes, its further development was discontinued.

Like the CAST trial described in Chapter 3, these trials represent a cautionary tale against being overly facile about leaping from finding an association in observational studies into assuming the efficacy of clinical interventions based on that association. But let us stop short of concluding that the concept of low HDL cholesterol as a target for intervention is a complete washout. The CETP inhibitors have taught us only the unhelpfulness of this particular mechanism of raising HDL cholesterol—i.e., by interfering with the normal pathway by which HDL particles rid themselves of cholesteryl esters, thereby perhaps creating engorged HDL particles that cannot function normally. The fact that some natural CETP mutations are not associated with decreased cardiovascular risk ought in retrospect to have alerted us to this possibility. It is still possible that raising HDL cholesterol by other mechanisms, such as stimulating the production of the A1 and A2 apoproteins that comprise the structural base of HDL, might prove beneficial. Before completely dismissing the HDL hypothesis, one should consider what dire fate might have befallen the LDL cholesterol hypothesis if the CETP inhibitors (and not the statins) were first introduced as LDL cholesterol-lowering drugs in the 1980s, rather than as HDL cholesterol-raising drugs in the 2000s. But be that as it may, the statin trials have firmly established the benefit of LDL cholesterol-lowering, while the trail to discover a drug that lowers cardiovascular risk by raising HDL cholesterol level has for now gone cold.

Impact of HDL on Decline in Cardiovascular Mortality

Clearly, HDL has played no role whatsoever in the observed decline in mortality from heart attacks and strokes since 1960. We have no safe, practical, and effective treatment for raising HDL cholesterol on a population scale, and it is far from certain that this hypothetical treatment would actually be beneficial.

9

THE MOTHER OF ALL TRIALS

Although we have always known that women are not immune from atherosclerotic cardiovascular disease, they clearly enjoy a distinct advantage over men. Heart attacks and strokes are roughly three times as common in men than women below age 50, and this difference narrows but does not disappear at older ages. The relative protection of women from heart attacks, strokes, and other adverse consequences of atherosclerosis accounts for much of their distinct advantage in life expectancy, which grew from two years (48.3 to 46.3) in 1900 to 7.4 years (74.0 versus 66.6) as the heart disease pandemic crested in 1968, and has fallen to 4.7 years in 2017 as the pandemic subsided.[1] This gender difference and the rise of heart attack rates in women after they reach the age of menopause raised the possibility that the female hormone estrogen might be useful in preventing or treating atherosclerotic heart disease as early as the 1960s when two doses of estrogen were tried (unsuccessfully) in men in the Coronary Drug Project.[2] Estrogen had no effect, other than to stimulate unwanted breast enlargement.

The relative protection of younger women from atherosclerosis also meant that they were excluded from most clinical cardiovascular trials in the 1960s and 1970s—at least those focused on patients without pre-existing cardiovascular disease. While this was understandable in view of the constraints on clinical trials to choose high-risk participants to keep the sample size and costs down, it meant that heart disease in women received little attention. However, by 1990, atherosclerosis was no longer seen as the natural and inevitable consequence of aging, and seniors—particularly older women—were increasingly viewed as prime targets for health interventions.

In the mid–1970s, analyses of epidemiologic studies began to report a strong association of menopausal hormone therapy and strikingly reduced rates of cardiovascular events and mortality.[3] In a meta-analysis of 16 studies, all but one (Framingham) found that post-menopausal estrogen users enjoyed significantly lower rates of cardiovascular events and deaths than non-users; the average estimated risk reduction was a whopping 44%.[4] While estrogen used by itself can cause uterine cancer, this risk does not exist in women who have undergone hysterectomy and can be mitigated in women who still have their uterus by co-administering progesterone.[5] Estrogen also has favorable effects on other cardiovascular risk factors, specifically HDL cholesterol, which is typically 10 mg/dL higher in White women than in White men below age 45, a difference that becomes less pronounced after age 50.[6] Now, I have already shown several examples illustrating the need for extreme caution in uncritically applying observational associations to clinical practice, especially when it comes to comparing persons who voluntarily decide to seek or not to seek a drug prescription for a particular condition. The NIH had appointed a task force to consider options for clinical trials of hormones and women's health as early as 1983. By 1990, the time was clearly ripe to put the hypothesis that menopausal hormone therapy could reduce cardiovascular risk to the test.

The politics were also ripe for clinical trials in women's health. In the late 1980s, Congress had grown justifiably critical of the NIH for neglecting women in its cardiovascular research portfolio and urged the development of new initiatives that focused on cardiovascular disease in women. Accordingly, one of my colleagues, Irma Mebane, developed the Postmenopausal Estrogen/Progestin Intervention Trial (PEPI), a short-term (three-year) trial in 875 healthy postmenopausal women, which compared the effects of five different combinations of estrogen and progestin and a placebo on a constellation of cardiovascular risk factors, notably HDL cholesterol.[7] In 1995, PEPI concluded that conjugated equine estrogen (Premarin) was optimal for women who had undergone a hysterectomy, and that cyclic micronized progesterone should be added for women who had not. In 1990, the NHLBI launched a two-year pilot study (under my lead) for a statin trial in seniors, the majority of whom would be women.[8] The Cholesterol Reduction In Seniors Program (CRISP) eventually led to the incorporation of a 10,000-patient statin trial as a partial factorial component in the ALLHAT BP trial (see Chapter 4).[9] Finally, and most importantly, another NHLBI colleague, Jacque Rossouw, developed an initiative for a new large primary clinical endpoint trial of menopausal hormone therapy in healthy postmenopausal women.[10] An investigator-initiated secondary prevention trial in women with pre-existing cardiovascular disease was being considered for funding at about the same time but was rejected and later picked up by Wyeth-Ayerst as the Heart and Estrogen/Progestin Replacement Study (HERS), which randomized 2763 women with known cardiovascular disease.[11] Then, in 1991, Bernadine Healy, who had just been appointed by President George H.W. Bush as the first female NIH Director, reassigned the primary prevention trial from the NHLBI to the Office of Disease Prevention in the Office of the Director of NIH. There it became the centerpiece of the $625 million Women's Health Initiative (WHI), which announced plans in 1992 to randomize 64,500 healthy postmenopausal women into a complex partial factorial trial, which incorporated a dietary and a calcium/vitamin D supplementation trial as well as an estrogen trial, and to recruit an additional 100,000 healthy postmenopausal women into a long-term observational epidemiologic study.[12]

In the late 1990s, the NHLBI developed its own portfolio of small short-term menopausal hormone trials in women with known coronary artery disease, in which progression would be measured by quantitative coronary angiography, a technique in which dye is injected into the coronary circulation and atherosclerotic plaques are visualized and measured with great precision. The Women's Angiographic Vitamin and Estrogen (WAVE) trial arose from an initiative that I developed, which also incorporated a trial of antioxidant vitamins C and E in a 2×2 factorial design.[13] Two similar concurrent trials—David Herrington's Estrogen Replacement and Atherosclerosis (ERA) trial in 309 women and Howard Hodis's Women's Estrogen-Progestin Lipid Lowering Hormone Atherosclerosis Regression Trial (WELL-HART) in 226 women—were conducted with NHLBI grants under my stewardship.[14]

Although these five trials used slightly differing drug regimens, all except HERS (which excluded women with hysterectomies) administered estrogen alone (usually Premarin) to women who had undergone hysterectomy and administered a combination of estrogen and progestin to women who still retained their uteri. The results of these trials, announced over an eight-year period from 1996 to 2004, were depressingly similar. The HERS trial announced in 1996 that menopausal hormone therapy produced no reduction in heart attacks despite an 11% mean reduction in LDL cholesterol and a 10% increase in HDL cholesterol.[15] It was noted that the null effect on cardiovascular events reflected an early adverse trend that appeared to improve and reverse over time; therefore, final judgment was withheld until additional follow-up data were available. Nevertheless, null findings for angiographic progression from the ERA (1998) and WAVE (2002) trials dampened expectations. Still, everyone eagerly awaited the results from the far larger WHI, which (unlike HERS) included women with prior hysterectomy who were treated with estrogen only and would be the first trial to address primary prevention in women who did not already have known cardiovascular disease.

The first shoe dropped in 2002 when the combined estrogen-progestin treatment component of the WHI in 16,608 women with intact uteri was stopped early, after completing 5.2 of its planned 8.5-year duration, due to a net adverse effect on health outcomes in the women who received active menopausal hormone therapy relative to placebo.[16] The significant adverse trends included not only a 29% *increase* in coronary events (mainly heart attacks), but also a 26% increase in breast cancer, a 41% increase in stroke, a 113% increase in pulmonary embolism (a life-threatening complication that occurs when a portion of a blood clot that forms in the deep calf veins breaks off and lodges in the pulmonary circulation), and a 22% combined increase in all adverse cardiovascular events. Partially offsetting significant beneficial trends were reported in the incidence of colorectal cancer (34% decrease), endometrial cancer (17% decrease), and hip fractures (34% decrease). Although menopausal hormone-treated women did not suffer a significant net increase in total cancers or deaths from all causes, they suffered a significant 15% worsening in their "global health index," a composite of major health outcomes selected for their gravity, which was defined in advance by the WHI investigators in their study protocol. Translating these results into absolute risk per 10,000 persons years of estrogen plus progestin exposure, seven extra coronary events, eight extra strokes, eight extra pulmonary emboli, and eight extra invasive breast cancers, but six fewer colorectal cancers and five fewer hip fractures were attributable to their menopausal hormone treatment. The net tradeoff was an increase of 19 global health index events—a bad deal by any reasonable accounting.

Still, the estrogen-only component of the WHI in in 10,739 post-menopausal women who had undergone hysterectomies continued, and there was still hope that estrogen would be beneficial in this setting. The HERS follow-up results, published in the same month (July 2002) as the first installment of the WHI, reported no continuation of the positive late trend seen in their 1998 report and thereby effectively put the final nail in the coffin of combined estrogen-progestin menopausal hormone therapy.[17] Negative results from the WELL-HART angiographic trial in 2003 were not encouraging. Finally, in April 2004, the second and last shoe dropped. The estrogen-only component of the WHI was stopped early after 6.8 of its planned 8.5 years of follow-up due to futility—meaning that the study's external data and safety monitoring board had determined that there was no discernable overall benefit or harm of estrogen therapy and that there was no realistic possibility that a significant trend would emerge in the remaining 1.7 years of planned follow-up.[18] The only statistically significant results (expressed as absolute attributable risk) were eight extra strokes and six fewer hip fractures per 10,000 person-years of exposure to estrogen, with no meaningful change in global risk index. However, estrogen-treated women had a nearly significant 23% *decrease* in breast cancer, in contrast to the significant 26% *increase* associated with combined estrogen-progestin treatment in the WHI cohort with intact uteri. This intriguing difference may represent the play of chance. So, from the perspective of cardiovascular and other major health outcomes, estrogen therapy after hysterectomy is a wash.

While these generally negative results sorely disappointed the many proponents of menopausal hormone therapy, their importance to the public health and to the cause of women's health ought not be underestimated. By the mid–1990s (before the HERS results were announced), as many as 40% of U.S. women were prescribed hormone therapy at menopause, in part because of its hypothetical cardiovascular benefits.[19] In addition, hormone therapy was increasingly being prescribed in women well past their menopause. In 2004, Buist et al. reported a 46% decline (14.6% to 7.9%) in the prevalence of women taking estrogen plus progestin and a 28% decline (12.6% to 9.1%) in the prevalence of women taking estrogen only between 1999 and 2002 in a cohort of 169,586 40- to 80-year-old women.[20] The decrease was driven mostly by 13.8% of women discontinuing their hormone therapy after the initial WHI results were announced in October 2002. Menopausal hormone use continued to decline rapidly over the next five years. A 2011 survey of office-based physicians reported a 63% decline in menopausal hormone use in the U.S. from 16.3 million women in 2001 to 6.1 million in 2009.[21] This decline was more reflective of the discontinuation of menopausal hormone therapy among older longtime users of than of reduced usage by younger newly menopausal women. A 2014 modeling study calculated that 126,000 breast cancers and 76,000 cardiovascular disease events were prevented because of the WHI.[22] Despite the 263,000 fractures that might have been prevented by hormone therapy, the

WHI results were estimated to have added 145,000 quality-adjusted years of life and saved more $37.1 billion in net costs—a 140-fold return on the investment in the WHI. In short, the WHI and other menopausal hormone trials had a profound effect on clinical practice. While short-term menopausal hormone therapy is still appropriate for women with significant vasomotor menopausal symptoms, especially following hysterectomy, long-term menopausal hormone therapy is no longer justified.[23]

The Women's Health Initiative did not end in 2004. The participants in both the randomized trial and observational studies continue to be followed. A 2013 report from the two menopausal hormone treatment trials confirmed the trends seen in the active treatment phase, albeit with some narrowing (as expected in any long-term follow-up) of the in-trial differences.[24] The results of the WHI diet trial will be covered in Chapter 14. The WHI has also spawned several spinoffs, like the WHI Memory Study (WHIMS) in the hormone trial cohort and the WHI Strong and Healthy (WHISH) exercise study, which also leverages the WHI observational study cohort.[25]

Impact of Menopausal Hormone Therapy on the Decline in Heart Attack Mortality

Menopausal hormone therapy offers no apparent cardioprotective effect and therefore has not contributed to the decline in cardiovascular mortality since 1960. One may speculate that the growing popularity of menopausal hormone therapy in 1975–95 may have acted as a slight drag on the early decline of heart attack and stroke mortality and that the subsequent fall-off in menopausal therapy prescriptions in 1995–2009 may have slightly accelerated this decline, but these offsetting effects are probably negligible. The peak popularity of menopausal hormone therapy was mainly in women in their 50s and early 60s (whose contribution to overall mortality is relatively small), and their absolute excess risk in WHI was only seven heart attacks and eight strokes per 10,000 women treated with estrogen plus progestin and zero for women treated with estrogen only. Ford et al. appropriately did not include menopausal hormone therapy in their IMPACT model of the decline in heart attack mortality.[26]

10

UNCLOGGING THE PIPES

Until now, I have focused primarily on advances in controlling risk factors to prevent adverse cardiovascular events, rather than on advances in treating these events. The priority of prevention reflects the fact that there is a ceiling on how much good one can do by treating heart attacks after they happen, since a substantial portion of heart attack victims die suddenly without surviving long enough to receive medical care. Still, spurred by spectacular advances in technology in the past half-century, we have witnessed a sea change in the treatment of heart attack since the 1970s, a change that is all the more remarkable because our initial therapeutic approach—i.e., to direct our attention to the arterial segments with the largest plaques and the most severe obstruction to blood flow—was based on a fundamental misconception of how heart attacks happen.

When I began my NHLBI career in 1977, atherosclerosis in the coronary arteries and elsewhere was viewed fundamentally as a plumbing problem. In this conceptualization (as applied to the heart), cholesterol and cellular debris accumulate as plaques in the walls of the coronary arteries, gradually narrowing their lumen (interior channel) until the circulation to a segment of heart muscle is cut off—usually by a blood clot—and an infarction (death of a segment of functioning heart muscle and its eventual replacement by a fibrous scar) or even arrhythmia and sudden death ensue. This theory did not tell us why plaques occur in some places but not others or what acute factors caused an occlusive clot to form in a particular place at a particular time. We did know that persons with large obstructive coronary plaques suffer a characteristic form of exertional chest pain called angina pectoris (or just angina, for short), which can be relieved by placement of a nitroglycerine tablet under the tongue, and that this syndrome is often a harbinger of the characteristic crushing chest pain of a full-blown heart attack. So we directed our efforts toward finding ways to open or bypass the most severe blockages, thereby reducing angina and hopefully the risk of heart attacks. Only much later did we learn that the stability rather than the size of plaques is the critical factor in infarction, and that the sudden rupture of a small but unstable plaque, which reduces blood flow through the affected artery from nearly 100% to zero in a matter of seconds, is far likelier to kill than a larger but stable plaque that has been gradually choking off blood flow and causing angina for years.

The History of Coronary Revascularization

During the past 50 years, procedures to "revascularize" the heart either by bypassing or dilating local blockages due to atherosclerosis have grown from nearly nothing to among the commonest and safest procedures in cardiovascular medicine. In the early 1970s, when our prototypical patient A.L. was hospitalized for a heart attack (Chapter 1), the treatments deployed were relatively low-tech—bed rest, intravenous medications for pain relief and arrhythmia, and an electronic monitor to alert nurses to changes in the pulse rate, BP, and electrocardiogram. Coronary artery bypass surgery (CABG) was first performed in the 1960s but carried a >10% mortality rate and was used only in patients with chronic intractable angina. Percutaneous coronary interventions (PCI) like coronary balloon angioplasty and stent placement, by which coronary blockages are opened via placement of an arterial catheter without opening the chest, did not even exist. By contrast, 337,444 CABG surgeries and 777,780 PCI procedures were performed in the U.S. in 2003.[1] Although these numbers fell to 201,840 CABG surgeries and 440,505 PCI procedures in 2016 (for reasons we will address later), they remain the bread and butter of cardiothoracic surgeons and interventional cardiologists—a medical subspecialty that did not yet exist in 1970. This exponential growth could not have happened without technological advances in diagnostic radiology, surgical techniques, and medical device development that date back as far as the late 19th century but converged in the 1970s and 1980s.

Since one cannot begin to "fix" coronary plaques with knowing where they are, let us begin with diagnostic radiology. To orient you, I have provided a diagram of the coronary circulation in Figure 10.1.

The left and right coronary arteries are the first arteries to branch off from the aorta above the valve that governs the exit of oxygenated blood from the left ventricle of the heart. The left coronary artery is responsible for most of the blood supply to the hard-working left ventricle, which pumps oxygenated blood at high pressure to every organ (including the heart itself) except for the lungs. After a short distance, the proximal segment of the left coronary artery (commonly called the left main coronary artery) divides into two large branches, the left anterior descending branch (also called the anterior intraventricular branch, which supplies blood to the front-facing portion of the left ventricle) and the circumflex branch (which circles behind the left ventricle). The right coronary artery is responsible mainly for the blood supply to the less hard-working right ventricle, which pumps de-oxygenated blood at low pressure only to the lungs, where it can take up oxygen. There are of course many additional branches downstream, but these four large coronary conduits—the left main, the left anterior descending, the circumflex, and the right—are where most fatal heart attacks originate and are the major targets for intervention. Blockages in the left main coronary artery—often called "the widow maker"—are especially dangerous.

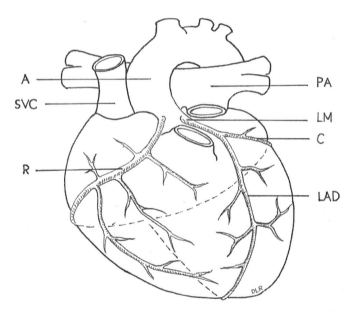

Anatomy of the coronary arteries. Drawing by Debra L. Roney. A = aortic trunk, C = circumflex coronary artery, LAD = left anterior descending coronary artery, LM = left main coronary artery, PA = pulmonary artery, R = right coronary artery, SVC = superior vena cava.

The science of diagnostic radiology dates back to 1895, when Wilhelm Röntgen took X-ray photos of his wife's hand; his discovery won him the 1901 Nobel Prize in Physics.[2] Although the injection of radio-opaque dyes to enhance contrast soon followed, the heart was considered off limits until a 25-year-old German surgical trainee, Werner Forssman, passed a venous catheter into his own right atrium in 1929.[3] Once practitioners recovered from their shock at what Forssman had dared to do, cardiac catheterization quickly became an important tool for diagnosing congenital heart malformations and cardiac valvular disease. However, well into the 1950s, selective injection of dye into the coronary arteries was considered too dangerous and likely to induce a fatal arrhythmia or to stop the heart entirely (asystole). The first injection of dye into the coronary arteries by Dr. F. Mason Sones of the Cleveland Clinic on October 30, 1958, happened by accident during a cardiac catheterization in a young man with rheumatic mitral valve disease, when a heartbeat displaced the catheter into the coronary root as dye was being injected.[4] When the man's heart beat normally after a cough or two, the taboo was broken, and Dr. Sones began to perform coronary angiography intentionally. Over the next decade, this procedure became a staple of the diagnosis and treatment of coronary artery disease.

Even after identifying and locating critical obstructions in the coronary circulation, performing delicate corrective surgical procedures on the heart represents a considerable challenge, since the heart is a constantly moving target that won't hold still voluntarily while a delicate surgery is performed. Cardiac surgeon John Gibbon's invention of the cardiopulmonary bypass machine, which was first used in human patients in 1953, allowed surgeons to operate on a still heart, while Dr. Gibbon's machine took over the heart's function of oxygenating blood and pumping it to the brain and other vital organs.[5] By the time the first CABG surgery was performed, cardiopulmonary bypass was already a staple of cardiothoracic surgery for many congenital heart defects, rheumatic valvular disease, and other conditions that had once been extremely risky or impossible to correct surgically.

Although animal experimentation on coronary bypass grafting dates back to 1910, the first CABG surgery in humans was performed in 1960 by Dr. Robert Goetz at the Albert Einstein Bronx Municipal Hospital Center in a man with a blocked right coronary artery by joining the right internal thoracic artery to the coronary artery downstream from the blockage.[6] The operation (which foreshadowed modern minimally invasive techniques) was done without cardiopulmonary bypass, and the grafting took only 17 seconds. The patient survived for 13 months and his graft remained open at autopsy. However, other attempts over the next five years to perform similar operations brought discouraging results. CABG surgery did not really catch on until 1967–68 at the Cleveland Clinic, when surgeons began using pieces of saphenous (leg) veins as conduits for bypassing obstructed segments of the coronary arteries. Although these vein grafts tended to be less durable than the bypasses constructed by joining the left internal thoracic artery to the left anterior descending coronary artery (the most common form of "arterial anastomosis" in current use), they have the important practical advantage of being able to provide multiple grafts for patients with multiple obstructions, while the arterial grafts can bypass only a single obstruction. Today, both types of graft are often used in conjunction in patients with multiple blockages. The early CABG surgeries carried a relatively high immediate mortality rate (up to 10%) and considerable long-term neurological morbidity (ranging from subtle cognitive changes to stroke) due to the formation of tiny air bubbles and clots during cardiopulmonary bypass. There have been many procedural advances in CABG surgery since 1970, which have shortened the time on cardiopulmonary bypass and reduced morbidity and mortality. A detailed exposition of these technical changes is beyond the scope of this chapter. However, the recent advent of minimally invasive CABG surgery, which is now used in about 25% of cases, is noteworthy. By using a thoracotomy (cutting through the ribcage) rather than a sternotomy (cutting through the breastbone) to access the heart and eschewing cardiopulmonary bypass, this procedure has shortened recuperation time and reduced neurological complications of conventional CABG surgery.[7] Currently, the operative mortality rate of CABG surgery is typically less than 3% in the non-emergency setting.

But in the 1970s, CABG surgery was still an ordeal, and there was a demand for kinder and gentler approaches to angina relief. This relief would take the form of coronary balloon angioplasty, a procedure in which a small catheter with an inflatable cuff is inserted via the femoral artery in the groin and guided under radiologic monitoring through the aorta to the coronary arteries and then to the targeted partially obstructed coronary arterial segment.[8] When the catheter reaches its destination, the cuff is inflated briefly to crush the obstructing plaque, then deflated and withdrawn, leaving behind an open channel. The first angioplasty (like the first coronary angiogram) was performed by accident in 1964 when Charles Dotter inadvertently recanalized an occluded right iliac artery as he was trying to pass a catheter for an aortic angiogram.[9] Andres Grüntzig performed the first deliberate femoral balloon angioplasty in 1974 and brought his technique to the coronary arteries in 1977. This achievement brought Dotter and Grüntzig the 1978 Nobel Prize in Medicine. Later, as techniques improved, angioplasty could be combined with diagnostic coronary angiography, and multiple obstructive lesions could be addressed during a single catheterization procedure. However, balloon angioplasty is not risk-free. The most serious potential complication is acute vessel closure, usually within 24 hours of the procedure, due to a combination of damage to the artery wall and clot formation. In the early days, this potentially lethal complication—the equivalent to an acute heart attack—occurred in 3–5% of cases. A more frequent and less dangerous complication was the gradual restenosis of the dilated coronary vessel over months due to fibrous scarring, which often left patients alive but no better off than they had been before the procedure.

The next major advance came in 1986 with the development of elastic wire mesh devices called stents, which could be put in place at the site of a balloon angioplasty to keep the newly dilated channel from narrowing or closing off.[10] Stents were actually invented by a 19th-century dentist named Charles Thomas Stent, who used them as an adjunct to root canal surgery.[11] In the first half of the 20th century, stent-like devices were frequently used in urological and biliary surgery to maintain the patency of ureters and bile ducts until they healed, although the term "stent" did not become standard for these devices until 1972. The cardiovascular application of stents began with their use in peripheral artery disease in the late 1970s, before they were adapted for coronary arteries. In any case, stent placement greatly improved the effectiveness and durability of angioplasty. However, stent thrombosis (clot formation) remained a significant and potentially life-threatening medium- and long-term risk. So in general, anti-platelet drugs, like clopidogrel (Plavix) and later variants, are prescribed in combination with aspirin for 1–2 years to stent recipients, which in turn raise the risk of serious bleeds. In the 1990s, the displacement of "bare metal" stents by new and improved drug-eluting stents, which are coated with drugs that inhibit the proliferation of the cells that form fibrous scars as they are slowly released in the artery wall. In a meta-analysis of 26.616 stent recipients, this and other improvements in stent design were shown effective in lowering rates of long-term stent thrombosis to about 1%.[12]

Randomized Trials of Revascularization to Prevent Heart Attacks in Stable Patients

So far, we have seen how technical advances in radiology, surgery, and medical technology have enabled surgeons and interventional cardiologists to make "plumbing repairs" that restore the coronary arterial circulation and mitigate angina pectoris for more than a million Americans every year. But the larger question, especially for the purpose of this book, is whether these plumbing repairs actually prevent heart attacks or prolong life. Although it seems logical to believe that this is the case, you must realize by now that what seems "logical" in medicine is not always true. After all, the application of leeches seemed logical to George Washington's physicians in 1799.

So let us begin with the clinical trials of CABG surgery and/or PCI in patients with stable coronary artery disease. Three largish, randomized trials were initiated in the 1970s to address this question—with lukewarm results:

- In 1982, the European Coronary Surgery Study (ECSS) reported a significant reduction in mortality after five to eight years of follow-up in 768 men with mild to moderate angina and > 50% stenosis in at least two coronary arteries.[13]
- In 1984, the Coronary Artery Surgery Study (CASS) reported a small reduction in mortality but no difference in the combined incidence of heart attack and death after five years of follow-up in 780 patients with stable ischemic heart disease.[14] A small reduction in mortality was offset by an equal increase in nonfatal heart attack.
- In 1992, the Veterans Affairs Cooperative Study of Coronary Artery Bypass Surgery, reported a small early reduction in mortality in 686 patients with stable angina and angiographically indicated coronary artery disease, but that reduction was reversed by the end of the planned 11-year follow-up.[15] The reversal was attributed to the rapid development of obstructive atherosclerotic plaques in the saphenous vein grafts.

However, despite these underwhelming results, a great deal of emphasis was placed on the subgroup results which showed favorable results in the highest risk subgroups—i.e., those with left main coronary obstruction and those who had three or more significantly obstructed coronary artery segments and left ventricular dysfunction.[16] Presumably, this reflected the relative infrequency of heart attacks and deaths in the low-risk subgroups and the consequent lack of statistical power to detect small differences between medically and surgically treated patients. Despite the limited usefulness of P-values when applied to subgroups identified after the fact, CABG surgery came to be recognized as the treatment of choice for the highest-risk subgroups of chronic coronary artery disease, and its primacy for treating left main coronary artery disease has rarely been challenged.

The government database ClinicalTrials.gov listed 665 completed clinical trials of stents in coronary artery disease as of July 2020.[17] That is probably an underestimate. I do not wish to overwhelm my readers—or myself, for that matter—with a detailed review of these trials. In general, the vast majority are trials sponsored by stent manufacturers to prove that their devices are at least as good as previously approved stents with regard to safety and short-term outcomes and may offer some advantage in reducing late stenosis. They focus mainly on patients with one- or two-vessel coronary artery disease and cede superiority of CABG surgery in patients with left main or more complex coronary artery disease. None of these studies really address the topic of interest here, namely long-term cardiac mortality. So, in 1999, the official ACC/AHA guidelines for intervention in chronic stable angina recommended CABG for patients with significant left main coronary disease and for most patients with 3-vessel or complicated 2-vessel disease (very strong evidence) and PCI for most other patients with significant angina (moderate evidence).[18] In my opinion, while these recommendations were not unreasonable given what was known at the time, the strength of the evidence supporting them was considerably overstated.

Let us now look at the results of more recent long-term outcome trials of coronary revascularization in chronic coronary artery disease. In 1988, the NHLBI initiated the Bypass Angioplasty Revascularization Investigation (BARI) trial, the first randomized trial to compare PCI and CABG head-to-head.[19] This trial, which began before stents were widely used, randomized 1819 patients who could be reasonably viewed as candidates for either procedure to receive either CABG surgery or angioplasty. Patients with left main coronary disease or complex triple vessel disease were excluded as inappropriate candidates for angioplasty, while patients with single-vessel disease were excluded as inappropriate candidates for CABG. After 5.4 years mean follow-up, overall survival and survival free of a heart attack were similar in patients who received angioplasty versus CABG. However, in a subgroup analysis of survival, diabetic patents did significantly better with CABG than angioplasty. The investigators drew the appropriate inference, not that CABG is preferable to angioplasty in diabetic patients, but that this finding was of sufficient interest to generate a new trial, which they called BARI-2D (where the D stands for diabetes).[20]

The new BARI 2D trial, which was sponsored by the NHLBI, with contributions from the NIDDK and Glaxo-Smith-Kline, included 2368 patients with type 2 diabetes and ran from 2000 to 2009. It differed from BARI in several respects:

- It did not compare CABG and PCI head to head but compared both to optimal medical care, which by this time included far more stringent control of BP and cholesterol than was practiced in BARI.
- The use of stents in PCI (including drug-eluting stents) was far more prevalent in BARI 2D than in BARI.
- BARI 2D also included a factorial component comparing insulin-providing and insulin-sensitizing strategies in type 2 diabetes (see Chapter 7).

After 5 years mean follow-up, BARI 2D patients who were randomized to revascularization plus optimal medical care fared neither better nor worse than patients randomized to optimal medical care alone with regard to the primary composite cardiovascular outcome or to heart attack or overall mortality. Since BARI 2D (like BARI) excluded high-risk patients with left main coronary and/or complex multivessel disease, it did not address the value of CABG in these patients. Still, the results gave pause to advocates of PCI and CABG in diabetic patients with chronic stable coronary artery disease.

Starting in 1999, while the BARI 2D trial was just getting underway, the Veterans Affairs Cooperative Study Group and the Canadian Institutes of Health Research co-sponsored the Clinical Outcomes Utilizing Revascularization and Aggressive Drug Evaluation (COURAGE) trial in 2287 patients with stable coronary artery (but not left main coronary artery) disease.[21] It was narrower than BAR 2D in that it addressed only PCI and not CABG, but also broader in that it included patients with and without diabetes. As in BARI 2D, there was no difference in adverse cardiovascular outcomes between patients randomized to PCI plus optimal medical care versus optimal medical care alone.

In 2005, Boston Scientific Corporation broke new ground by finally testing its TAXUS drug-eluting stent against CABG head-to-head in high-risk patients with left main coronary and triple-vessel disease, who had been considered the exclusive province of the surgeons.[22] The SYN-TAX trial randomized 1800 patients with severe coronary artery disease to receive either CABG or PCI with the TAXUS paclitaxel-eluting coated stent.[23] SYNTAX was designed as a "non-inferiority trial"—that is, its objective was to prove not that the stent was superior to CABG, but that it was no worse than CABG. This made sense clinically since most patients would prefer the less invasive procedure (PCI), other things being equal. (Also, a conventional superiority trial would have required many more patients and would have cost far more.) The inclusion of repeat revascularization in the primary outcome (along with death, heart attack, and stroke) was unwise, since CABG, in which long coronary artery segments are bypassed, has long been known to produce a more complete and lasting result than PCI, in which only the most severe blockages are fixed. The results confirmed this obvious and predictable fact, showing a significant advantage of CABG over PCI with respect to repeat revascularizations (5.9% versus 13.5%) and in the composite primary outcome (12.4% versus 17.8%) after one year of follow-up., However, there was virtually no difference between PCI and CABG for deaths, heart attacks, and strokes. A subgroup analysis suggested that CABG was superior to PCI in the subgroup with the highest "SYNTAX score," a risk score relating baseline coronary anatomy and function to adverse cardiovascular outcomes in the accompanying 1275-person SYNTAX registry. However, SYNTAX did not address whether either PCI or CABG was better than modern purely medical management.

The 2012–14 update to the ACC/AHA Guidelines, reflecting the results of COURAGE, SYNTAX and the two BARI trials, did not substantially change its recommendations, except for incorporating the SYNTAX score and diabetes in the decision tree of who should receive CABG versus PCI.[24] However, they were appropriately more circumspect in stating the strength of the evidence supporting their recommendations. After all, the only clinical trial evidence supporting the proposition that any form of revascularization intervention improved long-term outcomes relative to medical management dated back to subgroup analyses of randomized trials initiated in the 1970s, when CABG was performed mainly using saphenous vein grafts, coronary stents did not exist, and medical management did not include aggressive cholesterol and BP control. More recent trials showed that both CABG and PCI provided symptomatic relief of angina pectoris and that CABG was superior to stenting under some circumstances, but not that either reduced cardiovascular risk or prolonged life.

Even after the COURAGE, BARI 2D, and SYNTAX results were in, some continued to suggest that clinical trials were not a fair test of the long-term benefit of coronary revascularization since they excluded *de facto* many of the patients with the most clear-cut indications for the procedure, because their cardiologists simply went ahead and performed PCI as a continuation of their coronary angiography procedure, rather than stop to enroll them in a clinical trial. Thus, they argued, only the difficult or questionable cases were randomized into clinical trials. The NHLBI initiated the International Study of Comparative Health Effectiveness with Medical and Invasive Approaches (ISCHEMIA) in 2011 to address this criticism.[25] Rather than randomize patients after their coronary angiographic evaluation, which allows the angiographer/interventionist to immediately siphon off the "cleanest" cases for immediate PCI or referral to a surgeon for CABG, ISCHEMIA moved the randomization upstream to the identification of patients with cardiac ischemia (the medical term, derived from Greek, meaning inadequate blood supply), as determined by non-invasive diagnostic tests, *before* angiography. Thus, patients were randomized not to revascularization versus no revascularization, as in COURAGE or BARI 2D, but to either an invasive strategy beginning with coronary angiography or to a conservative strategy involving only optimal medical management (i.e., statins, BP control, aspirin, etc.) The downside to this design is that some patients who are randomized to the invasive strategy will turn out to have no treatable coronary blockages and thus receive no revascularization, and that some patients who are randomized to the conservative strategy will eventually require PCI or CABG due to worsening angina. Therefore, ISCHEMIA required a larger sample size to accommodate higher expected "crossover" rates.

The primary outcome results from ISCHEMIA (cardiovascular

ISCHEMIA Primary Composite Outcome

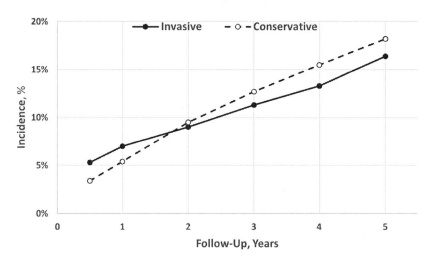

Primary composite outcome of ISCHEMIA trial, Invasive versus Conservative strategy. Data are from ISCHEMIA primary results paper, *N Engl J Med* **2020; 382:1395–1407.**

deaths, heart attacks, unstable angina hospitalizations, heart failure, and resuscitated cardiac arrest) are shown in Figure 10.2.[26]

Patients randomized to the conservative strategy did slightly better in the first two years, while patients randomized to the invasive strategy did slightly better thereafter. The overall difference between the two curves was not even close to statistically significant. The early increase reflected an increase in "procedural myocardial infarctions"—that is, damage sustained by a segment of heart muscle during the PCI procedure itself. Contrary to the general wisdom, there were no significant differences among subgroups; specifically, patients with more severe and widespread coronary artery disease benefited no more from the invasive approach than patients with one or two blockages. Unsurprisingly, patients with angina who were randomized to the invasive strategy had significant symptomatic improvement and required fewer anti-angina medications than patients randomized to the conservative strategy. No significant differences were seen in any secondary outcomes, including mortality.

So, at the end of the day, I draw the following conclusions about the use of revascularization in chronic coronary artery disease:

- Revascularization definitely offers symptomatic relief and improved quality of life to patients with significant angina, albeit at the cost of some short-term morbidity from the procedure.
- Based on early trial results, CABG probably improves long-term outcomes in patients with partial blockages of the left main coronary artery. Joining the left internal thoracic artery to the left main coronary artery achieves a more durable result than saphenous vein grafts. Ideally, one would like to see more robust clinical trial evidence on this point, but trials in which patients with known significant left main coronary artery disease can be randomized to conservative care have become ethically untenable.
- There is no good evidence that CABG or PCI offer any long-term survival advantage in patients without left main coronary disease. CABG offers more complete revascularization than PCI and is probably superior in patients with more severe disease, but PCI is a more benign procedure and is probably good enough in patients with lesser disease. New minimally invasive approaches to CABG may represent a good compromise. A recently funded follow-up to the ISCHEMIA trial may provide more answers.

Restoring Coronary Circulation in Acute Coronary Syndrome

The use of revascularization—particularly PCI—in the setting of an acute developing heart attack is a completely different story. When an unstable coronary plaque ruptures, its contents spill into the arterial channel (or lumen) and attract platelets, which form a clot (thrombosis) that partially or completely obstructs blood flow, abruptly depriving the downstream segment of heart muscle of oxygen-carrying blood. The ability of the heart to carry on pumping blood for a period of time depends on the location and degree of obstruction. If the obstruction is complete and cuts off the blood supply to a large and/or critical area of the heart, death may be virtually instantaneous, especially if the artery had not been significantly obstructed before the rupture. (Often, when obstructive plaques build up gradually over many years, collateral blood channels develop to augment blood circulation to the affected area.) Since the left main coronary artery supplies virtually the entire left ventricle (see Figure 10.1), plaque ruptures in this "widow maker" artery tend to be more lethal than similar ruptures downstream or in the right coronary artery. But even a small infarct in the wrong place can cause a fatal arrhythmia.

Let me pause here to make my terminology more specific than the familiar but imprecise term "heart attack," which I have tried to use (for simplicity) throughout the first nine chapters. The acute onset of persistent coronary pain is called acute coronary syndrome (ACS); this syndrome (which is also sometimes called "unstable angina") often signifies an impending or evolving myocardial infarction (or MI). When obstruction is severe, there is a window of perhaps three hours before the heart muscle downstream is irreversibly damaged and eventually replaced by scar tissue, which impairs its function of pumping blood. When a patient presents in the emergency room with ACS, the first step is to perform an electrocardiogram (ECG) and to draw blood to determine whether characteristic enzymes from heart muscle cells have leaked into the blood. An elevation of the ST-segment of the ECG and/or significantly elevated blood levels of cardiac enzymes (which have spilled out of damaged heart muscle cells into the bloodstream) are indicative of acute heart muscle damage or MI. For the purpose of this discussion, I will use the term MI to describe ACS patients who present with evidence of acute heart muscle damage, whether or not it is reversible. The acronym STEMI is often used to identify the subset of MI patients with ST elevation on their ECG; generally, they have sustained more widespread acute damage and have a worse prognosis than patients presenting with non–STEMI. The term "heart attack" may refer to any or all of these clinical situations.

Thrombolysis

Survival—or at least mitigation of the damages—of an acute MI requires urgent medical attention. The means of effectively treating these acute blockages and thus the sense of urgency in providing medical attention did not exist in the 1960s and early 1970s, when palliative treatments like bed rest and morphine were the order of the day. However, all this changed in the 1980s, with the development of "clot-busting" (thrombolytic) drugs, which could be administered intravenously at virtually any hospital.

The first thrombolytic drug used to re-open blocked arteries was streptokinase. Its medical use dates back to 1933 when William Smith Tillett noticed serendipitously that streptococcus bacteria made a substance that could digest fibrin, the essential structural protein of blood clots.[27] Streptokinase was used in a variety of medical conditions for several decades before being tried in acute coronary thrombosis. Several small trials in the early 1980s suggested that streptokinase improved survival in ACS if it was administered within six hours of onset of symptoms.[28] The results of the Italian megatrial Gruppo Italiano per la Sperimentazione della Streptchinasi nell'Infarto Miocardico (GISSI) trial, nailed it down.[29] Starting in February 1984, GISSI randomized 11,806 patients with the acute onset (< 12 hours) of MI symptoms in 176 coronary care units over a period of 17 months to receive an intravenous infusion of either streptokinase or a placebo. Patients receiving streptokinase had significantly improved in-hospital survival; mortality rate reductions were 26% for patients treated within three hours of onset of symptoms and 20% for patients treated within 3–6 hours of onset of symptoms. Longer delays in treatment resulted in no significant improvement. These survival differences persisted after one year of follow-up despite the occurrence of more re-infarctions in the streptokinase group.[30]

Several other randomized trials in 1985–92 built on the results of GISSI—the 290-patient NHLBI-sponsored Thrombolysis in Myocardial Infarction (TIMI) trial and two international megatrials, GISSI-2 (12,490 patients) and the 3rd International Study of Infarct Survival (ISIS-3, 41,299 patients).[31] These trials established the clear superiority of a newer synthetic thrombolytic drug called recombinant tissue plasminogen activator (tPA) to streptokinase in successfully restoring coronary blood flow. The benefits depended on rapid delivery of thrombolytic treatment, i.e., within six hours of symptom onset. In 1993, a third international trial called GUSTO (Global Utilization of Streptokinase and Tissue Plasminogen Activator for Occluded Coronary Arteries), which randomized 41,021 patients in 15 countries and 1081 hospitals, found that tPA, when given in an accelerated fashion (1.5 hours rather than 3 hours) with intravenous heparin significantly reduced 30-day mortality (6.9%) versus 7.8% in the streptokinase groups.[32] Thus, it had become clear that the timely delivery of thrombolytic therapy offered significant benefit to acute MI patients with regard to successfully restoring blood flow in clogged coronary arteries, re-establishing perfusion of the heart muscle, reducing rates of MI and improving survival. This major breakthrough in the treatment of patients experiencing acute MI symptoms began to blur the definition of a myocardial infarction, since thrombolytic treatment when delivered early enough could potentially prevent any lasting damage to the heart muscle, as if there had never been a heart attack at all.

Angioplasty, Stenting, and Surgery in the Acute Setting

By the late 1980s, coronary angioplasty and CABG had already come of age. However, unlike intravenous thrombolytic therapy, which could be administered at any hospital, these procedures were still available only at academic and major referral centers, with sophisticated coronary catheterization facilities and teams of interventional cardiologists and surgeons. A few early trials in the 1980s (before stents) comparing the efficacy of angioplasty versus thrombolysis in acute myocardial infarction found no difference.[33] However, the tide began to turn in the mid–1990s. In a 1995 review by Michaels and Yusuf of seven trials of primary angioplasty versus thrombolysis, angioplasty significantly reduced short-term (6 weeks) infarction and mortality by more than 40%.[34] These benefits were sustained after one year of follow-up. However, in 16 trials testing the efficacy of angioplasty after thrombolysis, mortality was not significantly reduced. In 1997, GUSTO IIb, a substudy of GUSTO, in which 1138 acute MI patients were randomized to primary coronary angioplasty versus tPA, showed a moderate short-term benefit of angioplasty as the initial treatment of acute MI.[35] In 1999, an NHLBI randomized trial called SHOCK (Should We Emergently Revascularize Occluded Coronary Arteries for Cardiogenic Shock) in 1492 patients with acute MI complicated by cardiogenic shock (inability of the damaged heart to sustain an adequate blood pressure), found no significant immediate benefit of emergency revascularization versus an initial strategy of medical stabilization, but a significant reduction in mortality after six months.[36] By 2003, Keeley, Boura, and Grines were able to incorporate 23 trials of primary angioplasty versus thrombolysis in a new meta-analysis, which demonstrated clear superiority of angioplasty over thrombolysis as the initial line of therapy in acute MI at hospitals where both were available.[37]

The sharp dichotomy between angioplasty in the acute versus chronic setting is illustrated by the results of the 2006 Occluded Artery Trial (OAT).[38] In this NHLBI-sponsored trial, 2166 stable patients who had

had a recent (within the preceding 3–28 days) MI that left them with persistent occlusion of the infarct artery were randomized to receive either PCI to open the blocked coronary artery or conservative (medical only) treatment. This was one of those trials that many practitioners considered unethical because they already "knew" that of course opening the blocked artery would improve cardiovascular outcomes. In fact, it did not. The incidence of the primary composite outcome of death, reinfarction, or heart failure was actually slightly higher in the PCI group (17.2%) than in the conservatively treated control group (15.6%). Revascularization clearly offered no survival advantage, even as few as three days after an infarction.

Since 2003, there have been many improvements in PCI, both in the technique itself (incorporation of stents, improvements in stent design) and in the expanding availability of antithrombotic and antiplatelet drugs (aspirin, heparin, clopidogrel, GPIIb/IIIa inhibitors, etc.) to minimize the rate of stent thrombosis. Two of these drugs, clopidogrel and aspirin, ranked as the 40th and 42nd most prescribed drugs in 2017, with 19.4 million and 17.3 million scripts, respectively.[39] A detailed review of the dizzying array of currently available options and the evidence supporting their use is beyond my scope here. The 2013 ACCF/AHA guidelines for the management of acute MI strongly recommend urgent revascularization (PCI, where feasible) as the first line of treatment.[40] In settings where the timely delivery of PCI is impossible, such as rural areas without rapid access to a tertiary medical center, thrombolysis is a viable alternative. And of course, proven risk factor management treatments like statins and antihypertensive drugs should be instated or re-instated as soon as the patient's condition has stabilized after the acute intervention.

Perhaps the most important change since 2003 is the increase in public awareness of the symptoms of acute MI and of the necessity of seeking immediate medical attention at their first onset and in the rapidity of the response once a patient arrives at the hospital. In 2011, Krumholz et al. report a marked improvement in door-to-balloon time (i.e., the time from arrival at the hospital to the angioplasty procedure) for U.S. hospitals between 2005 and 2010, based on a sampling of hospitals reporting to the Centers for Medicare and Medicaid Services, including roughly 50,000 cases per year.[41] During this period, the median door-to-balloon time decreased by one-third from 96 minutes in 2005 to 64 minutes in 2010. The percentage of patients with door-to-balloon time < 90 minutes (the maximal acceptable time) increased from under 45% in 2005 to over 90%

in 2010. Since the efficacy of PCI or thrombolysis in acute MI depends on delivery within 3–6 hours after onset of symptoms, time is of the essence.

Impact of Revascularization on the Decline in Heart Attack Mortality

So, at the end of the day, how did these spectacular technological advances, which have enabled us to intervene directly and decisively to restore blood flow in clogged coronary arteries, affect mortality from heart attacks in the U.S. since 1980? The answer is complicated. In their 2007 IMPACT model, Ford et al. attributed 5.5% of the decline in cardiac mortality between 1980 and 2000 to revascularization of patients with chronic stable angina (4.2% for CABG and 1.3% for angioplasty) and an additional 3.2% of this decline to revascularization and thrombolysis in the acute setting (acute coronary syndrome or MI).[42] I believe that both of these estimates are seriously flawed. The estimate for chronic stable angina assumes that CABG and angioplasty reduced mortality by 36% and 13%, respectively, in this setting. Neither of these figures is even remotely accurate. Recent clinical trials through ISCHEMIA (which exclude patients with left main coronary artery disease) suggest that CABG and PCI have little or no effect on CHD mortality in this setting.[43] While CABG may be helpful in patients with significant left main coronary disease, this condition is relatively uncommon; representing only 3.6% of patients in a recent report of a series of 13,228 consecutive coronary angiograms.[44] Similarly, 5.1% (434/8518) of patients screened by the ISCHEMIA trial were excluded due to left main coronary artery disease.[45] Thus, even if we grant that this subset of chronic patients receiving CABG enjoyed a 36% reduction in mortality, CABG in this setting can account for no more than 0.2% (5.1% times 4.2%) of the decline in heart attack mortality between 1980 and 2000. There is little evidence that angioplasty (with or without stents) accounts for any of this decline.

The real impact of revascularization on the CHD mortality has been in the acute setting, and nearly all of it has happened after 2000. This impact has almost certainly been driven by the growing use of PCI procedures (angioplasty plus stents), which have now largely superseded thrombolytic therapy and plain angioplasty and are far more commonly performed than CABG in the acute setting. Technological advances in the use and composition of stents, expanding PCI capability to many more hospitals, the increasingly sophisticated use of antiplatelet and other drugs to prevent stent thrombosis, and decreases in door-to-balloon time have brought about a sea change in the first decade of the 21st century—a period during which (not coincidentally) the most rapid decline in heart attack mortality has taken place (see Figure 1.2). So while the published IMPACT model results assumed that angioplasty reduced cardiac mortality by only a 7% in acute MI, a 2020 meta-analysis of recent PCI trials reports an overall 31% reduction in cardiac deaths in the acute scenario.[46] Furthermore, while Ford et al. also assumed that only 30% of unstable angina patients and 21% of acute MI patients received a PCI, a 2016 analysis of four national registries reported that more than 90% of STEMI patients who were brought directly to participating centers received a PCI within 90 minutes of arrival.[47] Also, Ford et al. incorrectly assumed a case-fatality rate of 9.4% in 2000 as the baseline case-fatality rate for acute MI, a figure that was already reduced by the use of thrombolysis and PCI. The actual in-hospital mortality rate for acute MI was 15% in 1980.[48]

Give all these flawed or outdated assumptions, I performed my own analysis of the contribution of improved treatment of acute MI (and acute coronary syndrome) based on the most current comprehensive data I could find, which covers the years 1970–2009 but does not include patents under age 45.[49] My calculation (the details of which are laid out in Table A.6 of the appendix) is based on the improvement of short term (in-hospital) survival of acute MI and does not try to dissect the separate contributions of PCI and the antiplatelet and other therapies that are initiated more or less simultaneously. The calculation is complicated by the fact that hospitalizations for MI have decreased because of our success in primary prevention (treatment of hypertension and high LDL cholesterol and smoking cessation). This decrease has been partially offset by the increased sensitivity of modern diagnostic criteria for acute MI (specifically the displacement of creatine phosphokinase by high-sensitivity troponin as the key diagnostic cardiac enzyme assay) and the greater proportion of MI patients reaching the hospital alive.[50] The consequent inclusion of milder cases has tended to artificially lower in-hospital case fatality rates. Thus, the profound drop in the in-hospital case fatality rate for acute MI from 23.9% in 1970 to 4.0% in 2009 reflects inflation of the proportion of milder cases, as well as actual improvements in treatment. For example, in a 2010 analysis of 46,086 Kaiser-Permanente patients hospitalized for acute MI between 1999 and

2008, the proportion of MI with ST segment elevation (STEMI), which have a worse prognosis than non–STEMI, decreased from 48% (133/274) in 1999 to 24% (50/208) in 2008.[51] However, when one multiplies case fatality rates by the number of incident cases to obtain the number of in-hospital deaths per 100,000 population-wide, this artificial inflationary effect washes out.

Taking all these factors into account, I have estimated that improvements in the treatment of acute MI, especially the rapid deployment of PCI, account for an estimated decrease of 45.2 in-hospital deaths per 100,000 annually after adjustment for the impact of primary prevention, which represents 13.7 % of the total decline in heart attack deaths between 1970 and 2009 (see Table A.5 in the appendix). I believe that this figure represents a far more current and accurate estimate of the contribution of acute MI interventions to the decline in CHD mortality than the IMPACT model's combined 2.8% estimate for thrombolysis, angioplasty, and CABG in the acute setting for 1980–2000. The impact of acute MI interventions has probably increased since 2009, due to continuing technological improvements and efficiency in delivering timely intervention.

11

SECONDARY
PREVENTION DRUGS

This chapter will review the impact of advances in "secondary pre-vention," defined here to encompass long-term medications prescribed to a patient who has already suffered a heart attack, which are intended to prevent another heart attack and to prolong life. These include aspi-rin, beta-adrenergic blockers, ACE inhibitors, as well as statins (which were discussed in Chapter 5). It will not address treatments like, nitrates, morphine, furosemide, and oxygen, which are given primarily to alleviate symptoms.

Aspirin

Acetylsalicylic acid (or aspirin), one of medicine's most ancient rem-edies, has been part of the medical pharmacopeia since the late 1890s.[1] It is derived from salicin, the active component of willow bark, which has been used for 4000 years to soothe pain and lower fevers. Although newer drugs like acetaminophen (Tylenol), ibuprofen (Advil, Motrin, Nuprin), and naproxen (Aleve) have displaced aspirin as the most popu-lar over-the-counter analgesic and anti-pyretic drugs, aspirin has enjoyed a renaissance in the past few decades as an anti-platelet drug to prevent clot-ting after a heart attack or a non-hemorrhagic stroke. Unlike many other anti-clotting drugs (clopidogrel heparin, etc.), which are used mainly in conjunction with PCI and whose clinical impact is inseparable from that of the PCI procedure, the importance of aspirin in secondary prevention pre-dates and extends well beyond its use as an adjunct to PCI.

The first reported trial of aspirin to prevent cardiac mortality was conducted in the UK in 1971–74.[2] In this trial, 1239 men with a recent MI were randomized to receive either a 300 mg daily dose of aspirin or a placebo. After two years of follow-up, mortality was 25% lower in the aspirin group than in the placebo group, with most of the divergence coming after eight months. Although this difference was not statistically significant because of the small number of deaths (108), and the results were clouded by high dropout rates, other investigators soon mounted bigger and better trials—and lots of them. By 1994, the Antiplatelet Trialists' Collaboration was able to identify and review 145 randomized trials of antiplatelet therapies—mostly using aspirin.[3] These included a large NHLBI-sponsored secondary prevention trial called Aspirin in Myocardial Infarction Study (AMIS) in 4524 post–MI patients.[4] They also included two large NHLBI-sponsored primary prevention trials—the Physician's Health Study (PHS) in 22,071 male physicians and the Women's Health Study (WHS) in 39,876 female health professionals.[5] Although the results of these three NHLBI trials were mixed, the Antiplatelet Trialists Collaboration found that antiplatelet therapy significantly reduced subsequent serious vascular events by 29% after an acute MI, by 25% after any MI, by 22% after a stroke, and by 32% in other high risk patients. However, it reduced cardiovascular risk by only 10% (borderline significant) in patients without prior cardiovascular disease. The impact on mortality was considerably smaller (17% in high risk groups and a non-significant 5% in patients without prior cardiovascular disease), since the benefit in atherothrombotic events was partially offset by an increased risk of fatal bleeds—particularly in the brain and gastrointestinal tract.

In 2009, a new updated meta-analysis—this time confined to aspirin—using individual patient data from six primary prevention trials (95,000 participants) and 16 secondary prevention trials (17,000 participants) reaffirmed and elaborated upon the 1994 analysis.[6] In the six primary prevention trials, aspirin significantly reduced major coronary events by 18%, but also significantly increased hemorrhagic stroke by 32% and gastrointestinal bleeds by 54%. The net effect was a significant 12% reduction in serious vascular events, and a non-significant 3% decrease in vascular deaths. In the 16 secondary prevention trials, aspirin similarly significantly reduced major coronary events by 20% and significantly increased hemorrhagic strokes by 67% and gastrointestinal bleeds by 169%. However, because heart attacks comprised a much higher proportion of serious vascular events in these patients, aspirin produced a significant 19% net reduction in serious vascular events and a significant 13%

net reduction in vascular deaths. This translates to 13 vascular deaths prevented per 1000 patients treated. With these results in hand, the U.S. Preventive Services Task Force recommended the use of aspirin in men age 45–79 and women age 55–79 in whom the potential risk reduction for a heart attack or atherothrombotic stroke is judged to outweigh the potential risk increase for a cerebral or gastrointestinal hemorrhage.[7] In practice, this would include nearly all patients with a prior heart attack and would exclude most patients without known prior cardiovascular disease. The Task Force recommended that aspirin not be prescribed in younger patients (where it is likely to do more harm than good) and in patients aged 80 and above (who are more susceptible to severe bleeds and in whom clinical trial evidence benefit is lacking).

Beta-Adrenergic Blockers

Since a heart attack is generally accompanied by a rush of adrenaline and similar hormones (catecholamines), which stimulate the heart and cause heart rate and BP to rise, the advent of beta-adrenergic blockers in the 1970s for treating hypertension naturally suggested a potential application in blunting the potentially harmful effects of catecholamine release in acute MI. However, because beta-blockers decrease the pumping efficiency of a damaged heart (a negative inotropic effect in medical parlance), patients with decreased ventricular function or heart failure were exempted.

The first randomized placebo-controlled trials to test this hypothesis were the 1884-patient Norwegian Multicenter Timolol trial in 1981 and the 3387-patient NHLBI Beta-Blocker Heart Attack Trial (BHAT) in 1982. In the Norwegian trial, the beta-blocker timolol produced a significant 39% reduction in mortality in 33 months of follow-up.[8] In BHAT, which was stopped early at 27 months, the beta-blocker propranolol significantly reduced mortality by 26%.[9] In 1986, the 16,027-patient First International Study of Infarct Survival (ISIS-1) megatrial looked at the short-term impact of the beta-blocker atenolol on in-hospital mortality and found a non-significant trend toward reduced mortality.[10] Based on these and other trials, beta-blockers became part of the standard therapy for uncomplicated acute MI with unimpaired ventricular function. Since beta-blockers lower BP, hypertensive patients often continued to take these drugs indefinitely after recovering from their acute MI.

Since the mid–1980s, many additional randomized trials have further explored the impact of beta-blockers on short- and long-term survival after an MI in various clinical settings. In 1999, Freemantle et al. published a meta-analysis of 82 such trials—51 of short-term survival (up to 6 weeks) and 31 of long-term survival (6–48 months)—in 54,234 MI patients randomized to a beta-blocker versus a placebo.[11] This meta-analysis included some trials that were conducted after thrombolysis and angioplasty became standard treatments for acute MI, but most studies pre-dated the widespread use of these treatments. They reported that beta-blockers brought about a nonsignificant 4% decrease in short-term mortality but a significant 23% reduction in long-term mortality. They estimated that treating 42 acute MI patients with a beta-blocker for two years—it didn't matter which one—would prevent one death.

In 2001, reports from a new beta-blocker trial called CAPRICORN (Carvedilol Post-Infarct Survival Control in Left Ventricular Dysfunction) revisited the question of using beta-blockers in acute MI patients with some left ventricular dysfunction—a group in whom beta-blockers were not ordinarily prescribed.[12] They were able to do this because it had become standard practice to treat all such patients with an angiotensin converting enzyme (ACE) inhibitor (see below) to ameliorate their risk of heart failure. CAPRICORN randomized 1959 patients with acute MI and left ventricular ejection fraction below 40% to receive the beta-blocker carvedilol or a placebo. Nearly all randomized patients received aspirin in addition to an ACE inhibitor, and nearly half received primary angioplasty before carvedilol was initiated. Carvedilol treatment brought about a significant 23% reduction in long-term mortality over and above the effects of their ACE inhibitor, aspirin, and angioplasty. In 2005, the CAPRICORN trial reported that carvedilol also cut the incidence of atrial fibrillation (a potential precursor of strokes caused by clots forming in the left atrium and travelling to the brain) by more than half.[13] Fast-forwarding to 2013–14, even after simple angioplasty had given way to PCI with drug-eluting stents, the latest ACC/AHA treatment guidelines for acute MI recommend oral beta-blockers for all MI patients without signs of heart failure, asthma, or heart block or risk factors for shock, although there is some question as to how long this treatment should continue.[14] Carvedilol was also one of three beta-blockers cautiously recommended in non–STEMI patients with "stabilized" HF (i.e., treated with an ACE inhibitor or angiotensin receptor blocker). In 2017, metoprolol (#6), carvedilol (#29), atenolol (#36), propranolol (#41), nebivolol (#144), and timolol (#146) were the most frequently prescribed beta-blockers, accounting for a combined 142.4 million prescriptions.[15]

Renin-Angiotensin-Aldosterone System (RAAS) Inhibitors

The kidneys (which secrete the enzyme renin) and adjacent adrenal glands (which secrete the hormone aldosterone) play a central role in regulation of blood volume and systemic vascular resistance.[16] Although the detailed physiology is beyond the scope of this book, I will provide a brief summary. Renin cleaves a protein called angiotensinogen (which is produced in the liver) to angiotensin-I, which is in turn converted (by an enzyme called angiotensin converting enzyme [ACE]) to its active form, angiotensin-II. Among other things, angiotensin-II causes arteries to constrict (raising blood pressure) and the kidneys to retain more sodium (raising blood volume and thereby increasing the heart's workload). Angiotensin-II also stimulates the adrenal cortex to release aldosterone, which further stimulates the kidneys to reabsorb sodium and lose potassium. The bottom line is that overactivity of the RAAS system is often a key player in the pathology of hypertension and congestive heart failure. So, naturally, this system has been a rich therapeutic target for these conditions.

The first RAAS-inhibiting drug, spironolactone, which dates back to 1960 but still ranks 69th with 11.6 million prescriptions in 2017, has enjoyed modest popularity as a second-line drug in treating hypertension and heart failure.[17] In hypertension, it has often been used in combination with thiazide diuretics because it preserves potassium and thereby counterbalances their potassium-wasting effect.[18] Since it is not used to treat acute MI and since we have already covered the benefits of BP control in Chapter 4, spironolactone will not be discussed further here. Instead, we will focus on the ACE inhibitors, which inhibit the activation of angiotensin, and the angiotensin receptor blockers (ARB) which block access of activated angiotensin to its target cells in the kidney, adrenals, and blood vessel walls.

The use of ACE inhibitors to treat hypertension and heart failure in the U.S. dates back to the FDA's approval of captopril in 1981 and enalapril and lisinopril shortly thereafter.[19] The Cooperative North Scandinavian Enalapril Survival Study (CONSENSUS, 1986), the NHLBI-sponsored

Studies of Left Ventricular Dysfunction (SOLVD, 1991), and the second Veterans Administration Cooperative Vasodilator-Heart Failure Trial (V-HeFT II, 1991) soon established the utility of ACE inhibition (by enalopril) in reducing mortality in patients with moderate to severe chronic congestive heart failure.[20]

In 1992, the Survival and Ventricular Enlargement (SAVE) trial was the first to report the efficacy of an ACE inhibitor to treat acute MI.[21] This trial randomized 2231 patients with acute MI and left ventricular dysfunction at 112 participating hospitals in the U.S. and Canada to receive either the ACE inhibitor captopril or a placebo 3–16 days after entering the hospital and followed them for an average of 42 months. About a third of patients received thrombolysis and another third received revascularization (mostly angioplasty) before they were randomized. Between 25% and 59% of patients in each treatment group also received aspirin, nitrates, calcium channel blockers, beta-blockers, diuretics, antithrombotic drugs, and digitalis (in decreasing order of frequency) in the first few days after their MI. In patients randomized to receive captopril, total and cardiovascular mortality and the worsening of heart failure were significantly reduced relative to placebo irrespective of other treatments they received. However, the incidence of myocardial re-infarction was similar in the captopril and placebo groups.

Two similar trials of ACE inhibition in acute MI reported similar results during the next five years. In the Trandolapril Cardiac Evaluation (TRACE) trial (1995), 1749 acute MI patients with significant left ventricular dysfunction (ejection fraction below 35%) were randomized to receive the ACE inhibitor trandolapril or a placebo within 3–7 days of hospitalization and followed for 24–50 months.[22] As in SAVE, mortality and progression to severe heart failure—but not myocardial re-infarction— were significantly reduced. Then, in 1997, the 2006-patient Acute Infarction Ramipril Efficacy (AIRE) trial re-iterated the positive findings for heart failure progression and mortality and the negative findings for myocardial reinfarction SAVE and TRACE, but also reported significantly (30%) fewer sudden cardiac deaths in the ramipril group than in the placebo group.[23] In retrospect, qualitatively similar reductions in sudden cardiac death were evident in SAVE and TRACE, but were ignored due to lack of statistical significance.

Having established the benefits of ACE inhibition in chronic heart failure and acute MI with impaired left ventricular function, the

117

international Heart Outcomes Prevention Evaluation (HOPE) trial set out to explore the potential benefit of ACE inhibition in 9297 high-risk cardiovascular patients (i.e., those with a prior history of heart attack or diabetes plus at least one other cardiovascular risk factor) but normal ventricular function.[24] The results were resoundingly positive. Ramipril treatment significantly reduced the combined incidence of MI, stroke, or death (the primary outcome) by 22%. Heart failure hospitalizations (of which there were many) and sudden cardiac deaths (of which there were few) were also significantly lower in the ramipril than in the placebo group. It is possible that some of the benefit was due to BP reduction, but fewer than 20% of HOPE participants had known hypertension.

Angiotensin receptor blockers (ARB) came into use in the late 1990s as better-tolerated alternatives to ACE inhibitors with a lower frequency of coughing and other side effects.[25] They have to some extent ridden on the coattails of ACE inhibitor trials like SAVE, TRACE, AIRE, and HOPE, in claiming efficacy for secondary prevention of cardiovascular events. The evidence supporting the use of ARB in secondary prevention is weaker than that for ACE inhibitors, but trials comparing ARB to ACE inhibitors head-to-head have not shown significant differences. The ACCF/AHA guidelines give the nod to ACE inhibitors as the first line of therapy in patients who can tolerate their side effects because of their longer track record, but treat ARB as an essentially equivalent alternative for patients who cannot tolerate an ACE inhibitor.[26] In 2017, 104.8 million prescriptions for lisinopril (plus another 16.7 million for a combination with hydrochlorothiazide) were written, making it the most prescribed drug in the U.S. Benazepril, enalapril, and ramipril are the only other ACE inhibitors in the top 200 prescription drugs of 2017, with about 21 million prescriptions combined.[27] Among the ARBs, losartan potassium ranks ninth with 52 million prescriptions (plus another 11.8 million for a combination with hydrochlorothiazide), and valsartan ranks 85th with 9.2 million prescriptions (plus another 5.3 million for a combination with hydrochlorothiazide).

Digitalis

Digitalis, the most venerable drug in cardiology, is a cardio-active glycoside extracted from a species of foxglove plant, digitalis purpurea.

Although the medicinal use of foxglove as an herbal remedy dates back to the ancient Greeks, the 18th-century Scottish physician William Withering is credited with the discovery and initiation of the modern use of digitalis extract to treat cardiac patients in 1775.[28] In the early 1970s, when I was a medical student and intern, digoxin (the chief active component of digitalis) was a mainstay first-line treatment for heart attack patients, especially those with signs of heart failure (like pulmonary congestion and edema) and/or atrial fibrillation. Its efficacy was thought to derive from its potent positive inotropic effect, which enables a damaged heart to pump blood more efficiently, and its stabilizing effect on the specialized cardiac cells that generate and conduct the electric impulses that sustain a regular heartbeat.[29] The main problem with digitalis has always been its extremely narrow therapeutic margin between the dosage required for efficacy and a toxic dose, which makes it a favorite poison among murder mystery authors. I learned about digitalis and foxglove from Agatha Christie long before attending medical school.

In February 1991, the NHLBI initiated the Digitalis Investigation Group (DIG) trial, a randomized placebo-controlled trial of digoxin in 6800 patients with chronic heart failure, as defined by left ventricular ejection fraction (the proportion of blood ejected by the left ventricle when it contracts) below 45%. In about 70% of the DIG patients, coronary ischemia was the cause of heart failure; 65% had had a prior heart attack, and 27% had angina pectoris. The results, published in 1997, indicated that mortality (the primary outcome) was totally unaffected by digoxin.[30] However, digoxin did significantly reduce the rate of hospitalization for worsening heart failure. Today, digoxin is no longer recommended in the treatment of acute MI but is still viewed as a secondary treatment option for heart rate control in atrial fibrillation and to alleviate symptoms and reduce the need for hospitalization in congestive heart failure.[31] The number of digoxin prescriptions in the U.S. has fallen by 78% from nearly 17 million in 2007 (42nd) to 3.74 million (168th) in 2017.[32]

Contribution of Secondary Prevention to the Decline in Heart Attack Mortality

We can dispense with digoxin right away because its usage has trended downward since 1970 and because it has no discernible effect on mortality. However, statins, aspirin, beta-blockers, and ACE inhibitors—and by extension angiotensin receptor blockers—all came on the scene for secondary prevention of heart attacks in the 1980s and have been staples of secondary cardiovascular prevention ever since. In their IMPACT model, Ford et al. attribute 8.5% of the observed decline in heart attack deaths between 1980 and 2000 to the use of statins, 8.0% to aspirin, 6.1% to beta-blockers, and 4.3% to ACE inhibitors (and other RAAS inhibitors) to treat patients who have already had a heart attack or other manifestation of atherosclerotic coronary heart disease (CHD).[33] I derived these figures by combining the separate estimates for the impact of these treatments in acute MI, unstable angina, non-acute secondary prevention post–MI, secondary prevention post–PCI/CABG, chronic angina, heart failure (hospitalized and non-hospitalized), and hypertension. I have applied the method explained in the appendix and applied in Chapters 4–6 and to extrapolate these results to the current usage of these four treatments.[34] Based on these increases in usage of these three secondary prevention treatments, I have estimated that 8.2% of the 81% decline in heart attack mortality rate could be attributed to statins, 8.1% to aspirin, 4.3% to beta-blockers, and 5.0% to RAAS inhibitors (see Table A.4 in the appendix). Note that, strictly speaking, some of this reduction in mortality (especially that attributed to RAAS inhibitors) might reflect prevention of heart failure deaths, which might be counted as other heart disease, rather than heart attack deaths. When we combine these four estimates to get a global estimate for secondary prevention (as we did for BP, LDL cholesterol, and smoking interventions in the primary prevention setting), we estimate that secondary prevention accounts for 23.3% of the of the 80.7% decline in heart attack mortality since 1968 (Table A.4). Although this figure represents less than half the contribution of primary prevention—reflecting the fact that these interventions apply only to the fraction of the population that has suffered and survived a heart attack or other CHD manifestation—these treatments still represent an important factor in the decline of heart attack mortality.

12

SUDDEN CARDIAC ARREST

Perhaps the most difficult manifestation of atherosclerotic coronary heart disease to prevent or treat is sudden cardiac arrest (SCA), which describes an abrupt disruption of the heartbeat (arrhythmia) that disables the capacity of the heart to pump blood. This may happen without warning to a seemingly healthy person, who is carrying on his or her normal life one minute and is dead minutes later. Death may come while the unfortunate victim is engaged in strenuous activity, but just as often when he or she is sleeping, reading, watching TV, or even while he is shaving in his hospital room (as was the case for A.L. in Chapter 1). SCA may be the final assault to a damaged or failing heart but is just as often the first and only symptom of a sudden and catastrophic plaque rupture and thrombosis occluding a critical coronary artery in an otherwise healthy heart. According to the 2020 AHA statistical report, which uses data from the Cardiac Arrest Registry to Enhance Survival (CARES), approximately 90% of persons brought to the hospital after suffering an SCA die before leaving the hospital; most are either dead on arrival or die in the emergency room.[1] In 2017, there were 379,133 sudden cardia deaths in the U.S. or 97.1 deaths per 100,000. However, nearly half of this total (46%) are of non-cardiac origin (trauma, respiratory failure, etc.), while only 28% are known to be due to heart disease; the remaining 26% are due either to multiple or unknown causes. Thus, if one assumes that half of the SCD with multiple or unknown causes are attributed to heart disease, SCD accounted for about 41% of the 647,457 heart disease deaths in the U.S. in 2017. Only 16% of all SCD (22% of those with a single known cause)—or 21 SCD per 100,000—were due to acute rupture of a coronary plaque. This represents approximately 23% of the 92.9 heart attack deaths per 100,000 in 2017. Thus, the old saw that attributes roughly half of all heart attack deaths to SCD is probably exaggerated.[2] But the truth is bad enough.

Whatever the precipitating event, the timeline for responding to sudden cardiac arrest is far shorter than for an "ordinary" myocardial infarction, in which the non-infarcted portion of the heart muscle continues to function. In sudden cardiac arrest, the entire body is suddenly deprived of oxygen—most critically the brain, which can survive for only about 10 minutes in that state. In an ordinary myocardial infarction, the damaged segment of the heart muscle can recover much of its function if the circulation is restored within 3–6 hours. So, given the impossibly short time window for intervention, the only sensible strategy for addressing sudden cardiac arrest is to prevent it; intervening after the fact can only scratch the surface. Prevention of sudden cardiac arrest can be subdivided into primary and secondary prevention. The strategies for primary prevention of sudden cardiac arrest in persons without known cardiovascular disease are the same as those for primary prevention of myocardial infarction and need not be rehearsed here. The same is generally true for secondary prevention in patients without known ventricular dysfunction. So most of this chapter will focus on preventing sudden cardiac arrest in patients with known left ventricular dysfunction.

Let us begin by reviewing how a normal heartbeat is generated and propagates through the heart. Each heart muscle cell contains a metabolic pump that moves potassium ions into the cell and sodium ions out of the cell through specialized channels in the cell membrane. This process creates an electrochemical polarization of the cell membrane, in which the interior has a higher potassium concentration, a lower sodium concentration, and a net negative charge relative to the exterior.[3] A heartbeat is initiated by a wave of depolarization that begins in the sinoatrial (SA) node in the right atrium, near the inlet from the superior vena cava, and propagates to the atrioventricular (AV) node near the tricuspid valve between the right atrium and right ventricle, then travels down the ventricular septum via the Bundle of His, which divides into left and right bundle branches which divide into smaller branches that propagate the impulse throughout the left and right ventricles (Figure 12.1).

When this electrical wave reaches a heart muscle cell, it momentarily allows sodium to rush into the cell and potassium to rush out, depolarizing the cell membrane and causing the cell (which is packed with filaments of the contractile proteins actin and myosin) to contract. When the wave passes, the cell relaxes and the sodium-potassium pump gets back to work to repolarize the membrane. (This wave of depolarization and repolarization is what an electrocardiogram records.) The ability of the heart to

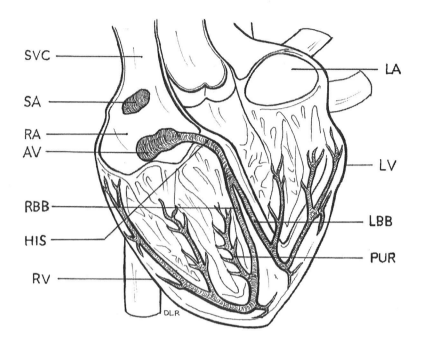

Anatomy of the cardiac conduction system. Drawing by Debra L. Roney. AV = atrioventricular node, HIS = Bundle of His, LA = left atrium, LBB = left bundle branch, LV = left ventricle, PUR = Purkinje fibers, RA = right atrium, RBB— right bundle branch, RV = right ventricle, SA = sinoatrial node, SVC = superior vena cava.

pump blood effectively depends on the ability of the specialized conduction system to generate and propagate regular electrical impulses—60–80 per minute—which permit the heart muscle cells to discharge, contract, and recharge in a coordinated rhythmic fashion.

Any disruption of that rhythmic heartbeat is called an arrhythmia. Arrhythmias originating above the AV node may require an implantable pacemaker or other treatment but do not generally cause sudden cardiac arrest. The most serious of these "supraventricular" arrhythmias is atrial fibrillation (AF), in which the atria do not beat effectively and just allow random impulses to reach the ventricles. The most serious complication of AF is the formation of atrial blood clots, pieces of which may break off and travel to the brain, causing small strokes. Treatments for AF include anti-coagulants, drugs that control heart rate (beta-blockers calcium channel blockers, digoxin, etc.) drugs that control rhythm (amiodarone, flecainide, etc.), electrical shock (cardioversion), and surgical or chemical ablation of abnormal sources of electrical impulses.[4] But none of this has much to do with heart attack deaths, sudden or otherwise.

From the SCD perspective, ventricular arrhythmias are the problem. Many adults—especially older ones—have the occasional premature ventricular contraction without suffering any ill effects. Impairments of the ventricular conduction system are more serious and may require treatment. However, the lethal ventricular arrhythmias (in order of increasing direness) are ventricular tachycardia (in which the heart beats too rapidly to maintain an adequate BP), ventricular fibrillation (in which the ventricles merely quiver without pumping blood), and asystole (in which electrical activity has ceased); these are the arrhythmias that cause SCA.

Since at least one in every five heart attack deaths presents as sudden death without prior warning, the best way to reduce the toll of SCD—at least the portion that is due to atherosclerotic coronary artery disease—is to prevent the underlying coronary disease by controlling BP, cholesterol, smoking and other risk factors, rather than to wait until after a heart attack occurs. We know that this is already occurring. Zheng et al. reported parallel declines in SCD and overall cardiac deaths between 1989 and 1998; the proportion of cardiac deaths that were sudden did not change.[5] In the more recent AHA report, SCD declined by 25% from 130.1 per 100,000 in 2000 to 97.1 per 100,000 in 2017 while heart attack deaths fell by 50%.[6] We also know that two of the drug classes that have proven effective in the secondary prevention setting—the beta-blockers in post–MI patients and the ACE inhibitors in patients with impaired ventricular function— reduce risk for subsequent SCD. These drugs have been covered in Chapter 11. The present chapter will focus on treatments that are specifically intended to prevent SCD in patients who have suffered a SCA or who are at particularly high risk of SCD due to severe left ventricular dysfunction.[7] Specifically, I will review the evidence concerning the use of amiodarone, implantable cardioverter defibrillators, and cardiopulmonary resuscitation.

Amiodarone

After the failure of the sodium channel blockers in the 1989 Cardiac Arrhythmia Suppression Trial (CAST), in which these drugs increased mortality despite suppressing premature ventricular contractions, amiodarone became the drug of choice for treating ventricular arrhythmias.[8] Actually, the clinical trial evidence supporting its efficacy in preventing SCA is mixed. A 2004 meta-analysis of 13 small amiodarone trials in patients with acute MI or congestive heart failure showed a significant reduction in SCD.[9] Also, in the Optimal Pharmacological Therapy in Cardioverter Defibrillator Patients (OPTIC) trial in patients with an implantable cardioverter defibrillator (ICD), the combination of beta-blocker and amiodarone was far more effective than beta-blockers alone in reducing the frequency of shocks delivered when the ICD detects a potentially life-threatening ventricular arrythmia.[10] However, in the NHLBI-sponsored three-armed Sudden Cardiac Death in Heart Failure Trial (SCD-HeFT), mortality in the 845 patients who received amiodarone plus conventional heart failure treatment was not reduced relative to the 847 who received only conventional heart failure therapy.[11] The use of amiodarone has declined rapidly in the past decade due to the recognition of a 5% incidence of potentially life-threatening pulmonary toxicity. It has been overtaken by beta-blockers as the first-line drug for patients at high risk for SCD and now ranks only 196th among all drugs with 2.9 million prescriptions in 2017, which represents a 25% drop since 2012.[12]

Implantable Cardioverter Defibrillators (ICD)

Ultra-high-tech niche devices like ICDs are too labor-intensive and expensive to have had a noticeable impact on national mortality trends but are a godsend for the roughly 60,000 patients who receive them each year.[13] The basic idea is for patients who are known to be at very high risk for sudden cardiac arrest (usually because they have already survived a similar episode) to have a device implanted in their chest that senses the onset of a life-threatening ventricular arrhythmia (tachycardia or defibrillation) and automatically delivers an electrical shock that jolts the heart back to a normal rhythm. So each device has internal electrodes to constantly monitor the patient's electrocardiogram and to deliver a high-voltage shock directly to the heart when needed, a capacity to record and store when and why each shock is delivered, and a lithium battery (implanted under the skin of the chest and replaced every 5–10 years) to provide power. Usually an antiarrhythmic drug (a beta-blocker and/or amiodarone) is given to minimize the number of electrical shocks delivered, which are very unpleasant and disconcerting. Although not all the arrhythmias detected and shocked by an ICD would have otherwise been lethal, the net intended effect is to substantially reduce sudden cardiac deaths and improve survival.

ICDs have been proven more effective in preventing SCD than antiarrhythmic drugs alone in several randomized trials. The 1016-patient NIH-sponsored Antiarrhythmics Versus Implantable Defibrillators (AVID) trial in the U.S., the 659-patient Canadian Implantable Defibrillator Study (CIDS), and the 288-patient Cardiac Arrest Study Hamburg (CASH) trial in Germany each compared ICD placement versus amiodarone and/or metoprolol in resuscitated survivors of sudden cardiac arrest.[14] Mortality was reduced in the ICD group relative to antiarrhythmic drugs by 28% in AVID (P=0.02), 20% in CIDS (P=0.14), and 23% in CASH (P=0.08).[15] Although only the AVID result surpassed the threshold for statistical significance, the consistency of the three trials is compelling. The 1996 Multicenter Automatic Defibrillator Implantation Trial (MADIT) found an even greater (46%) survival advantage over conventional medical therapy in heart attack survivors with ventricular dysfunction and a documented history of ventricular tachycardia but not SCA.[16]

Two additional trials in the early years of the 21st century expanded the indications for an ICD beyond patients with known prior episodes of ventricular tachycardia or fibrillation, to all patients with advanced ischemic heart failure. In the MADIT-II trial in 1232 patients with advanced heart failure, mortality was significantly reduced by 69% in the group randomized to receive an ICD versus those randomized to receive only antiarrhythmic drugs.[17] In the 3-armed SCD-HeFT, mortality was 23% lower in the 829 patients assigned to receive an ICD than in the 847 patients assigned to receive only conventional heart failure therapy (P=0.007).[18] Thus, it seems fair to conclude that ICD placement significantly improves survival by at least 20–30%—perhaps a good deal more—in all patients who are at high risk for sudden cardiac death due to advanced ischemic heart failure and/or a prior life-threatening arrhythmic episode.

Cardiopulmonary Resuscitation (CPR)

The immediate goal of CPR is to quickly establish sufficient cardiac function to sustain a blood pressure that is adequate to perfuse the brain. This is done by using an external defibrillator to administer a high-voltage shock to jolt the heart back to a functional rhythm and by periodically compressing and releasing the chest and inflating and deflating the lungs until a functional spontaneous heartbeat is established. Successfully bringing someone back from the brink of death by CPR is very dramatic—even miraculous—when portrayed on television or in the movies. But the reality is more sobering. Only 10.4% of patients who suffer out-of-hospital SCA survive to hospital discharge, and only 8.2% are discharged without significant neurological impairment.[19] And this does not even count many persons who are already dead and cold before a first responder arrives on the scene. To be sure, the 25.9% survival rate for the 18% of patients who have a "shockable" heart rhythm (ventricular tachycardia or fibrillation) when the first responder arrives is far better than the 6% survival rate for the remaining patients who have no electrical activity at all (asystole). Also, survival is far better for patients who have their SCA in a hospital (25.8%) or public place (40%) than for patients having their SCA at home, where they are often unwitnessed by anyone trained in CPR. The hard fact is that anyone who suffers an unwitnessed SCA or in whom more than 10 minutes or so has elapsed before resuscitation is initiated is beyond the reach of CPR.

One does not need a controlled clinical trial to establish that cardiopulmonary resuscitation reduces mortality, since the outcome of sudden cardiac arrest is uniformly fatal without it. However, in the past two decades, there has been intensive research aimed at improving CPR techniques and extending their reach. The NHLBI has been at the center of these efforts. In 2000, the NHLBI initiated a randomized community-based trial called the Public Access Defibrillator (PAD) trial in 993 communities with a combined 19,000+ volunteer responders.[20] Lay volunteers were trained in CPR in all 993 communities. Then the communities were randomized to two groups. In one group (496 communities), automated external defibrillators (AED) were placed in public sites like shopping malls, community centers, and apartment complexes. In the control group (497 communities), no AEDs were placed. After four years, there were significantly more survivors of SCA in the AED communities (30 survivors out of 128 SCA) than in the control communities (15 survivors among 107 SCA).

As the PAD trial was winding down, the NHLBI initiated the Home Automated External Defibrillator Trial (HAT) to explore the value of providing 7001 high-risk MI survivors who were not candidates for an ICD with an AED for home use.[21] Unfortunately, the group who received a home AED did not show any reduction in mortality. The main reason that the home AED strategy was ineffective is that only 117/160 instances of SCA occurred at home, only 58 of these at-home SCA were witnessed, and the home AED was used in only 32 instances. It would seem that only an ICD can provide useful protection for these patients.

In 2007–15, the NHLBI supported a clinical trial network called the Resuscitation Outcomes Consortium (ROC) which conducted a series of randomized trials designed to optimize resuscitation protocols and techniques.[22] Among the issues explored were the optimum ratio of chest compressions to respirations, the use of an impedance device to regulate airflow, and whether it was better to defibrillate 30 seconds or 3 minutes after initiating CPR. These nuances had only a minor impact on SCA survival. The bigger public health issue is how to reach more SCA victims in time, rather than tweaking the process itself.

Impact of Prevention of SCD on Decline in Heart Attack Mortality

In their IMPACT model, Ford et al. attribute 2.5% of the decline in heart attack mortality between 1980 and 2000 to CPR—1.3% for out-of-hospital SCA and 1.2% for in-hospital SCA—and none to amiodarone or ICDs.[23] I would quibble with these estimates because the numerators and denominators are mismatched. About half of the SCD prevented by CPR (the numerator) are of non-cardiac etiology (trauma, respiratory failure, etc.) and half the remainder are due to non-atherosclerotic heart disease (cardiomyopathies, genetic conduction disorders, etc.). It is incorrect to represent these prevented SCD as a fraction of the decline in heart attack deaths. Although CPR has improved and reaches more people that it did in 2000, I am skeptical that it accounts for more than 1% of the observed decline in *heart attack deaths* since 1970. I do agree that amiodarone and ICDs have had a negligible impact on the overall decline in heart attack deaths. Amiodarone usage is declining and has not been proven to actually reduce the incidence of SCD. The impact of ICDs is limited by their rarity—60,000 per year (including replacements). Based on the mortality rate (10% per year) and risk reduction (23%) in SCD-HeFT, ICDs can account for only 1380 SCD prevented annually.[24]

13

THE FIRE WITHIN

Although the dominant mid–20th century paradigm viewed atherosclerosis primarily as an obstructive disease caused by the deposition of cholesterol and proliferation of smooth muscle cells in the artery wall, the inflammatory nature of atherosclerosis is not a new concept.[1] Even the great 19th century pathologist Rudolf Virchow, who first described atherosclerosis, once wrote that "the softening manifests itself even in the arteries not as the consequence of a really fatty process, but as a direct product of inflammation."[2] But it was not until the 1990s that modern medical scientists began to fully appreciate the active role of the arterial wall in atherosclerosis. Atherosclerosis is not merely a passive cholesterol storage disease but an active inflammatory process involving hormone-like molecules called cytokines that recruit white blood cells and scavenger cells called macrophages that try to clear cholesterol and calcium deposits from the plaque but instead get trapped inside and contribute to its growth.[3] Some plaques become very fibrous, with calcium deposits and thick caps that contain this material within the plaque. These fibrous plaques rarely cause heart attacks. But others contain abundant cholesterol and soft inflammatory cellular debris and have thin fragile caps. When the cap is breeched, the plaque contents spill into the artery lumen and attract clot-forming platelet cells, blocking the flow of blood through the artery. In a coronary artery, this causes a heart attack; in a cerebral artery, this causes a stroke. The detailed biology of inflammation is complex and beyond the scope of this book. Here we will focus only on how our new understanding of atherosclerosis as a dynamic inflammatory process has led us to explore the potential role of anti-inflammatory drugs in the prevention of heart attacks.

An important catalyst of the paradigm shift in our understanding of atherosclerosis was the recognition of circulating biological markers that signaled the presence of active inflammation somewhere in the body.

One of the oldest of these nonspecific inflammatory biomarkers (but by no means the only one) is C-reactive protein (CRP), which was discovered in the 1930s and is elevated in diverse inflammatory diseases, ranging from rheumatoid arthritis to tuberculosis.[4] In the 1990s, the development of a high-sensitivity CRP assay let to the realization that modest elevations of CRP, heretofore considered within the "normal range," were associated with atherosclerotic cardiovascular disease, independently of the conventional cardiovascular risk factors enumerated in Chapter 2.[5] A later study, which included a review of CRP analyses on stored samples from several statin trials confirmed this result.[6] However, while it appeared that CRP and other known markers of inflammation were moderate predictors of future heart attacks and strokes, it was not clear whether these molecules were active agents or mere bystanders in the inflammatory process and whether inflammation itself was a cause or effect of atherosclerosis. Therefore, the 2009 U.S. Preventive Services Task Force did not recommend routine screening for CRP levels.[7]

The interest in CRP as a cardiovascular risk factor was further piqued by the results of a large statin trial called JUPITER (Justification for the Use of Statins in Primary Prevention: An Intervention Trial Evaluating Rosuvastatin) in 2008.[8] This 17,802-patient randomized trial was unique in that it specifically targeted healthy volunteers with elevated CRP (> 2.0 mg/L) but *not* elevated LDL cholesterol levels. JUPITER participants were randomized to receive the highly potent statin rosuvastatin (Crestor) or a placebo. The trial was stopped early after 1.9 years of treatment because of a highly significant 44% reduction in the combined incidence of MI, stroke, revascularization, unstable angina, and death from cardiovascular causes (the prespecified primary outcome). While the outcome could readily be attributed to the 50% mean reduction in LDL cholesterol in the rosuvastatin group, rosuvastatin also reduced CRP levels by 37%. Further analysis showed that reductions in CRP were as predictive of a favorable outcome as reductions in LDL cholesterol.[9] Participants who experienced large reductions in both LDL and CRP had fewer adverse cardiovascular outcomes than those who experienced large reductions in only one of these two risk factors, who in turn experienced fewer adverse cardiovascular outcomes than those whose LDL and CRP responded minimally to rosuvastatin. These results prompted medical scientists to look at statins not merely as potent cholesterol-lowering drugs but also as anti-inflammatory drugs that could spearhead a two-pronged attack on atherosclerotic cardiovascular disease. Two years later, the FDA extended their indications for rosuvastatin to include healthy persons with normal LDL cholesterol but increased risk based on a combination of age, CRP, and at least one other risk factor.[10] The 2018 ACC/AHA Guideline on the Management of High Blood Cholesterol has also incorporated CRP as a risk factor to consider in primary prevention.[11]

The post–JUPITER controversy about whether to put inflammatory markers like CRP on an equal footing with conventional cardiovascular risk factors like LDL cholesterol led to a push, spearheaded by lead JUPITER investigator Paul Ridker, to test the "inflammation hypothesis" in a randomized clinical trial using an anti-inflammatory drug with no measurable effect on LDL cholesterol or other risk factors that might affect outcomes. This rules out statins and aspirin (which has both anti-inflammatory and anti-thrombotic activity). Two such trials have recently been completed. The four-armed Canakinumab Anti-inflammatory Thrombosis Outcome Study (CANTOS) randomized 10,161 patients with a prior MI and a CRP > 2 mg/L to receive 0 (placebo), 50, 150, or 300 mg subcutaneous dose of canakinumab, a monoclonal antibody targeting interleukin-1β (an inflammatory cytokine), at 3-month intervals.[12] The 150 mg dose (but not the other two doses) brought about a significant reduction in the combined incidence of nonfatal MI, stroke, and cardiovascular death (the primary outcome). Total mortality was not reduced. An increase in fatal infections in the combined treated groups relative to placebo was offset by an equal decrease in cancer deaths. While the CANTOS results were promising, their clinical application is uncertain due the small absolute reduction in cardiovascular outcomes and uncertain adverse risks of canakinumab.[13]

However, the results of the second large trial, the NHLBI-sponsored Cardiovascular Inflammation Reduction Trial (CIRT), were disappointing. In this trial, 4786 patients with stable coronary artery disease were randomized to receive an established anti-inflammatory drug—low-dose methotrexate—or placebo.[14] There was no difference in the combined incidence of MI, stroke, cardiovascular death, or hospitalization for unstable angina leading to urgent PCI (the primary outcome). Surprisingly, methotrexate treatment did not reduce mean levels of inflammatory markers like CRP, interleukin-1β, or interleukin-2 in CIRT participants, although it is a proven anti-inflammatory drug for treating rheumatoid arthritis. So the CIRT results do not disprove the "inflammation hypothesis" but merely leave us back at square one.

Impact of Anti–Inflammatory Treatment on Decline in Heart Attack Mortality

While it is possible that the anti-inflammatory properties of statins and aspirin have contributed to the decline in heart attacks since 1980, such effects have been inadvertent and unquantifiable. The deliberate use of specific anti-inflammatory drugs to quell atherosclerosis and prevent cardiovascular deaths is in its infancy. Such treatments have not yet been proven effective and are not in wide use but may hold promise for the future.

14

DIET, EXERCISE,
AND OBESITY

Throughout history, poverty has always been and still is bad for your health. Even as the technological advances of the late 19th century lessened the burden of labor and lengthened life expectancy, it was still the poor, living in crowded slums, where infections disease flourished, or on rural dirt farms with barely enough to eat, who suffered the brunt of disease and early death. However, atherosclerosis in general, and coronary heart disease in particular, was a notable exception. As the 20th century began, coronary heart disease was viewed as a disease of affluence and was relatively rare among the poor.[1] However, as the 20th century brought less oppressive working conditions, better nutrition, a higher general standard of living, and longer life to the U.S. population at large, it also brought coronary heart disease to the masses. As more and more Americans grew able to enjoy a middle-class lifestyle and extreme poverty grew relatively rare, atherosclerosis coronary heart disease became the leading cause of death among all strata of American society. By the end of the century, it was those at the bottom of the socioeconomic ladder, who suffered the most from this disease. This chapter will explore the role of the elements of the emerging middle-class lifestyle—specifically an abundant diet, a shrinking necessity for vigorous physical inactivity, and the increasing prevalence of obesity—in the rise and decline of heart disease from 1900 to the present.

In the previous chapters, I have tried to present an orderly progression of evidence-based advances informed by epidemiology and confirmed by randomized clinical trials. However, we must rely mostly on epidemiological observations for evidence of the impact of lifestyle on cardiovascular disease.

- In prospective epidemiologic studies like Framingham, diet, physical inactivity, and obesity are not independently associated with subsequent risk of cardiovascular events. Their impact on cardiovascular risk seems to operate substantially through their effects on more proximate risk factors like BP, cholesterol, and diabetes.

- Measuring diet and exercise accurately and controlling behavior are next to impossible in free-living volunteers. Few people are willing and able to keep a detailed and accurate diary of their food intake or physical activity over any length of time. Instruments like the 24-hour dietary recall, which are often the best one can do in these studies, provide an incomplete and sometimes skewed version of the participant's typical daily diet.

- Since everyone must eat something, it is difficult to separate the effects of specific dietary components on the outcome of interest. For example, if one wants to reduce the percentage of caloric intake from fat while maintaining overall caloric balance, the percentage of other dietary components—most often, carbohydrate—must go up. So, if LDL cholesterol falls, how can one be certain whether the reduction in dietary fat or the complementary increase in dietary carbohydrates is responsible? If one simply reduces fat and does not replace the calories with something else, how can one be certain whether any observed fall in LDL cholesterol is due specifically to the reduced intake of fat or to the general reduction in caloric intake?

- Randomized clinical trials of the direct impact of diet, exercise, and obesity on cardiovascular disease outcomes require very large numbers of participants (10,000 or more) and 7–10 years to complete. Maintaining compliance over the full duration of such a trial is all but impossible outside of a prison or institution. Very few such trials have been successful.

There is certainly no shortage of scientific and popular books and articles on diet, exercise, obesity and cardiovascular disease. Indeed, a bewildering array of popular books have been written, especially on diet, each offering detailed (and sometimes conflicting) guidance for attaining a svelte physique and cardiovascular health. Even the scientific literature on this subject is rather contentious. A detailed review of this diverse literature is beyond my scope or expertise. I will simply confine myself to acquainting you with the consensus lifestyle recommendations of the mainstream medical experts and their rationale.

Without embarking on a lengthy review, I will cite three examples of unsuccessful attempts to show that lifestyle interventions improve cardiovascular outcomes. In the late 1990s, the Women's Health Initiative (WHI) randomized 48,835 postmenopausal women to receive either a control diet in which fat comprised at least 32% of the caloric intake or a diet designed to reduce fat intake to 20% by limiting meats and fatty foods and adding fruits, vegetables, and grains.[2] After 8.1 years mean follow-up, there were only modest differences in cardiovascular risk factors and no differences in the incidence of heart attack, stroke, or cardiovascular mortality between the two groups. I have already commented on the NIDDK's Look-AHEAD Study, a dietary weight loss study in 5125 obese type 2 diabetic patients, in Chapter 7.[3] In that study, patients on the active diet successfully lost 8.6% of total body weight in year 1 (versus 0.7% in the control group) but could not sustain this weight loss over time. After nine years of follow-up, there was no difference in mortality between the two groups. Finally, the 1976–79 National Exercise and Heart Disease Project (NEHDP) trial randomized 651 male heart attack survivors to a supervised exercise program versus usual care.[4] After 19 years, mortality was not significantly reduced. A 1989 overview of 22 similar cardiac rehabilitation trials also showed no net reduction in mortality.[5]

So, the 2013 AHA/ACC Lifestyle Management Guidelines, which acknowledge that "RCTs examining the effects on hard outcomes (myocardial infarction, stroke, heart failure, and CVD related death) are difficult if not impossible to conduct," are based on studies of the impact of these interventions on cardiovascular risk factors rather than health outcomes.[6] Here are the key recommendations of this panel and of a separate AHA/ACC Panel on Managing Obesity[7]:

Dietary recommendations:

- Consume a dietary pattern that emphasizes vegetables, fruits, and whole grains, includes low-fat dairy products poultry, fish, legumes, non-tropical vegetable oils, and nuts, and limits sweets, sugar-sweetened beverages and red meats.
- For LDL cholesterol lowering, reduce intake of saturated fats (5–6% of calories) and trans fats.
- For BP lowering, reduce daily intake of sodium below 2400 mg; below 1500 mg is even better.

Physical Activity:

- Adults should engage in aerobic physical activity, 3–4 sessions per week, lasting on average 40 minutes per session and involving moderate- to vigorous-intensity physical activity.

Obesity

- Body Mass Index (BMI), which is calculated by dividing body weight in kilograms by the square of the height in meters, is the standard criterion. BMI > 25 indicates overweight, BMI > 30 indicates obesity, and BMI > 35 indicates morbid obesity. Body waist circumference is another useful measurement.
- Caloric restriction—< 1500 Cal per day in women and < 1800 Cal per day in men—is the preferred method of weight reduction in those who are overweight or obese.
- Bariatric surgery (in which a portion of the stomach is stapled to reduce its capacity) may be warranted in morbidly obese high-risk patients.

Diet and Cardiovascular Risk Factors

In the absence of direct evidence linking lifestyle interventions to cardiovascular outcomes, expert panels have relied mainly on studies linking these interventions to established cardiovascular risk factors—specifically LDL cholesterol, BP, and type 2 diabetes. There have been many small but rigorous studies, performed under controlled conditions in metabolic wards, of the influence of dietary fats on serum cholesterol level. Two classic examples, a study by Ancel Keys and another by David Hegsted, both published in 1965, developed linear regression models showing that (in descending order of strength of association) higher intake of saturated fat (found in animal fat and tropical oils), lower intake of polyunsaturated fat (found in corn, sunflower, safflower, and other plant oils), and higher intake of cholesterol (found in animal and dairy fat and eggs) each raised serum cholesterol levels.[8] Their work has held up well in subsequent studies. In my own master's thesis, for example, I found similar (but weaker) relationships of changes in dietary composition (as derived from 24-hour dietary recall data) to changes in LDL cholesterol in the run-in phase of the Lipid Research Clinics Coronary Primary Prevention Trial.[9] In my analysis, weight loss was an even stronger predictor of a fall in LDL cholesterol, but this may reflect the greater precision of measuring weight than dietary composition in this study.

The most important studies of the impact of diet on cardiovascular risk factors are the two Dietary Approaches to Stop Hypertension (DASH) trials, (both supported by the NHLBI) in which all meals were prepared for study participants to rigorous specifications and sample meals were sent to a laboratory for nutrient analysis.[10] In the first DASH trial, after a three-week run-in period in which all 464 participants received a control diet designed to reflect a "typical American diet" containing 36% fat, they were randomized to three groups: (1) a control group who continued to receive the typical American diet, (2) a diet enriched in fruit, vegetables, and whole grains but in which fat content and total calories were similar to the control diet, or (3) a diet similar to #2 but with replacement of dairy products with their low-fat counterparts and overall reduction of fat content to 26%.[11] After eight weeks, diet #2 significantly reduced both systolic and diastolic BP by 2.8 and 1.1 mmHg, respectively, relative to the control diet, and diet #3 reduced systolic and diastolic BP by 5.5 and 3.0 mmHg. In a subsequent analysis, diet #3 (but not diet #2) also significantly reduced LDL cholesterol by 10.7 mg/dL.[12] Diet #3 is now known as the DASH diet.

Upon the completion of the first DASH trial, a second 2×3 factorial trial was undertaken in which 412 participants were randomized to the DASH or control (typical American) diet and to either high (3.3 g/day), intermediate (2.5 mg/day), or low (1.5 g/day) sodium content.[13] At the end of 30 days, systolic and diastolic BP both fell significantly as sodium intake was reduced and were significantly lower in the group receiving the DASH versus control diet at every level of sodium intake. Mean BP was 133/84 mmHg in the group receiving the control high-sodium diet and 124/79 in the group receiving the DASH low-sodium diet. Thus, the DASH low-sodium diet became the standard dietary recommendation for treating hypertension.

In view of the worsening problem of obesity, insulin resistance, and type 2 diabetes since the 1970s, dietary plans employing the "glycemic index," a quantitative scale of the glycemic load imposed by the consumption of different carbohydrates, have gained popularity.[14] Sugars, refined carbohydrates (like white bread), and potatoes are among the foods with a high glycemic index, while whole grains, fresh produce, and fructose are among the foods with a low glycemic index. While the standard DASH diet tends to be high in foods with a low glycemic index, an NHLBI controlled feeding trial called OmniCarb (Effect of Amount and Type of Dietary Carbohydrates on Risk for Cardiovascular Heart Disease and Diabetes Study), which specifically compared a low-glycemic index version of the DASH diet with a high-glycemic index version of the DASH diet, found no significant improvement in insulin sensitivity or other risk factors.[15]

Recently, a dietary model based on the diet of Mediterranean countries like Spain, Italy, and Greece (which enjoy relatively low rates of heart attack and stroke) has gained increasing currency.[16] Like the DASH diet, the "MED" diet emphasizes fruits, vegetables, and whole grains and reduced intake of red meats. But unlike the DASH diet (which replaces sources of saturated fat with carbohydrates), the MED diet calls for increased intake of sources of unsaturated fat (like olive oil and nuts) to compensate for lost saturated fat calories. In 2013, a 7447-participant Spanish randomized trial called Prevención con Dieta Mediterránea (PREDIMED) compared two versions of the MED diet—one involving supplementation with extra virgin olive oil and the other involving supplementation with nuts—versus a control diet recommending reduced fat intake.[17] Although the first version of their article had to be retracted due to data irregularities, the revised corrected version still showed a significant 30% reduction in the combined incidence of heart attack, stroke, and cardiovascular death (the primary outcome measure) in both MED groups versus the control groups after a mean 4.8 years of follow-up. Unlike DASH, PREDIMED was conducted in free-living people and did not report dietary compliance or actual nutrients consumed. So the actual specifications of the MED diet and the control are difficult to pin down. The results of PREDIMED are consistent with other published studies (mostly observational) of the Mediterranean diet.[18] Because of the success of PREDIMED where prior diet-heart trials had failed, the Mediterranean diet will likely be put on an equal footing with the DASH diet in future AHA/ACC guidelines.

Exercise and Cardiovascular Risk Factors

Exercise is one of those virtuous behaviors that everyone knows is good for you, but it is best not to rely on epidemiologic cohort studies like Framingham, to support this hypothesis. People who exercise regularly are undoubtedly healthier than those who do not, but there is a chicken-and-egg factor here. Is it lack of exercise that causes poor health, or is it poor health that limits a person's capacity to exercise? The best epidemiologic evidence that exercise lowers cardiovascular disease outcomes comes from classical occupational studies going back to the 1950s and 1960s, which compared seat-bound London coach drivers with conductors who walk the aisles, sedentary postal office workers versus mailmen who walk a delivery route, sedentary railroad workers versus active longshoremen. Each of these studies showed that people of comparable socioeconomic status with more active jobs had lower rates of heart attack and other cardiovascular events than those with sedentary jobs in the same sector.[19]

The evidence linking exercise with improvement in known cardiovascular risk factors is more robust. A 2003 overview of exercise studies reported that regular exercise is associated with improved exercise tolerance, reduced body weight, reduced BP, reduced LDL cholesterol, increased HDL cholesterol, and increased physical activity.[20] The first two benefits are obvious, although they are not among the traditional Framingham independent risk factors. However, getting more exercise clearly helps lower BP and LDL cholesterol and curb the development of insulin resistance—the precursor of type 2 diabetes. These benefits may be mediated at least in part by the importance of exercise in maintaining a healthy body weight. The increase in HDL cholesterol, which was touted in 2003 as a major benefit of exercise, has lost some of its luster in view of the recent negative CETP trial experience (see Chapter 8).

The specific benefits of exercise in patients with metabolic syndrome (a constellation of metabolic risk factors that includes insulin resistance) were explored in a 2013 meta-analysis of seven randomized clinical trials.[21] Significant reductions in BMI, waist circumference, systolic and diastolic BP, LDL cholesterol, plasma glucose, and cardiovascular fitness (as measured by peak oxygen consumption) and a significant increase in HDL cholesterol were observed. Again, the extent to which the beneficial effects of exercise on BP, cholesterol, and insulin resistance are mediated by weight control is uncertain.

Obesity and Cardiovascular Risk Factors

Although obesity is generally not an independent predictor of future heart attacks and other adverse cardiovascular events in Framingham and other epidemiologic studies, there is no doubt that obesity is bad for the heart.[22] There are two major problems with epidemiologic studies of obesity. First, obesity is a major contributing cause of type 2 diabetes, hypertension, and hypercholesterolemia. So epidemiologic models that include these more proximate causes of cardiovascular disease tend to drown out the impact of obesity acting through these risk factors. Second, significant weight loss ("wasting") is a frequent pre-terminal accompaniment of failing health—not just in cancer patients, but in patients with advanced heart failure or dementia and for very elderly and frail persons in general. This phenomenon gives rise to the "obesity paradox" in which persons at the far low end of the BMI distribution—especially those who have lost weight recently—tend to exhibit the *highest* rates of cardiovascular disease and mortality in epidemiologic studies. The 2006 updated AHA Scientific Statement on Obesity and Cardiovascular Disease sums up the evidence very nicely, including the direct cardiovascular adverse effects of obesity and its contribution to increased morbidity and mortality during cardiovascular surgery.[23] But most of all, the alarming rise in obesity in the U.S. during the last three decades, as shown in Figure 14.1, is certainly the major cause of the explosive rise in type 2 diabetes during this period (see Figure 7.1 in Chapter 7) and has been a drag on progress in controlling BP and LDL cholesterol.[24]

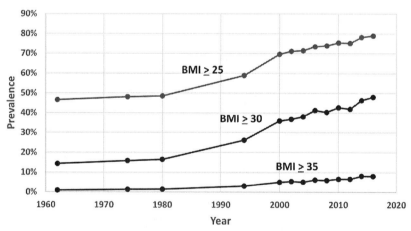

U.S. obesity trend, 1960–2016. Data are from NHANES surveys. National Center for Health Statistics. Health E-Stats, September 2018.

A 2019 article projecting recent obesity trends forward predicts that the prevalence of obesity (BMI > 30 kg/m^2) among U.S. adults will stabilize at 50% but that the prevalence of severe obesity (BMI > 35 kg/m^2) will triple to 24% in 2030.[25]

A History Lesson: The Role of Changing Lifestyle in the Heart Attack Pandemic

As we have said earlier, the 20th-century cardiovascular disease pandemic was actually a pandemic of atherosclerotic coronary heart disease or, more simply put, heart attacks. Mortality from heart attacks, all heart diseases, and all cardiovascular diseases rose during the first 60 years or so of the 20th century then declined steadily thereafter, falling well below the 1900 mortality rates (Figure 1.1). Stroke mortality, on the other hand, was already declining in 1900 and declined steadily throughout the 20th and early 21st century. In the previous chapters we have addressed the role of smoking in explaining about 28% of the doubling of heart disease mortality between 1900 and 1960 and the role of a variety of medical advances in the > 80% decline in heart attack deaths since then. So where do diet, exercise, and obesity come in?

We must begin with a summary of the profound social and cultural developments that had already taken hold in 1900 and accelerated over the course of the 20th century, transforming every aspect of American life. These developments include:

- The industrial revolution of the late 19th century sparked a mass migration from farms to cities. The proportion of Americans living on farms which had been 94% in 1800, declined to 39% by 1900, and continued to decline to 16% in 1950, and 1% in 1990.[26] Meanwhile, the proportion of Americans living in cities increased from 40% in 1900 to 64% in 1950 to 75% in 1990.
- In the late 19th and early 20th centuries, waves of immigration from Ireland, Italy, Germany, China, Eastern Europe, and Latin America and of migration of southern rural Blacks to northern cities brought greater diversity to American cities.
- Automation and the union movement reduced the burden of

physical labor and afforded average Americans more leisure time for recreation.

- Advances in public hygiene and the development of vaccines and (much later) antibiotics reduced infant and maternal mortality and extended life expectancy. In 1900, for every 1000 live births, 100 infants did not live to see their first birthday and six to nine women died of pregnancy-related complications.[27] By 1997, infant mortality had fallen by 93% to about 7 per 1000, and maternal mortality was less than 5 in 100,000. Mean life expectancy increased from 49 years in 1900 to nearly 80 years today.[28]
- The invention and popularization of the automobile around the turn of the century made it possible to perform daily errands without physical exertion.
- The popularization of television in the 1950s and personal computers in the late 1990s has contributed mightily to Americans' increasingly sedentary lifestyle and the acceleration of our epidemic of obesity.

One thing that has changed less than you might think since 1900 is the American diet. The popular myth in some circles is that the doubling of heart disease deaths in 1900–60 reflects our straying from the pristine heart-healthy diet of our agrarian forbearers and succumbing to the charms of red meat, butterfat, salty, fatty convenience foods, and general overindulgence. The truth is more complicated. Deprivation and malnutrition were widespread in the inhabitants of rural backwaters and crowded city slums at the turn of the century; their lean dietary intake was dictated by necessity, not by choice. The elites and the prosperous farmers of that time ate very well indeed, as illustrated in the following literary descriptions of Sunday dinner on the farm in the late 19th century—the first from Laura Ingalls Wilder's *Farm Boy* and the second from Willa Cather's *My Antonia*.

> Mother sliced the hot rye'n'injun bread on the bread-board by her plate. Father's spoon cut deep into the chicken-pie; he scooped out big pieces of thick crust and turned up their fluffy yellow under-sides on the plate. He poured gravy over them; he dipped up big pieces of tender chicken, dark meat and white meat sliding from the bones. He added a mound of baked beans and topped it with a quivering slice of fat pork. At the edge of the plate he piled dark-red beet pickles. And he handed the plate to Almanzo. Silently Almanzo ate it all. Then he ate a piece of pumpkin pie, and he felt very full inside. But he ate a piece of apple pie with cheese.[29] A few hours earlier, before church, the family had consumed a breakfast consisting of pile

after pile of pancakes with butter and molasses, sausage cakes, oatmeal, and apple pie.

On Sundays she [Mother] gave us as much chicken as we could eat, and on other days we had ham or bacon or sausage meat. She baked either pies or cake for us every day, unless, for a change, she made my favorite pudding, striped with currents and boiled in a bag.[30]

This was clearly not the DASH or MED diet; fresh fruits and vegetables and low-fat dairy products are mentioned nowhere. Lest you think I am cherry-picking, check out the menus from popular early 20th century cookbooks, which feature meats three times a day, sometimes including mutton chops or fried chicken for breakfast, lots of fried potatoes and vegetables, and helpings of cake, pie, ice cream, puddings, etc. for dessert at all the noon and evening meals.[31]

Table 14.1. Changes in American Diet in 20th Century

Dietary Component	1909–19	1960–69	1990–99
Total Calories	3400	3100	3600
Fat, g	120	143	151
Saturated, g	50	54	48
Monounsaturated, g	47	56	64
Polyunsaturated, g	13	22	31
Carbohydrate, g	487	383	481
Protein, g	96	93	109
Cholesterol, mg	440	470	400
Fiber, g	28	18	24
Meats, %Cal	14.7	18.9	13.7
Beef/Pork	13.3	16.2	8.9
Poultry	0.9	2.2	4.2
Fish	0.6	0.5	0.6
Dairy, %Cal	8.5	11.6	9.6
Whole Milk	5.1	6.1	1.6
Low-Fat	0.8	0.7	2.1
Cheese	0.6	1.6	3.2
Other	2.1	3.1	2.7
Eggs, %Cal	1.8	2.1	1.4

Dietary Component	1909–19	1960–69	1990–99
Fats & Oils, %Cal	12.6	16.8	19.4
Butter	4.4	1.8	1.1
Margarine	0.6	2.8	2.4
Shortening	3.1	5.1	6.7
Lard, Beef Tallow	3.8	2.2	0.9
Vegetable Oils	0.7	4.8	8.3
Grain Products, %Cal	37.5	21.1	24.6
Legumes, nuts, & soy, %Cal	2.3	3.0	3.1
Vegetables, %Cal	6.5	5.6	5.2
Potatoes	4.0	2.7	2.5
Green/Yellow	0.9	0.4	0.4
Tomatoes	0.4	0.6	0.6
Other	1.3	1.8	1.6
Fruits, % of Calories	2.9	2.8	3.3
Sugars & Sweeteners, %Cal	12.9	17.8	18.8
Sodium, mg	920	1270	1290

Turning to less anecdotal data, Table 14.1 (above) shows U.S. Department of Agriculture data on U.S. consumption of key nutrients in 1909–19, 1959, and 1999 at the early, peak and decline phases of the heart attack pandemic.[32] If you study this table (which covers all socioeconomic classes), several important points stand out:

- Mean daily caloric intake did not change very much. Indeed, daily caloric consumption was higher in 1909–19 than in 1960–69. However, daily calorie expenditure fell far more, as jobs required less strenuous physical labor and shorter hours. Then, daily caloric intake rose by 17% between the 1960s and 1990s while jobs became even more deskbound and obesity began to take off (Figure 14.1). Indeed, the popularization of personal computers and email in the 1990s and smart phones in the 2000s made it possible to communicate with co-workers without even leaving one's chair.
- The mid–20th century diet derived a higher proportion of its calories from fat—particularly saturated fat—and less from carbohydrates than the 1909–19 diet. The rise in fat consumption

largely reflects the greater annual consumption of beef, which grew from a steady 40–50 pounds per capita before 1950, peaked as high as 90–95 pounds per capital in the late 1970s, and then fell back to about 60 pounds per capita at the end of the century. Annual pork consumption was relatively stable at 40–50 pounds per capita throughout the century, while annual poultry consumption steadily rose from 10 to 50 pounds per capita.[33] Increased consumption of dairy products also contributed to the rising fat content of the American diet. The fall in carbohydrates largely reflects the drop in grain and potato consumption, although this is offset partially by the increased consumption of sugars and sweeteners, which in turn reflects the growing popularity of carbonated soft drinks.

- The cholesterol and sodium content of the diet also increased between early and mid-century. The sodium figures reported by Hiza and Bente reflect the natural salt content of foods and salt added in canning vegetables and does not include salt added at the table or in home-cured meats (ham, sausage, etc.), which were prominent in the early part of the century.[34] Therefore, the reported increase in dietary sodium (which reflects mainly increased cheese consumption) may not be real.

- Many of the qualitative dietary changes in the last three decades of the 20th century—the shift from butter, lard and beef tallow to margarine, shortening and vegetable oils; the shift from beef to poultry; the shift from whole to low-fat milk; the fall in egg consumption; the increase in dietary fiber—appear to reflect the influence of the AHA and other medical experts. However, these ostensible improvements came in the context of rapidly increasing caloric intake, insufficient consumption of fresh fruits and vegetables, unhealthy consumption of sugar and corn syrup, in the form of soft drinks, and exploding rates of obesity and type 2 diabetes.

Impact of Changes in Diet, Execrcise, and Obesity on the Rise and Fall of Cardiovascular Diseases

While acknowledging the paucity of hard evidence from randomized controlled trials (or even compelling prospective epidemiologic studies) demonstrating the quantitative relationship of diet, exercise, and obesity to heart attack and other cardiovascular diseases, I believe that the circumstantial evidence strongly supports a major role of these important lifestyle factors in the doubling of heart disease mortality between 1900 and 1960. Clearly, the disconnect between how much we eat and how many calories we burn daily must have been a major factor. Even the rich and abundant meals described by Laura Ingalls Wilder and Willa Cather, must be viewed in the context of the extreme caloric demands of farm work, which far exceeded the demands on modern physical laborers. Qualitative changes in how those calories were distributed among saturated fats, unsaturated fats, and carbohydrate probably contributed to the increase in heart attacks by raising LDL cholesterol levels, but there were no national surveys of cholesterol levels until the first National Health and Nutrition Examination Survey (NHANES) in 1960.[35] I am skeptical about the role of salt consumption and BP in this doubling of heart attack mortality, because the prevalence of "malignant hypertension" and incidence of strokes (a frequent consequence of this disease) have been in decline at least since 1900 (see Chapter 4). In any case, other than the rise of cigarette smoking, which may explain about 28% of the rise in heart attacks between 1900 and 1960, there are few other candidates, other perhaps than the increased stress associated with the urbanization of America. But make no mistake, life in 1900 was hardly stress-free.

Might changes in the U.S. lifestyle since 1970 have contributed to the 81% decline in heart attack mortality since the 1960s? Again, I am skeptical—*not* because I believe that diet and lifestyle are unimportant, but because they have continued to trend mostly in the *wrong* direction. Indeed, I believe that if Americans were becoming fitter instead of fatter, there would be far less need for the other interventions described in this book. Ford et al. do not include diet explicitly in their IMPACT model of the changes between 1980 and 2000, although favorable changes in the consumption of meat and dairy products and of saturated fat may have contributed to the model's estimated impact of LDL cholesterol reduction and BP control on the decline in heart attack mortality.[36] However, the contributions of these favorable dietary changes to this model were likely far smaller those of cholesterol- and BP-lowering drugs. I am also highly skeptical of the IMPACT model's attribution of 5% of the decline in mortality to changes in physical activity, given our increasingly sedentary culture.[37] I assume that the authors must have been thinking of the increasing popularity of leisure exercise programs (gym memberships, yoga classes, etc.) among the affluent, rather than the increasingly sedentary American workplace and the popularity of video games and online activity among the young. The estimated 7.6% *negative* impact of changes in BMI in the IMPACT model probably overlaps heavily with the negative impact of the rise in type 2 diabetes (see Chapter 7).[38] The prevalence of obesity in the U.S. has only grown since 2000 (see Figure 14.1). Thus, the combined contribution of post–1968 trends in diet, exercise, and obesity on the decline in heart attack deaths has probably been a wash at best; they have been more a continuing part of the problem than part of the solution.

15

RACIAL CARDIOVASCULAR HEALTH DISPARITIES

In 1932, the U.S. Public Health Service, with the cooperation of the Tuskegee Institute (now Tuskegee University), initiated a natural history study called the Tuskegee Study of Untreated Syphilis in the Negro Male.[1] They enrolled 600 poor Black Alabamans, mostly sharecroppers, 399 of whom had latent syphilis, a venereal disease that progresses slowly over decades and if untreated can eventually lead to severe neurological complications, blindness, dementia, and death. They enticed the participants (most of whom had rarely if ever seen a doctor) with the promise of free medical care, but that free care did not include any education about their condition and included only sham or placebo treatments. Although no safe and effective treatments for syphilis existed until well after the study began, the study doctors actively lobbied local physicians and military physicians (for those who enlisted during the war) not to offer Tuskegee study participants the best treatments available at the time. When penicillin was proven to be a safe and effective cure for syphilis in 1947, it was deliberately withheld from study participants, and the study continued unchanged, despite its violation of the Nuremberg Code for human research, which had been newly adopted as a consequence of the horrific human experiments conducted in Nazi concentration camps. Throughout the Civil Rights movement of the 1950s and 1960s—from the historic Brown v Board of Education decision in 1954 to the assassination of Martin Luther King in 1968—the Tuskegee Study continued to deny its hapless participants access to proven efficacious treatment for syphilis. It was not until July 1972, when a whistleblower named Peter Buxton and an enterprising reporter named Jean Heller exposed what had been going on in Tuskegee in the guise of medical research, that an act of Congress finally ended the study. By this time, 128 Tuskegee study participants had died of syphilis or related complications, at least 40 of their spouses had contracted the disease, and 19 of their children had been born with the disease.

Although we have discussed trends in cardiovascular risk factors and mortality in the previous chapters as if all of us equally enjoy the fruits of the advances in biomedical research, this is clearly untrue. While the appalling Tuskegee study represents the nadir and not the norm for medical research, it is but one of many instances in which medical scientists have ignored the rights of Blacks. For example, consider the story of Henrietta Lacks, an indigent Black Virginia mother whose cervical cancer cells were cultured and shared worldwide without her consent while she died of her cancer in the Johns Hopkins paupers' ward.[2] Poor rural southern Blacks are at the intersection of groups who have historically gotten the short end of the stick in healthcare as in other aspects of life in America. Unfortunately, this too has been the case for cardiovascular disease. While cardiovascular health disparities may not rank high among the many hardships and injustices afflicting Blacks in America, the story of the American front in the battle against cardiovascular disease is incomplete without addressing this topic.

Racial Differences in Mortality

Figure 15.1 shows the U.S. trends in age-adjusted mortality for coronary heart disease (CHD)—i.e., heart attacks—from 1968–2017 and for all heart disease (which include rheumatic heart disease, heart failure, etc., as well as heart attacks) from 1950 to 2017.[3]

Before we begin discussing these curves, let me point out two technical issues with the heart attack mortality data for Blacks before 1968. First, the mortality rates for Blacks were not separated from other non–White racial groups until 1968; in 1950–67, mortality data were reported only for Whites and non–Whites. Second, when the coding system for classifying heart disease deaths as due to heart attack versus other causes was revised in 1968, some deaths for which hypertensive heart disease and heart failure were contributing causes were newly classified as heart attack deaths.[4] This revision affected Blacks more than Whites and led to an abrupt jump in heart attack mortality in non–Whites from 322.6 per 100,000 in 1967 (77% of the rate in Whites) 468.5 per 100,000 in 1968 (97% of the rate in Whites). Neither this coding change nor the separation of Blacks from

US Trends in Heart Disease Mortality

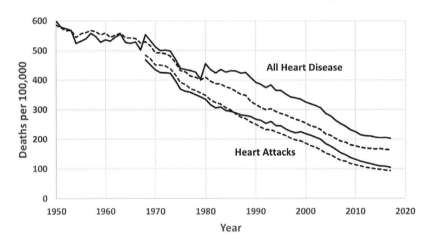

U.S. trends in coronary heart disease (CHD) and all heart disease mortality by race, 1950–2017. From published CDC Vital Statistics compilations. Blacks are represented by solid lines, and Whites by dashed lines. Pre–1968 heart disease mortality rates for Blacks include all non–Whites.

other non–White racial groups caused a similar discontinuity in the mortality trends for all diseases of the heart or for stroke (see below). Therefore, I have discarded the pre–1968 heart attack mortality data from this analysis but have retained the pre–1968 total heart disease and stroke mortality data. The coding system was revised again in 1979, but this change caused only a small blip in the mortality trends.[5]

Heart disease mortality was roughly similar among racial groups before 1980, but mortality has been higher in Blacks than Whites from 1980 going forward (Figure 15.1). Similarly, heart attack mortality was slightly lower in Blacks than Whites in 1968 and remained so through 1986, but the curves eventually crossed over in 1986. From 1986 to 2017, mortality rates for heart attack and well as total heart disease have been higher in Blacks than Whites. The Black-White disparity in excess mortality reached as high as 21% for heart attacks and 32% for all heart disease in 2003–04 but has narrowed since then to 12% and 23%, respectively in 2017. Since 1968, mortality rates from heart attacks and all heart diseases have declined steadily in both Blacks and Whites, but more rapidly in Whites. After starting at similar levels in 1968, annual heart disease mortality declined to 164.4 per 100,000 (93.5 due to heart attacks) in Whites versus 202.4 per 100,000 (104.7 due to heart attacks) in Blacks in 2017. Thus, African Americans have not consistently enjoyed the full fruits of the advances we have made toward controlling the heart attack pandemic.

Figure 15.2 shows the U.S. trends in age-adjusted heart attack mortality from 1968 to 2008 broken down by both race and sex.[6]

In 1968, heart attack mortality was 12.3% lower in Black than White men and 8.6% higher in Black than White women. However, heart attack mortality fell more steeply in White versus Black men (74% versus 67%) and in White versus Black women (75% versus 71%) during the four decades following the 1968 peak. From 1987 to 2008 heart attack mortality was higher in Blacks than Whites of both sexes. By 2008, heart attack mortality was 13.6% higher in Black than White men and 25.8% higher in Black than White women.

Unlike heart disease mortality, stroke mortality rates (Figure 15.3) have always been 35–50% higher in Blacks than Whites—231.3 versus 175.5 per 100,000 in 1950 and 51.2 versus 36.3 per 100,000 in 2017.

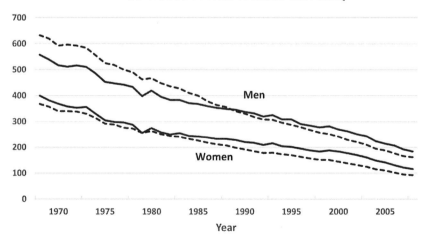

U.S. trends in heart attack mortality by race and sex, 1968–2017. From published CDC Vital Statistics compilations. Blacks are represented by solid lines, and Whites by dashed lines.

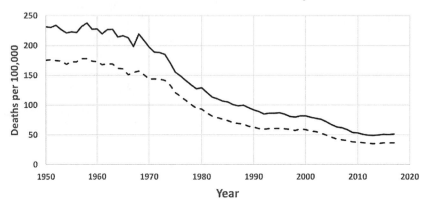

U.S. trends in stroke mortality by race, 1950–2017. From published CDC Vital Statistics compilations. Blacks are represented by solid lines, and Whites by dashed lines. Pre–1968 stroke mortality rates for Blacks include all non–Whites.

This reflects, no doubt, the longstanding Black-White disparity in the prevalence and severity of hypertension. The percent decline in stroke mortality between 1950 and 2017 has been similar (close to 80%) in Blacks and Whites, although the absolute decline in stroke mortality has clearly been higher in Blacks. In the remainder of this chapter, some reasons for the trends in these three figures will be explored. I will draw heavily on an ongoing long-term NIH-funded prospective epidemiologic cohort study called the Reasons for Geographic and Racial Differences in Stroke (REGARDS) study, which was initiated in 2003 to study racial, socioeconomic, cultural, and regional health disparities in the U.S.[7]

What Is Race?

Let us first stipulate that race in the United States is more of a sociocultural than a biological construct. While most modern-day African Americans are the descendants of people who were brought to the Americas in bondage from sub-Saharan Africa (specifically the present-day countries of Senegal, Gambia, Guinea-Bissou, Mali, Angola, Congo, the Democratic Republic of Congo, Gabon, Ghana, and the Ivory Coast) during the 16th to 19th centuries, some are also the descendants of intermarriages and of

White slave masters who sexually misused their female slaves. So many who identify as African Americans today are a biological mixture of Caucasian and African.[8] What makes them *African* American is not their African genes as much as their 400-year shared history of oppression in the United States, including 246 years of slavery in the south and another century of *de jure* segregation in the rural south and *de facto* segregation in large U.S. cities like New York, Chicago, Detroit, and Los Angeles, to which many fled between World War I and the 1970s. Even today, the African American community continues to endure discrimination, widespread poverty, high rates of unemployment and incarceration, and permanent underclass status. Obviously, there are general biological distinctions between the Black and White racial groups; however, there is far more biological diversity within than between racial categories. For example, the greater skin content of melanin in African Americans is obviously biological, as is their propensity for sickle cell trait, a genetic hemoglobin mutation which was preserved evolutionarily because of the protection it offers against malaria (which is endemic in their tropical countries of origin). But White persons of Mediterranean descent have more melanin in their skin than those of Nordic descent and also have a propensity for certain genetic hemoglobin disorders like thalassemia. Biological differences among the races loom far larger in the collective imagination than in reality.

To bring this discussion closer to cardiovascular disease, the well-known but poorly understood Black-White disparity in the prevalence of hypertension is probably a complex mixture of biological and sociocultural factors. On the one hand, comparative studies of Black (B) and White (W) Americans showing racial differences in salt retention (B > W), response to diuretics (B > W), and response to ACE inhibitors and beta blockers (W > B) have often been cited as evidence of a biological basis for the higher prevalence of hypertension in Black than White Americans.[9] Some have even theorized—with no historical basis—that this may be an evolutionary adaptation to a (non-existent) scarcity of salt in central Africa.[10] However, there are also important environmental differences. In the REGARDS study, in which half of the 30,000 participants live in the southeastern "Stroke Belt" states of Georgia, the Carolinas, Alabama, Mississippi, Tennessee, Arkansas, and Louisiana, the leading predictor of hypertension among 12 clinical and social variables examined was their *diet*; participants with a high "southern diet score"—Black or White—had the highest prevalence of hypertension. Given the high fat and salt content of the traditional southern diet, which southern Blacks carried with them as "soul food" when they migrated northward, this is hardly surprising.[11] The fact that hypertension is not especially prevalent in rural sub–Saharan African countries where American slaves originated (but where the diet is quite different) also argues that the high rate of hypertension in African Americans has more to do with diet than biology.[12] Another possible environmental source of the Black-White difference in BP is the chronic psychosocial stress associated with poverty and racism, which induces elevated levels of vasoactive hormones like adrenaline.[13] The elevated prevalence of hypertension among rural Black migrants to large crowded African cities supports the possible contribution of chronic stress to the high prevalence of hypertension in African Americans.[14] A recent genetic analysis of participants in the NHLBI's SPRINT study showed that West African ancestry was not associated with BP, response to antihypertensive medications, and end organ damage (i.e., heart and kidney failure) after adjustment for behavioral/cultural risk factors like diet and obesity.[15] Thus, although the particular causes of the known Black-White differences in BP in America remain somewhat uncertain, environmental factors likely play a more important role than biology.

Socioeconomic Disparities

To a large extent, the health disparities between Black and White Americans reflect the vast socioeconomic gulf between the races in the U.S. Cross-cultural comparisons reinforce this association. Abdel Omran and others have described the "epidemiologic transition" from low-income countries, where life is short and diseases of undernutrition and poor sanitation dominate the leading causes of death, to middle- and high-income countries, where improvements in nutrition and sanitation prolong life-expectancy and where degenerative diseases of overnutrition and underactivity emerge as the leading causes of death (or the cardiovascular disease pandemic, as I have called it).[16] The U.S. underwent its epidemiologic transition in the late 19th and early 20th century, before we had systematic surveillance data, but late 20th-century China is a good recent example of this phenomenon. In the 1960s, China suffered several years of widespread famine during Mao's "Great Leap Forward."[17] As recently as 1983, when I visited China with an American medical group, diseases of undernutrition dominated the leading causes of death, and heart attacks were uncommon. When a man with a myocardial infarction was presented to us on morning rounds in a hospital in Shanghai, he might have been a novelty to the Chinese, but we American doctors had each seen a thousand like him. The average serum cholesterol level in China in the 1980s was only 4.2 mmol/L (162 mg/dL), which corresponds roughly to the bottom decile of American MRFIT screenees a decade earlier.[18] Mean cholesterol levels in China would climb to 4.73 mmol/L (183 mg/dL) in 2004—far closer to the U.S. average of 196 mg/dL reported in 2010 by NHANES.[19]

In the last three decades of the 20th century, America and other affluent countries across the globe have successfully used their science and technology to respond to the epidemiologic transition, as we have recounted in Chapters 4 through 14. But this success was uneven, with the lion's share of benefit accruing to the highest socioeconomic classes. It is the affluent in the U.S. who have access to the best medical care, to the most healthful food choices, to gym memberships and yoga classes to compensate for their sedentary jobs, and to the education to make the best health-related decisions. So, in the latter decades of the 20th century, the relationship of socioeconomic status to cardiovascular risk factors and deaths became inverted.[20] By 1990, as we have seen when comparing Black versus White Americans in Figure 15.1, atherosclerotic coronary heart disease had transitioned from a disease of affluence to just another disease of poverty. Today, coronary heart disease mortality is highest in Russia, the Middle East, northern Africa, and south Asia and lowest in former coronary heart disease epicenters like the U.S., Canada, western Europe, and Australia.[21]

Racial Disparities in Cardiovascular Risk Factors

The data on racial disparities in risk factors is somewhat scattered; I have been unable to find a comprehensive analysis of changes in risk factors by racial group during a common time frame. However, I have cobbled together Table 15.1, from multiple recent sources. The hypertension figures come from a CDC posting of 2013–16 NHANES data.[22] The total and HLD cholesterol figures come from a 2013 NCHS data brief.[23] The smoking figures come from a current American Lung Association website.[24] The obesity figures come from a 2017 American Heart Association Task Force report.[25] The diabetes figures come from the CDS 2020 National Diabetes Statistics Report.[26]

Table 15.1: Racial Disparities in Cardiovascular Risk Factors in the U.S.

Characteristic	Sex	Blacks	Whites
Hypertension, Yes/No	Men	42%	31%
	Women	42%	27%
Cholesterol > 240 mg/dL	Men	7%	12%
	Women	12%	15%
HDL Cholesterol < 40 mg/dL	Men	19%	25%
	Women	8%	9%
Smoking, Yes/No	Men	21%	17%
	Women	14%	16%
BMI > 30 kg/m²	Men	38%	34%
	Women	58%	33%
Diagnosed Diabetes, Yes/No	Men	12%	8%
	Women	12%	6%

*U.S. adults, age >20 years.

Clearly, the cardiovascular risk profiles of Blacks and Whites differ substantially—especially with respect to the higher prevalence of hypertension and diabetes in Blacks of both sexes and the enormous prevalence of obesity in Black women. Rates of awareness and treatment of hypertension among are similar among White and Black men and have improved over time—from 17% to 30% in Black men and from 22% to 39% in White men between 1988–94 and 1999–2004—and are even better among Black women.[27] However, the proportion of hypertensive patients whose BP is controlled is significantly lower in Blacks than Whites—a finding that may reflect their lesser responsiveness to ACE inhibitors and beta-blockers. Similarly, in the REGARDS study, awareness and treatment of hypertension were actually higher in Blacks than Whites in all regions, but rates of BP control were lower in Blacks.[28] This suggests an issue with finding the right drugs and dosages for Black patients, rather than just a failure to recognize and treat the problem.

The large and growing Black-White disparity in the prevalence of obesity, especially among women, and the resulting disparity in type 2 diabetes is also clearly manifest in Table 15.1. The easy availability of fried foods and fatty snacks from convenience stores and fast-food restaurants and the relative paucity of grocery stores selling fresh produce in urban Black neighborhoods ("food deserts") have undoubtedly contributed to this disparity.[29] Black-White disparities in physical activity may also contribute to the growing disparity in obesity.

Returning to the question raised earlier about the biological underpinning of Black-White racial differences, the data from the international Modeling the Epidemiological Transition Study (METS) are illuminating (Table 15.2).[30]

Table 15.2: International Differences in Cardiovascular Risk Factors Among Black Populations

Characteristic	Sex	Ghana	South Africa	Jamaica	Seychelles	Chicago
UN Human Development Index	All	Low-Middle	Middle	High	High	Very High
BP, mmHg	Men	119/68	129/80	122/71	123/75	128/81
	Women	110/66	118/76	115/72	112/73	117/80
Hypertension, Yes/No	Men	7%	28%	12%	28%	35%
	Women	7%	21%	28%	17%	27%
LDL Cholesterol, mg/dL	Men	92.2	82.6	94.1	112.7	112.4
	Women	103.4	98.1	105.9	109.1	107.3
HDL Cholesterol, mg/dL	Men	44.7	56.7	47.1	47.4	50.1
	Women	47.2	46.2	46.1	47.9	51.7
Smoking, Yes/No	Men	4%	63%	26%	25%	55%
	Women	2%	33%	13%	13%	42%
BMI, kg/m²	Men	22.2	22.4	23.6	26.5	29.7
	Women	25.5	31.9	29.5	27.6	34.1
Obesity, Yes/No	Men	2%	6%	8%	21%	35%
	Women	16%	56%	46%	32%	64%
Diabetes, Yes/No	Men	1%	2%	0%	7%	9%
	Women	1%	3%	1%	3%	13%

This study compared the cardiovascular risk profiles of Blacks in four countries ranging in wealth on the UN human development index scale from low-middle to high with the U.S. Unfortunately, the METS population was confined to the 25- to 45-year age range and cannot be compared directly to the far broader age range in Table 15.1. However, it is clear that the prevalence of hypertension, obesity, and diabetes among U.S. Blacks is far higher than among the non–American Black populations, particular those from Ghana, one of the countries from which American slaves originated. Indeed, the Black-Black differences between Chicago and Ghana (Table 15.2) are far larger than the Black-White differences among Americans (Table 15.1).

In addition to the Black-White disparities in risk factors, there is also evidence that African Americans who have had a heart attack—especially without electrocardiographic ST segment elevation (non–STEMI)—are less likely than White Americans to receive the recommended treatments.[31] Hospitalized Black non–STEMI patients were less likely than their White counterparts to receive aspirin (85% versus 92%), other antiplatelet therapy (45% versus 60%), beta-blockers (85% versus 88%), and cholesterol-lowering medications (68% versus 76%). Blacks were also 29% less likely than Whites to undergo coronary angiography and 45% less likely to undergo revascularization. This racial disparity represents more than just the reduced access to the health care system associated with poverty. After all, nearly all the patients studied had health insurance, and all had made it into the hospital. A recent study of attitudes and beliefs of trained medical personnel about how Blacks and Whites experience pain suggests a more insidious explanation—a tendency of health care providers to downplay the pain of Black patients.[32] This would be bad enough if it were manifested only in withholding pain medications, but in the context of non–STEMI, where chest pain is a critical factor in the diagnosis and the efficacy of potentially life-saving treatments depends upon their rapid delivery, it is entirely unacceptable. The denial of proven treatments to the least favored segment of our population echoes the crime of the infamous Tuskegee study, which has left an enduring residue of mistrust of the medical establishment among African Americans. Whatever else is going on around us, medical caregivers must work diligently to restore this trust rather than allow their racial biases to further erode it.

The Impact of Racial Disparities on the Decline in Heart Attack Mortality

The impact of racial disparities is complicated because so many risk factors and because so many racial and ethnic groups are involved. Health disparities affect many groups not discussed here—American Indians, Hispanics, South and East Asians, Appalachian Whites, etc.—each with its own story. Focusing on Black-White health disparities has allowed me to develop some of the driving factors in greater depth, but I have still barely scratched the surface. From 1968 (when heart attack rates were 15% lower in Blacks than Whites) through 2007 we saw a reversal of race-specific heart attack death rates over the rest of the 20th century and into the 21st century (Figure 15.1–2). As of 2017, heart attack mortality is 12% higher in Blacks than Whites, while overall heart disease mortality is 23% higher in Blacks than Whites. Since Black-White differences in BP (favors Whites), HDL and LDL cholesterol (favor Blacks), and cigarette smoking (similar in Blacks and Whites) have not really changed much during this period, the growing prevalence of obesity and type 2 diabetes in Blacks and racial biases in the delivery of effective heart attack treatments that have come on the scene since 1980 are the most likely culprits for the observed Black-White difference in the decline in mortality rates. If we ask simplistically, how many more heart attack deaths could have been prevented if we had achieved the same (73%) mortality reduction in Blacks that we achieved in Whites between 1980 and 2017, the answer is only about an extra 1%, since African Americans comprised only 12–14% of the U.S. population during this period.[33] One could perhaps double this estimate by also considering the other racial groups who have lacked equal access to optimal health care, but all this is beside the point. All U.S. taxpayers have invested in the research that has advanced our understanding of cardiovascular disease and led to new and better treatments; all of us own the fruits of this investment. That all should share in its benefits is a matter not of numbers but of simple equity and justice.

159

16

Wrap-Up

In the preceding pages I have taken you on a guided tour of how America's epidemiologic transition of the early 20th century brought a steep rise in mortality due to atherosclerotic heart disease and how the medical advances in many disciplines during the past six decades have helped us turn the curve and bring cardiovascular mortality down to levels well below what they were in 1900. From a health care consumer's perspective, here are the practices that will minimize your risk of suffering and dying from atherosclerotic cardiovascular event:

1. If you have no cardiovascular disease or risk factors:

   - Don't smoke cigarettes. As an added bonus, you will also minimize your risk of dying from respiratory (and some non-respiratory) cancers and other lung diseases.
   - Don't eat more calories than you can burn. Avoid caloric fatty snacks and sugary drinks, and exercise regularly.
   - Types of food: Get your calories from fresh fruits and vegetables, whole grains, and unsaturated vegetable oils. Minimize saturated fats and salt.

2. If you have cardiovascular risk factors, you should also:

   - Lower your blood pressure to < 130/80 mmHg. Thiazide diuretics, ACE inhibitors (and angiotensin receptor blockers), calcium channel blockers, and (to a lesser extent) beta blockers are safe and effective antihypertensive drugs.
   - Lower your LDL cholesterol to < 130 mg/dL—or to < 100 mg/dL if you have atherosclerotic cardiovascular disease, diabetes, or other risk factors. Statins are the drug of choice.
   - If you smoke cigarettes, stop.

3. If you are experiencing the symptoms of a heart attack, you should receive urgent medical attention to include:

   - Cardiopulmonary resuscitation (CPR) if there is no heartbeat.
   - Coronary angiography and stent placement to open up acutely blocked coronary arteries.
   - Aspirin and other antiplatelet drugs to prevent stent thrombosis.
   - If a cardiac catheterization lab is unavailable, intravenous thrombolytic therapy is a viable alternative.

4. If you have had a heart attack in the past and/or have symptoms of advanced atherosclerotic heart disease, you should:

   - Take a statin, aspirin, an ACE inhibitor, and a beta blocker, whether or not you have specific indications (high LDL cholesterol, hypertension, heart failure) for those drugs.
   - If you have angina or other signs of cardiac ischemia, get evaluated by coronary angiography and consider coronary artery bypass surgery (CABG) if your left main coronary artery is significantly obstructed. The internal thoracic artery is superior to venous grafts as a conduit.
   - If you are at high risk for sudden cardiac arrest due to a known ventricular arrhythmia or significant ventricular dysfunction, consider an implantable cardioverter defibrillator (ICD).

The impact of an intervention on the public health depends not only on its efficacy when it is implemented, but on how broadly and well it is implemented. The first set of recommendations, for what is sometimes called "primordial prevention," is aimed to prevent the emergence of cardiovascular risk factors like high BP, high LDL cholesterol, smoking, obesity, and diabetes by promoting a healthy lifestyle starting in childhood. In theory, this should have been the keystone of our efforts to reverse the rise of cardiovascular mortality in the first half of the 20th century, since adverse population changes in diet, physical activity, and cigarette smoking are what caused it in the first place. Unfortunately, the U.S. population as a whole has continued to grow fatter and more sedentary, and the rise in our prevalence of type 2 diabetes has accelerated.

From a public heath perspective, our crowning achievement has been our success in implementing the second set of interventions, for primary prevention. Although the impact of these treatments is delayed and undramatic, more than half of all American adults had one or more of these risk factors when heart attack mortality peaked in the 1960s. The third set of recommendations, which are aimed at increasing survival of an acute life-threatening coronary artery blockage or arrhythmia, are the most dramatic and spectacular, but their impact has been limited by the stubborn reality that many of these patients die before any medical help can arrive. The fourth set of recommendations, for secondary prevention, though quite successful, has also been limited by the fact that they are applicable only to survivors of an acute MI. Thus, although high-tech interventions like CPR, ICD placement, and coronary revascularization may be dramatically and immediately beneficial in those who receive them, it is the less dramatic but more sustainable low-tech interventions for controlling BP, LDL cholesterol and cigarette smoking that have made the biggest difference.

I have attempted to parse out the relative contributions of the major advances of the past 50 years to the 81% decline in heart attack mortality since 1968.

- I attribute 55.7% of the decline to primary prevention—specifically, cholesterol lowering (mainly statins), treatment of hypertension, and smoking cessation, in that order—perhaps, with a 2–3% offset for the rising prevalence of type 2 diabetes,
- I attribute 13.7% of the decline to advances in the treatment of acute myocardial infarction (mainly to urgent angioplasty and stent placement in conjunction with anti-platelet drugs) and perhaps 2–5% to other acute interventions
- I attribute 23.3% of the decline to secondary prevention in MI survivors—specifically, statins, aspirin, RAAS inhibitors (mostly ACE inhibitors), and beta blockers, in that order.

Of course, these are only estimates, relying on many assumptions and approximations. Since these interventions apply to different patient populations, their estimated contributions to the decline in heart attack mortality may be combined by simple addition. Although they do not quite add up to 100%, some of these figures may underestimate the true impact of these trends for reasons explained in the preceding chapters.

You may notice that there is a natural hierarchy in the four groups of recommendations I have presented. In the best of all worlds, people would adopt and sustain a healthy lifestyle that would keep them fit and healthy and would obviate much of the need for primary prevention drugs. Unfortunately, human nature being what it is, nothing short of poverty, war, and famine have curbed on our growing tendency toward dietary excess over the past century. Given the draconian nature of these "cures," we have successfully pursued primary prevention as a fallback plan to mitigate the harm done by unhealthful lifestyle choices. When primary prevention fails and a myocardial infarction or arrhythmia occurs, acute intervention followed by secondary prevention in the survivors is the final fallback. But our success in primary prevention, which has prevented 45% of the heart attacks that would have happened in 1968 from happening in 2017 has limited the scope and impact of these secondary strategies. Just as our lack of success in primordial prevention has amplified the need for primary prevention, our success in primary prevention has lessened the need for acute and secondary intervention. If our primary prevention efforts had prevented only 10% of heart attacks, acute and secondary interventions would have assumed a far greater significance.

While the four sets of recommendations listed above demonstrably save lives, many other cardiac interventions are also useful even if they have not been proven to prevent heart attack deaths. For example, a wide selection of drugs is available to control blood glucose and HbA1C levels in type 2 diabetes and thereby reduce microvascular complications like blindness, neuropathy, and kidney failure. Oral nitrates and non-urgent angioplasty and stent placement can alleviate angina symptoms and improve quality of life. Judicious use of estrogen therapy can alleviate vasomotor and other debilitating symptoms following menopause, especially in women whose ovaries have been surgically removed. Other once promising interventions, like CETP inhibitors to raise HDL cholesterol and certain anti-arrhythmic drugs, have turned out to be useless or worse.

I have focused primarily on atherosclerotic coronary heart disease (heart attacks) because that is the chief driver of the 20th-century cardiovascular disease pandemic. I have not addressed the enormous advances in treating congenital heart disease and the near elimination of rheumatic heart disease during this period. I have also not focused on heart failure, which is often the end stage of atherosclerotic coronary vascular disease but also has many non-atherosclerotic causes (especially hypertension). These deaths are generally tallied as "heart disease deaths" but not necessarily as "coronary heart disease" or "heart attack" deaths, and their trends are more difficult to parse. I have not discussed heart transplants, ventricular assist devices, and other treatments for end-stage heart failure. I have also not focused on stroke, for which we lack reliable data as to which are caused by atherosclerosis and which by bleeding (usually due to hypertension).

I have focused here on interventions that have been proven efficacious and have been sufficiently impactful to influence the course of the cardiovascular pandemic. I have recounted a few important "dry wells" that cardiovascular researchers have come across during their 50-year fight to curb the heart attack pandemic—specifically, cholesterol ester transfer protein inhibition (Chapter 8) and menopausal hormone therapy (Chapter 9). However, I have deliberately omitted many other less important blind alleys and dead ends in the interest of not bogging my readers down unnecessarily. For example, I have said little about the many clinical trials of the efficacy of the anti-oxidant vitamins C and E and beta-carotene in the prevention of heart attacks, none of which demonstrated any benefit. Many of these trials were factorial add-ons to trials of other more promising interventions like aspirin, ACE inhibition, and menopausal hormone therapy. I have also said little about omega-3 fatty acids (fish oils), since clinical trial evidence for their efficacy in preventing or treating heart disease is lacking.

Looking to the future, one can find cause for both optimism and concern. Our pharmacology and technology continue to advance rapidly. New avenues for intervention (e.g., anti-inflammatory drugs) hold promise. However, the U.S. is not doing well in the lifestyle arena, as evidenced by the rapidly rising tide of obesity and type 2 diabetes. Although we have been extraordinarily resourceful in finding drugs and medical procedures to compensate for our shortcomings in this area, it seems foolhardy to rely on drugs and technology to continue to bail us out from our continuing unhealthy lifestyle choices. Taking care to choose healthful foods and not to eat more calories than you can burn is tedious and less gratifying than placing a stent to restore blood flow in a blocked coronary artery or bringing someone back from the brink of death by a well-timed electrical shock. But the tedious course is more rewarding and sustainable. If we do not at least hold the line on diet and exercise and stem the rising tide of obesity and diabetes, cardiovascular mortality rates may begin to rise once again.

Appendix

Details of Calculation
of Attributable Declines in Mortality

Estimating the contribution of the medical advances described in this book to the decline in heart attack mortality has been one of my recurring themes in this book. Ford et al. devised a model called IMPACT for this purpose, but the published results are now 20 years old and out of date.[1] Given the continuing advances in treatment and the continuing decline in heart attack mortality since 2000, it was imperative to extrapolate these results forward to a more current date, within the limitations of publicly available national health statistics. The year for which the necessary data were available ranged from 2009 for the in-hospital mortality data for acute myocardial infarction to 2017 for smoking and secondary prevention. I will provide the details of how these calculations were done in this appendix for those with a working knowledge of algebra, including natural logarithms (ln) and exponentials (exp).

I have made the following assumptions for these calculations:

1. I can identify a reported health statistic that can serve as a credible surrogate for the national state of treatment/control of each risk factor. For example, the percent of hypertensive patients whose BP is treated to < 140/90 mmHg for blood pressure treatment, the proportion of people on statins for cholesterol lowering, etc.

2. I have assumed a log-linear relationship between the surrogate metric and CHD mortality. In other words,

3. ln (CHD mortality ratio) for a given year versus baseline = β times the change in the surrogate metric

Table A.1 shows the national CHD (heart attack) mortality rates for the years that I used in my calculations.[2] The percent decline in mortality from 1968 and 1980 (the starting point for the published IMPACT model) are also shown.

Table A.1: Selected U.S. CHD Mortality Rates

Year	CHD Deaths per 100,000	% Decline from 1968	% Decline from 1980
1968	482.6		
1980	345.2	28.5%	
2000	186.8	61.3%	45.9%
2009	117.7	75.6%	65.9%
2011	109.2	77.4%	68.4%
2014	98.8	79.5%	71.4%
2017	92.9	80.7%	73.1%

Approximately 41% ((345.2–186.8)/(482.6–92.9)) of the total decline in U.S. CHD mortality since 1968 took place in the period (1980–2000) covered by the published IMPACT analysis.

Primary Prevention

Table A.2 shows the how the national health statistics for hypertension control, statin use, and cigarette smoking were used to extrapolate the published IMPACT data to five decades of decline in cardiovascular mortality. The top line shows the proportion of the 46% decline in CHD mortality (from 345.2 deaths per 100,000 in 1980 to 186.8 deaths per 100,000 in 2000) attributed in the IMPACT publication to interventions for high LDL cholesterol, high BP, and cigarette smoking.[3] The second line (which is obtained by multiplying the top line by 46%) is the actual decrease in CHD mortality attributable to improvements in each of these risk factors. We know from the literature that the improvement in statin use, BP control, and smoking since 1968 exceeded that for the 1980–2000 period covered by the published IMPACT results by a factor ("change ratio") of 2.05 for statins, 2.46 for BP, and 2.57 for smoking.[4] The log-linear relationship of CHD mortality to each of our surrogate risk factors allows us to multiply the natural log of the CHD risk ratio for 2000 versus 1980 by the change ratio, take the exponential to convert the result back to a mortality ratio, and subtract from 100% to obtain the percent mortality reduction. For smoking, as an example, one calculates

$$100\% - \exp\left(2.57{*}\ln\left(1 - .45\right)\right) = 13.2\%$$

to obtain the percent of CHD deaths prevented by smoking in 2017 relative to the number who would have died if smoking had remained unchanged since 1968. Dividing this number by the observed 81% decline in CHD mortality, one calculates that 16.4% of this decline was due to smoking. Similarly, 27.7% of the total decline through 2011 was attributable to LDL cholesterol lowering and 26.7% to BP control.

Table A.2. Contributions of Primary Prevention to the Decline in CHD Mortality, 1968 to present

Steps in Calculation	*LDL Cholesterol*	*Blood Pressure*	*Cigarettes*
IMPACT Model	24.2%	20.1%	11.7%
Attributable percent CHD Deaths Saved, 1980–2000[†]	11.1%	9.2%	5.4%
Surrogate Indicator	On a statin	Under 140/90 mmHg	Current smoker
1968	0.0%	0.0%	39.4%
1980	0.0%	10.0%	33.2%
2000	8.5%	31.8%	23.3%
Current	17.4%	53.8%	14.0%
As of	2011	2014	2017
Change ratio[^]	2.05	2.47	2.57
Attributable percent CHD Deaths Saved, 1968–present[†]	21.4%	21.2%	13.2%
Modified IMPACT Estimate[◊]	27.7%	26.7%	16.4%
Combined Primary Prevention[~]	55.7%		

*The IMPACT model estimate of the percent of decline attributed to the risk factor times the 45.9% decline in CHD mortality in 1980–2000.

^The change in the risk factor surrogate from 1968 to the present divided by the change from 1980 to 2000.

†The exponential of the product of the change ratio times the natural log of the attributable percent of deaths saved in 1980–2000.

◊The ratio of the attributable percent of CHD deaths saved in 1968–present to the total percent decline in CHD mortality during that period.

~Removes the overlap in deaths prevented by treating each of the three risk factors

The last line of Table A.2 shows the combined contribution of these three primary prevention risk factors to the decline in CHD mortality. One cannot simply add the three contributions (which total 71%) without subtracting the overlap. For example, if the 27.7% impact of LDL cholesterol lowering and the 26.7% impact of BP lowering are independent, there is a 7.4% overlap (27.7% times 26.7%) of the CHD deaths prevented. The easiest formula for calculating the combined impact of the three primary preventions in Table A.2 without the overlaps is:

$$100\% - (100\% - 27.7\%) * (100\% - 26.7\%) * (100\% - 16.4\%) = 55.7\%$$

This means that primary prevention has reduced CHD mortality by 45% (55.7% of 80.7%) since 1968.

Since we have reliable cigarette smoking data going back to 1900, we can use the same logic to estimate its contribution to the rise of cardiovascular mortality in 1900–68.[5] For this purpose, we have to shift from CHD to all heart disease (HD) mortality, since pre–1950 national mortality statistics do not distinguish between CHD, heart failure, and congenital, rheumatic, hypertensive, and other forms of heart disease.[6] We must also correct the IMPACT estimate of the relative risk associated with not smoking versus smoking from 0.72 to 0.50, since the former figure applies to smoking cessation, rather than the initiation of smoking.[7] Table A.3 shows the result.

Table A.3: Contributions of Cigarettes to the Rise in Heart Disease (HD) Mortality, 1900 to 1968

Steps in Calculation	Cigarette Smoking	HD Mortality
1900	0.0%	265.4
1968	39.4%	531.0
1980	33.2%	412.1
2000	23.3%	257.6
Change Ratio—(1900–68)/(1980–2000)*	−4.0	
IMPACT Model	11.7%	
Corrected to assume reversion to pre-smoking risk^	15.9%	
Attributable percent of HD Deaths Saved, 1980–2000†	6.0%	
Attributable percent of HD Deaths Caused, 1900–68†	27.7%	

The ratio of changes in smoking during 1900–1968 versus 1980–2000.
  ^Assumes that HD mortality in non-smokers is 50% (not 72%) of that in smokers.
    †The IMPACT model estimate of the percent of decline attributed to smoking times the 37.5% decline in HD mortality in 1980–2000.
      ◊The exponential of the product of the change ratio times the natural log of the attributable percent of deaths saved in 1980–2000.

This calculation estimates that smoking may have been responsible for 27.7% of the doubling of HD mortality between 1900 and 1968.

Secondary Prevention

Table A.4 shows the calculation of the contributions of the four major secondary prevention drugs to the 81% decline in CHD mortality between 1968 and 2017. I have assumed that none of these drugs were in significant use in heart attack survivors before 1980; indeed statins and ACE inhibitors had not yet been invented. I have taken the 2000 drug usage data from the Ford IMPACT paper for secondary prevention after MI; the 2017 drug usage data are projections from a 2012 analysis of NHANES data by Shah, et al.[8] The logic of the table follows that of Table A.2, and I will not repeat it here.

Table A.4. Contributions of Secondary Prevention to the Decline in CHD Mortality, 1968 to Present

Steps in Calculation	Statins	Aspirin	Beta Blockers	RAAS Inhibitors
IMPACT Model	8.5%	8.0%	6.1%	4.3%
Attributable percent CHD Deaths Saved, 1980–2000[†]	3.9%	3.7%	2.8%	2.0%
1968	0.0%	0.0%	0.0%	0.0%
1980	0.0%	0.0%	0.0%	0.0%
2000	45%	38%	29%	26%
2017 (projected)	77%	69%	36%	54%
Change ratio^	1.71	1.82	1.24	2.08
Attributable percent CHD Deaths Saved, 1968–present[†]	6.6%	6.6%	3.5%	4.1%
Modified IMPACT Estimate[◊]	8.2%	8.1%	4.3%	5.0%
Combined Secondary Prevention~	23.3%			

The IMPACT model estimate of the percent of decline attributed to the risk factor times the 45.9% decline in CHD mortality in 1980–2000.

^*The change in the risk factor surrogate from 1968 to the present divided by the change from 1980 to 2000.*

†*The exponential of the product of the change ratio times the natural log of the attributable percent of deaths saved in 1980–2000.*

◊*The ratio of the attributable percent of CHD deaths saved in 1968–present to the total percent decline in CHD mortality during that period.*

~*Removes the overlap in deaths prevented by each of the four treatments.*

The modified IMPACT estimates are quite similar to the published ones for statins and aspirin, indicating that their usage has increased more or less in parallel to the continuing decline in CHD mortality since 2000. The usage of beta-blockers has not kept pace with the other drugs, while increases in the use of RAAS inhibitors have modestly outpaced those in statins and aspirin. These four secondary prevention drugs, considered together, account for 23.3% of the 81% decline in CHD mortality since 1968—i.e., a net 18.8% reduction in CHD mortality. As for primary prevention (Table A.2), this is less than the sum of their individual contributions (25.7%); the difference reflects the overlap of deaths prevented by each drug.

I do not have confidence in the IMPACT model's estimates of the contribution of improvements in the treatment of acute myocardial infarction and diabetes, and the (negative) contribution of the rapid increase in the prevalence of type 2 diabetes, since both occurred largely after 2000. Instead, I have made my own estimates.

Type 2 Diabetes

I have assumed that type 2 diabetes still confers a threefold increase in risk of CHD mortality relative to non-diabetics and that the prevalence of type 2 diabetes was 8.2% in U.S. adults as of 2017.[9] Note that the threefold relative risk reflects similar and substantial reductions in CHD mortality of diabetic and non-diabetic persons due to the use of statins, BP drugs, etc., that were unavailable in 1968. So let us use M to symbolize the CHD mortality in deaths per 100,000. p to symbolize the prevalence of diabetes, X to symbolize the CHD mortality rate in non-diabetic persons, and 3x to symbolize the CHD mortality rate in diabetics. We can write the following equation and solve for x:

$M = (1-p)*x + 3px$

$x = M/(2p+1)$

The results for 1968 and 2017 are tabulated in lines 2–3 of Table A.5.

Table A.5. CHD Mortality
Projections for Diabetes

Scenario	*Prevalence of Diabetes*	*CHD Deaths per 100,000*	
		1968	*2017*
Actual CHD Mortality		482.6	92.9
Non-Diabetics		467.6	79.8
Diabetics		1402.8	239.4
Calculated CHD Mortality			
1968 Diabetes %	1.6%	482.6	82.4
2017 Diabetes %	8.2%	544.3	92.9
Circa 2040??	40.0%		143.7

In the last three lines of the table, the CHD mortality rates for 1968 and 2017 are recalculated under three hypothetical scenarios. First, if the prevalence of diabetes had been 8.2% (instead of 1.6%) in 1968 and nothing else changed, the CHD mortality rate would have been 544.3 instead of 482.6 deaths per 100,000. Conversely, if the prevalence of diabetes had remained at 1.6% (instead of 8.2%) in 2017, the CHD mortality rate would have been 82.4 instead of 92.9 deaths per 100,000. Thus, if the prevalence of diabetes had not changed between 1968 and 2017, CHD mortality decreased by 82.9% (from 482.6 to 82.4 or from 544.3 to 92.9 deaths per 100,000), rather than by 80.7%.

Finally, in the last line of Table A.5, we imagine a worst case scenario, in which the prevalence of diabetes stays on its current trajectory and reaches 40% sometime around 2040, while nothing else changes. In that scenario, CHD mortality would increase by 55% of its 2017 rate to reach 143.7 deaths per 100,000 annually.

Acute MI

Table A.6 lays out the calculation of the contribution of PCI and other acute interventions to the 73.7% decline in CHD between 1970 and 2009, the timespan for which published in-hospital case-fatality ratios for acute MI are available.

Table A.6. Contribution of Improved In-Hospital Survival to the Decline in Heart Attack Mortality, 1970–2009

Outcome*	1970	2009	Difference
Heart Attack Deaths per 100,000	448.0	117.7	330.3
Adjusted for Impact of Primary Prevention^	264.1	117.7	146.6
Acute MI Hospitalizations (age 45+)	268.4	179.7	88.7
Adjusted for Impact of Primary Prevention^	219.0	179.7	39.3
In-Hospital Case Fatality Rate (age 45+)	23.9%	4.0%	
In-Hospital MI Deaths per 100,000	64.1	7.2	57.0
Adjusted for Impact of Primary Prevention^	52.3	7.2	45.2

Age-adjusted to the U.S. population in 2000.
^*Assumes that 55.7% of the decline in heart attack deaths and acute MI hospitalizations in 1970 could have been prevented if the primary prevention measures in effect in 2009 had been available in 1970.*

The first line of Table A.6 shows the national heart attack death rates for 1970 and 2009 from Table A.1, which decreased from 448.0 to 117.7—a decline of 330.3 deaths per 100,000. In the second line, I have adjusted the 1970 rate to remove the impact of primary prevention by subtracting 55.7% of this 330.3 deaths per 100,000 decline—the proportion attributable to primary prevention in Table A.2—from the unadjusted 448.0 figure, to obtain adjusted rate of 264.1 deaths per 100,000 in 1970. This figure represents what the mortality rate would have been if the 2009 levels of smoking and BP and LDL cholesterol treatment had prevailed in 1970. The third line shows the national incidence rates of hospitalized acute MI, adjusted to the 2000 U.S. Population using census data for persons over age 45, which have decreased by 88.7 cases per 100,000 between 1970 and 2009.[10] You will note that this decrease between 1970 and 2009 is far smaller than the decrease in CHD mortality rates; this reflects the use of more sensitive diagnostic criteria for acute MI—specifically high-sensitivity serum troponin levels—in 2009.[11] In line 4, I subtracted 55.7% of the 88.7 case difference in acute MI hospitalizations from 268.4 to obtain an adjusted rate of 219.0 cases per 100,000 for 1970. Now, applying the reported age-adjusted case-fatality rates for ages > 45 (line 5), which dropped from almost 23.9% in 1970 to only 4.0% in 2009, to the adjusted incidence rates (line 4), one calculates a decrease of 45.2 deaths per 100,000 (line 7) in the national in-hospital mortality rate after adjustment for primary prevention.[12] This represents 13.7% of the 330.3 deaths per thousand unadjusted difference in overall CHD mortality between 1970 and 2009.

Glossary of Medical Terms and Acronyms

Acute Coronary Syndrome (ACS)—Acute cardiac pain and ECG changes due to a developing myocardial infarction. Also called unstable angina.

American Cancer Society (ACS)—National volunteer organization promoting cancer research and education. Instrumental in campaign to reduce cigarette smoking.

American College of Cardiology (ACC)—National professional society of cardiologists. Co-sponsors national treatment guidelines in heart disease.

American Heart Association (AHA)—National volunteer organization promoting heart disease research and education. Co-sponsors national treatment guidelines in heart disease.

American Lung Association (ALA)—National volunteer organization promoting pulmonary disease research and education. Instrumental in campaign to reduce cigarette smoking.

Amiodarone—A drug used to treat arrhythmia. Its use has declined due to significant pulmonary toxicity

Angina Pectoris—Exertional chest pain due to coronary atherosclerosis, limiting the blood supply to the heart muscle.

Angiography—A radiologic (x-ray) procedure in which dye is injected to visualize the contours of blood vessels and their target organs. Coronary angiography is the primary diagnostic procedure for assessing potential targets for revascularization procedures.

Angioplasty—A procedure in which a balloon catheter with an inflatable cuff is threaded into an artery that is partially obstructed by atherosclerotic plaque and the cuff is inflated to compress the plaque and restore blood flow.

Angiotensin Converting Enzyme (ACE) Inhibitors—A class of drugs that block the conversion of the inactive to the active form of angiotensin, used to treat hypertension, myocardial infarction, and heart failure

Angiotensin Receptor Blockers (ARB)—A class of drugs that block the action of angiotensin and have fewer side effects than ACE inhibitors. They are used as an alternative to ACE inhibitors to treat hypertension, myocardial infarction, and heart failure.

Glossary of Medical Terms and Acronyms

Antiplatelet Drugs—A class of drugs that includes aspirin, clopidogrel, and others, that inhibits clotting by blocking the action of platelets.

Antithrombotic Drugs—A class of drugs that includes warfarin, heparin, and others, that inhibits clot formation by interrupting the cascade protein reactions that result in the conversion of fibrinogen to fibrin.

Arrhythmia—Disruptions of the regular heartbeat, ranging from benign premature atrial contractions to life-threatening ventricular fibrillation.

Aspirin—A salicylate, initially derived from willow bark and used to treat pain and fever, which is now a staple of secondary prevention because of its inhibition of clot-forming platelets.

Asystole—Absence of any electrical activity in the heart. Usually irreversible.

Atherosclerosis—The pathological chronic inflammatory process in which cholesterol, calcium, and cell debris are deposited in arterial walls, eventually obstructing blood flow. Their sudden rupture and resulting clot formation is the immediate cause of most heart attacks and many strokes.

Atherothrombotic Stroke —The acute deprivation of blood flow and oxygen to a portion of the brain following a rupture of an atherosclerotic plaque in one of the cerebral arteries.

Atrial Fibrillation—Total disruption of electrical conduction in the heart's atrial chambers leading to inability to actively pump blood into the ventricles. Not immediately fatal, but stagnation of blood in the left atrium may lead to the formation of blood clots that may travel to the brain and cause strokes.

Beta Adrenergic Blockers—Drugs that block the action of epinephrine (adrenaline) and are useful in treating hypertension, arrhythmia, and myocardial infarction.

Biguanides—Antidiabetic drugs that reduce insulin resistance

Bile Acid Sequestrant Resins—Pre-statin cholesterol-lowering drugs that block the reabsorption of bile acids in the large intestine.

Blinded Clinical Trial—A clinical trial in which the patients (single-blind) and sometimes the treating medical practitioners (double-blind) are kept unaware of which treatment each participant receives. Also called "masked."

Blood Pressure (BP)—The pressure within the arteries when the left ventricle is contracted (systole) or between contractions (diastole), as measured by the height (in millimeters) of a column of mercury (Hg) will be supported when a cuff around the arm is inflated to impede blood flow in the arm.

Body Mass Index (BMI)—Weight in kilograms divided by height in meters. In general, a BMI < 30 kg/m² is considered healthy.

Calcium Channel Blockers—A class of drugs used to treat high blood pressure by impeding the flow of calcium across membranes.

Carbohydrates—Sugars and sugar polymers.

Cardiac Enzymes—Protein catalysts of muscle energy metabolism in the heart that leak into the bloodstream in a myocardial infarction and the measurement of which are useful in diagnosis.

Cardiopulmonary Bypass—A machine which takes over the function of the heart by oxygenating blood and returning it to the circulation while the heart is stopped for a surgical procedure.

Cardiopulmonary Resuscitation (CPR)—A method of buying time for a patient who has suffered a cardiac arrest by rhythmically compressing the chest and inflating the lungs until the heartbeat can be restored by defibrillation.

Cardiovascular Disease—All diseases of the heart and blood vessels supplying the heart, brain, limbs, kidneys, and other organs.

Cardiovascular Risk Factors—Attributes and behaviors (age, male sex, BP, LDL cholesterol, smoking, diabetes, etc.) that predict the risk of future adverse cardiovascular events.

Centers for Disease Control and Prevention (CDC)—The branch of the U.S. Department of Health and Human Services responsible for tracking and fighting infectious diseases and for maintaining national health statistics.

Cholesterol—A fat-soluble organic animal sterol that is a structural component of cell membranes, the precursor of steroid hormones, and is also a major component of atherosclerotic plaques.

Cholesteryl Ester Transfer Protein (CETP)—A protein that assists the transfer of cholesterol from HDL to LDL and was therefore once thought to be a promising target for intervention to raise circulating HDL cholesterol levels.

Confounding Variables—Variables than are correlated both with the treatment and outcomes of interest and which may confuse the results of clinical trials if they are imbalanced among treatment groups.

Congenital Heart Disease—A group of structural heart malformations of varying severity caused by in utero disruption of cardiac development.

Coordinating Center—An organization that provides essential statistical and logistic support for the conduct of large blinded randomized clinical trials.

Coronary Artery Bypass Graft (CABG) Surgery—A surgical procedure in which obstructed segments of coronary arteries are bypassed by grafting segments of the superficial saphenous (leg) veins or joining an internal thoracic artery to the coronary artery distal to the obstruction.

Coronary Heart Disease (CHD)—The disease caused by obstruction of the coronary arteries by atherosclerotic plaques potentially leading to angina, myocardial infarction, and death. I have used the terms CHD death, IHD death, and heart attack death interchangeably.

Cytokines—A broad category of small proteins important in cell signaling

DASH Diet—A diet based on low intake of fat and high intake of grains and vegetables, which is proven to reduce BP and LDL cholesterol.

Diabetes Mellitus (or Diabetes)—A metabolic disease caused either by insulin deficiency (type 1) or insulin resistance (type 2), which disrupts glucose metabolism and is associated with life-threatening ketoacidosis (in type 1), disease of the small blood vessels of the eyes, kidneys and other organs, and with a threefold increased risk of CHD.

Diastole—The period between heartbeats when BP is at its lowest.

Digitalis—A drug derived from the foxglove plant that was once a mainstay for treating myocardial infarction and heart failure but is now used mainly to treat atrial fibrillation.

Door-to-Balloon Time—The time between the arrival of an acute MI patient in the emergency room and revascularization by PCI.

DPP4 Inhibitors—Antidiabetic drugs that inhibit dipeptidyl Peptidase-4 (DPP4) and stimulate insulin secretion

Electrocardiogram (ECG)—An external recording of voltages associated with the electrical depolarization and repolarization of the heart in the course of a heartbeat. Sometimes abbreviated EKG from the German.

Endpoints—The pre-defined patient outcomes (heart attack, death, etc.) upon which the success of a treatment will be judged in a clinical trial.

Estrogen—The primary female hormone secreted by the ovaries, which is responsible (with progesterone) for the menstrual cycle and the development of female secondary sexual characteristics, and whose abrupt decline after menopause is responsible for the adverse vasomotor symptoms of menopause.

External Defibrillator—A device that is applied externally to the chest of a person in ventricular fibrillation to deliver a high-voltage shock to try to restore a normal heart rhythm.

Ezetimibe—A second-line LDL cholesterol-lowering drug often used in conjunction with a statin or instead of a statin in statin-intolerant patients.

Factorial Trial—A trial in which patients are simultaneously randomized with regard to two or more independent treatments (see Figures 3.1–2 in Chapter 3).

Familial Hypercholesterolemia—An autosomal dominant genetic condition characterized by defective or absent LDL receptors. Patients who inherit a defective gene from both parents (homozygotes) suffer severe coronary atherosclerosis and often die before adulthood. Patients who inherit a defective gene from one parent and a normal gene from the other survive to adulthood but are at elevated risk for heart attacks in middle age.

Fibrates—Second-line cholesterol-lowering drugs that modestly raise HDL cholesterol and lower LDL cholesterol and triglyceride levels.

Food and Drug Administration (FDA)—The federal agency in the Department of Health and Human Services that responsible for approving (or disapproving) new drugs and for monitoring their safety after they are approved.

Framingham Heart Study (FHS)—The first large cardiovascular epidemiologic study, founded by the NHLBI in 1948 in Framingham, Massachusetts.

Global Health Index—A composite endpoint used in the Women's Health Initiative to assess the overall harm or benefit of menopausal hormone therapy.

Glucagon-like Peptide-1 (GLP-1) Receptor Antagonists—Antidiabetic drugs that reduce glucose reabsorption by the kidneys.

Glucose—The simplest sugar, which is the fundamental substrate of energy metabolism in humans and other animals.

Glycemic Index—A metric for rating of carbohydrates by their tendency to raise blood glucose levels.

Heart Attack—A popular term for the symptoms produced by acute blockage of a coronary artery (myocardial infarction) and the resulting deprivation of oxygen (ischemia) of the heart muscle downstream. I have used the term "heart attack deaths" interchangeably with CHD or IHD deaths, to signify deaths due to coronary atherosclerosis.

Heart Disease (HD)—All diseases of the heart including those from non-atherosclerotic causes (congenital, rheumatic, cardiomyopathy, etc.) as well as atherosclerotic CHD.

Heart Failure—Decreased ability of the heart—most often the left ventricle—to pump blood to the body. Related terms include left ventricular dysfunction, congestive heart failure, and reduced ejection fraction.

Hemoglobin A1c (HbA1c)—A circulating glycated hemoglobin molecule whose concentration in the blood is superior to the level of glucose itself as a stable measure of the state of glucose metabolism.

Hemorrhagic Stroke—A sudden often lethal bleed into the substance of the brain often associated with hypertension. Less commonly the source of bleeding may be the rupture of a small congenital aneurysm (a bulging and weakened arterial wall) in a small artery at the base of the brain.

High-Density Lipoprotein (HDL)—A protein-rich cholesterol-carrying particle, associated with reduced cardiovascular risk.

HMG CoA Reductase—3-hydroxy-3-methylglutaryl coenzyme A (HMG CoA) reductase, the key rate-controlling enzyme in the synthetic pathway for cholesterol

Hypertension—Elevated blood pressure, defined until recently as > 140/90 mmHg, but now defined as > 130/80.

Hysterectomy—Surgical removal of the uterus (and sometimes the Fallopian tubes and ovaries).

Glossary of Medical Terms and Acronyms

Implantable Cardioverter Defibrillator (ICD)—A device inserted in the chest of patients who have survived a sudden cardiac arrest (SCA) or are at high risk for an SCA to detect life-threatening ventricular arrhythmias and to deliver a corrective electrical shock to the heart when such an arrhythmia is detected.

Insulin—A peptide (short protein) hormone, made in the pancreas, which is essential for the utilization of glucose by fat and muscle cells. Absence of or resistance to insulin is the underlying metabolic defect in diabetes.

Ischemia—Deprivation of oxygen-carrying blood to an organ due to obstruction of the blood vessels supplying that organ.

Ischemic Heart Disease (IHD)—Used interchangeably with coronary heart disease (CHD)

Isolated Systolic Hypertension—Elevation of systolic BP without elevation of diastolic BP. Most often seen in older patients, as a manifestation of arterial stiffening.

Left Main Coronary Artery Disease—Significant atherosclerotic obstruction of blood flow in the proximal section of the left coronary artery before it bifurcates into the anterior descending and circumflex branches. Associated with the highest risk of a fatal MI.

Low-Density Lipoprotein (LDL)—The particle typically containing 60–70% of circulating cholesterol, associated with elevated cardiovascular risk.

Malignant Hypertension—An increasingly uncommon condition, featuring systolic BP levels exceeding 200 mmHg, retinal hemorrhage, and heart and kidney failure.

Mediterranean Diet—A diet based on dietary patterns in Italy, Greece, and other Mediterranean countries, which is characterized by high intake of olive oil and other unsaturated fats and relatively low intake of carbohydrates and has recently been shown to lower cardiovascular risk.

Meglitinides—Antidiabetic drugs that stimulate insulin secretion

Meta-Analysis—A statistical method to combine the results of clinical trials to produce more reliable estimates of overall benefit and more robust subgroup results.

Myocardial Infarction (MI)—An acute blockage of an atherosclerotic coronary plaque and subsequent clot formation, which causes measurable ischemic damage to the segment of heart muscle downstream.

National Center for Health Statistics (NCHS)—The CDC Center that is responsible for tracking national vital statistics and conducting national health surveys.

National Health and Nutrition Survey (NHANES)—A biennial survey conducted by the NCHS to track national trends in BP, cholesterol, diet, smoking, and other attributes and behaviors related to cardiovascular risk.

National Heart Lung and Blood Institute (NHLBI)—The NIH institute responsible for reviewing and supporting grants and contracts for basic and applied research in non-cancer diseases of the heart, lungs, and blood.

National Institute of Diabetes and Digestive and Kidney Diseases (NIDDK)—The NIH institute responsible for reviewing and supporting grants and contracts for basic and applied research in diabetes and in digestive and kidney diseases.

National Institutes of Health (NIH)—The agency within the Department of Health and Human Services that is responsible for reviewing and supporting grants and contracts for basic and applied biomedical research.

Niacin—A B vitamin (B-3), which when given in in high doses (150–400 times the 14–16 mg recommended daily intake), modestly raises HDL cholesterol and lowers LDL cholesterol and triglyceride levels.

Obesity—Defined here as having a BMI > 30 kg/m². Overweight is defined as BMI between 25 and 30 kg/m², and severe obesity is defined as BMI > 35 kg/m².

P-Value—The probability that a treatment effect at least as large as the one observed in a clinical trial could have occurred by chance. P < 0.05 (i.e., one in 20) is generally accepted as the threshold for statistical "significance."

Pandemic—A worldwide outbreak of a disease. An epidemic refers to an outbreak in one country or geographic region.

PCSK9 Blockers—Injectable monoclonal antibodies that block proprotein convertase subtilisin kexin 9 (PCSK9), a natural membrane protein that interferes with LDL receptors

Percutaneous Intervention (PCI)—The combination of angioplasty and stent placement via arterial catheter to produce a lasting re-establishment of blood flow in a partially obstructed coronary (or other) artery.

Placebo—An inactive drug provided to the control group of a clinical trial to achieve "blinding."

Plaques—Gruel-like deposits of cholesterol, calcium, and cellular debris within artery walls that may partially obstruct blood flow and may cause an acute occlusion and ischemia of the tissue downstream—i.e., a heart attack, a stroke, etc.—when they rupture and a blood clot forms See Figure 5.2.

Primary Prevention—Treatments designed to prevent an initial heart attack or other cardiovascular event, in persons who have not already had a prior event.

Progesterone—The female hormone secreted by the ovaries, which is responsible (with estrogen) for the menstrual cycle. Progesterone mitigates the stimulatory (and pro-carcinogenic) effect of estrogen on the uterus.

Proteins—Large amino acid polymers, which comprise many of the cell's structural elements, hormones, and enzymes.

Randomized Clinical Trial—An experiment conducted in human volunteers in which the allocation of participants among treatment and control groups is random. Randomization ensures that the treatment groups are similar at the start of the trial.

Glossary of Medical Terms and Acronyms

Renin-Angiotensin-Aldosterone System (RAAS)—An interconnected group of vasoactive proteins and hormones involved in regulating sodium excretion and reabsorption in the kidneys and affect BP (see Chapter 11).

Revascularization—A procedure in which circulation is re-established to an ischemic area of the heart (or other organs) either by reopening or bypassing the obstructed arterial segment(s).

Rheumatic Heart Disease—A form of heart disease, manifested mainly in damage to the heart valves, caused by a hyperimmune response to an infection by certain strains of streptococcus bacteria.

Saturated Fat—Hard fats found mostly in animals and tropical plants, which are defined chemically by the absence of carbon-carbon double bonds.

Secondary Prevention—Treatments designed to prevent a recurrent heart attack or other adverse cardiovascular event, in persons who have already had a prior event.

Statins—Drugs that inhibit HMG CoA reductase, the rate-limiting enzyme for cholesterol synthesis, and thereby stimulate the productions of LDL receptors and lower circulating LDL cholesterol levels. Statins are first-line drugs for treating patients with high LDL cholesterol, diabetes, and prior heart attacks.

Statistical Power—The probability that a trial will obtain a positive result if the treatment does in fact have the hypothesized beneficial effect. Power depends on the size of the hypothesized effect, the number of patients enrolled, and the incidence rate of the primary endpoint.

Stent—A thin wire-mesh tube—often impregnated with a drug that inhibits scarring—that is inserted to keep an arterial channel open after an angioplasty.

Streptokinase—An enzyme produced by streptococcal bacteria than digests fibrin, the structural protein of blood clots. Can re-establish coronary circulation when administered intravenously to patients with acute MI.

Stroke—A sudden blockage of circulation to a portion of the brain either by rupture of an atherosclerotic plaque in a cerebral artery or a sudden bleed into the brain, resulting in a loss of neurologic function or death.

Sudden Cardiac Arrest (SCA)—A stoppage of the heart due to an acute MI, arrhythmia, or non-cardiovascular cause, which results in an immediate loss of consciousness and brain death within 10 minutes if the heartbeat is not restored.

Sulfonylureas—Antidiabetic drugs that stimulate insulin secretion

Systole—The portion of the cardiac cycle when the heart is maximally contracted and BP is at its highest.

Thiazide Diuretics—A class of diuretics—including chlorothiazide and hydrochlorothiazide and closely related to chlorthalidone—used as first-line drugs to treat hypertension.

Thiazolidinediones—Antidiabetic drugs that reduce insulin resistance. Associated with increased risk of heart failure.

Thrombolytic Therapy—Treatment of acute MI with drugs that dissolve fibrin (the structural protein of blood clots) and re-establish circulation after an arterial thrombosis. Thrombolysis has been largely been replaced by PCI but is still of value in hospitals that lack facilities to perform angiography and PCI.

Tissue Plasminogen Activator (tPA)—A synthetic intravenously administered thrombolytic drug, which replaced streptokinase as a first-line treatment.

Trans Fats—Harmful fats containing trans carbon-carbon double bonds produced by processing polyunsaturated oils to produce margarine that is sold at refrigerator temperatures.

Unsaturated Fats—Fats, found largely in plants and seafood, containing one (mono) or more (poly) carbon-carbon double bonds, which are liquid at room temperature. Examples are olive and canola oil (mono) and corn, safflower, and sunflower oil (poly). Oils derived from fish and certain plants contain double-bonds at a specific location (omega-3) in the carbon chain.

Ventricular Fibrillation (VF)—A ventricular arrhythmia in which the heart muscle cells are bombarded with uncoordinated electrical impulses, and the ventricles cannot pump blood. VF is lethal if not reversed rapidly by a high-voltage shock (defibrillation).

Ventricular Tachycardia—A potentially life-threatening ventricular arrhythmia in which the heart beats too fast to pump blood efficiently. A high-voltage electric shock (defibrillation) is often needed to prevent VF and death.

CHAPTER NOTES

Preface

1. Proceedings of the Conference on the Decline in Coronary Heart Disease Mortality: National Heart, Lung, and Blood Institute, National Institute of Health, Bethesda, Maryland. NIH publication no. 79–1610, 1978. Bethesda, MD: National Heart, Lung, and Blood Institute, NIH, 1979, Oct 24–25.

Chartbook for the Conference on the Decline in Coronary Heart Disease Mortality. Hyattsville, MD: NCHS, 1978. National Center for Health Statistics.

2. C Dampier. At age 100, the father of preventive medicine is going strong—as living proof that he was right all along. *Chicago Tribune*, December 26, 2019. https://www.chicagotribune.com/lifestyles/ct-life-100-year-old-scientist-stamler-20191226-jeprzoeqazha7nuvs2prfcndwy-story.html.

3. Centers for Disease Control and Prevention (CDC), National Center of Health Statistics. Leading Causes of Death, 1900–1998.

4. National Archives, Vietnam War U.S. Military Fatal Casualty Statistics, Electronic Records Reference Report, https://www.archives.gov/research/military/vietnam-war/casualty-statistics.

5. MD Ritchie, HK Wall, MG George, JS Wright. U.S. trends in premature heart disease mortality over the past 5 years: Where do we go from here? *Trends in Cardiovascular Medicine* 2020, 30:364–374. Doi: org/10.1016/j.tcm.2019.09.005. https://reader.elsevier.com/reader/sd/pii/S1050173819301343?token=7F40CE582 41E384675154F72DB6A47DA204635A A02005A37DE85A7A8ED4F1F679D9F 00D9FDE3E1D64DC89666494E1ED0.

6. GA Mensah, GS Wei, PD Sorlie, LJ Fine, Y Rosenberg, PG Kaufmann, ME Mussolino, LL Hsu, E Addou, MM Engelgau, D Gordon. Decline in Cardiovascular Mortality: Possible Causes and Implications. *Circ Res* 2017:366–380. doi:10.1161/CIRCRESAHA.116.309115.

7. AZ Quotes—Alexander Pope. https://www.azquotes.com/author/11775-Alexander_Pope.

8. A Christie. *Murder on the Orient Express*. London: Collins Crime Club, 1934.

Chapter 1

1. JM Barry. *The Great Influenza: The Story of the Deadliest Pandemic in History*. New York: Penguin Random House, 2004, 2005, 2009, 2018.

2. RJ Myerburg, J Junttila. Sudden cardiac death caused by coronary heart disease. *Circulation* 2012; 125:1043–1052.

3. Chartbook for the Conference on the Decline in Coronary Heart Disease Mortality. Hyattsville, MD: NCHS, 1978. National Center for Health Statistics, https://www.cdc.gov/nchs/data/misc/corltrtacc.pdf, pp. 12–13, Tables 3A-3B. IHD death rates for 45–54, 55–64, and 65–74 age groups were multiplied by age-specific population data from U.S. Census for 1960–1974 (extrapolated back to 1955) obtained from Centers for Disease Control and Prevention (CDC), National Center of Health Statistics. Population by age groups, race and sex for 1960–97.

4. Centers for Disease Control. Age-adjusted death rates for 69 selected causes by race and sex using year 2000 standard population: United States, 1950–59.

183

https://www.cdc.gov/nchs/data/dvs/hist293_1950_59.pdf, 1960–67. https://www.cdc.gov/nchs/data/mortab/aadr6067.pdf, 1968–78. https://www.cdc.gov/nchs/data/mortab/aadr6878.pdf.

5. *Ibid.*

6. Centers for Disease Control (CDC). Leading Causes of Death, 1990–1998. Data provided to NIH by the National Center for Health Statistics.

7. CL Beale. A century of population growth and change. *Food Review* 2000; 23:16–22. https://wayback.archive-it.org/5923/20110903152144/http://ers.usda.gov/publications/foodreview/jan2000/frjan2000c.pdf.

8. CDC, Leading Causes of Death.

9. Achievements in Public Health, 1900–1999. Healthier Mothers and Babies. *MMWR Weekly* 1999; 48:849–858. https://www.cdc.gov/mmwr/preview/mmwrhtml/mm4838a2.htm.

10. Life Expectancy in the USA 1900–98, https://u.demog.berkeley.edu/~andrew/1918/figure2.html.

11. Centers for Disease Control and Prevention (CDC), National Center of Health Statistics Mortality Data, HIST293. Age-adjusted death rates for selected causes by race and sex using year 2000 standard population: death registration states, 1900-32 and United States, 1933-49, Diseases of the Heart. https://www.cdc.gov/nchs/data/dvs/hist293_1900_49.pdf.

Centers for Disease Control. Age-adjusted death rates for 69 selected causes by race and sex using year 2000 standard population: United States, 1968–78. https://www.cdc.gov/nchs/data/mortab/aadr6878.pdf.

12. W Osler. *Lectures on Angina Pectoris and Allied States.* New York: D. Appleton and Company, 1897, pp. 22–23.

13. Wikipedia. The free encyclopedia. www.wikipedia.org.

14. CDC Age-adjusted death rates, 1900–49.

Morbidity and Mortality. 2012 Chartbook on Cardiovascular, Lung and Blood Diseases, NIH-NHLBI. Chart 3-24. https://www.nhlbi.nih.gov/files/docs/research/2012_ChartBook_508.pdf.

Centers for Disease Control. Age-adjusted death rates for 69 selected causes by race and sex using year 2000 standard population: United States, 1950–59. https://www.cdc.gov/nchs/data/dvs/hist293_1950_59.pdf, 1960–67. https://www.cdc.gov/nchs/data/mortab/aadr6067.pdf, 1968–78.

Centers for Disease Control and Prevention (CDC), National Center of Health Statistics. Mortality Data Finder. Table 5: Age-adjusted death rates for selected causes of death by sex, race and Hispanic origin: United States, selected years 1950–2017, https://www.cdc.gov/nchs/hus/contents2018.htm#Table_005 (Excel spreadsheet link).<U></U>S Sydney, CP Quesenberry, MG Jaffe, M Sorel, MN Nguyen-Huynh, LH Kushi, AS Go, JS Rana. Recent trends in cardiovascular mortality in the United States and public health goals. *JAMA Cardiology* 2016; 1:594–599. Doi:10.1001/jamacardio.2016.1326.

15. Centers for Disease Control and Prevention. Heart Disease Facts, https://www.cdc.gov/heartdisease/facts.htm.

16. J Lennon and P McCartney. When I'm Sixty-Four, Sergeant Pepper's Lonely Heart Club Band, 1967, https://www.songfacts.com/lyrics/the-beatles/when-im-64.

17. Getty Images. B/W 1955 Dwight Eisenhower smiling in wheelchair surrounded by doctors and nurses after heart attack. https://www.gettyimages.com/detail/video/news-footage/2034-252.

18. Mortality and Top 10 Causes of Death, USA, 1900 vs 2010, https://www.ncdemography.org/wp-content/uploads/2014/06/All-Cause-Mortality-and-Top-10_USA-e1402597040445.png.

19. Life Expectancy in the USA 1900–98.

20. Macrotrends, U.S. Life Expectancy 1950–2020, https://www.macrotrends.net/countries/USA/united-states/life-expectancy.

Chapter 2

1. SS Mahmood, D Levy, RS Vasan, TJ Wang. The Framingham Heart Study and

the Epidemiology of Cardiovascular Diseases: A Historical Perspective. *Lancet* 2014 March 15; 383 (9921): 999–1008; doi 10.1016/S0140–6736(13)61752–3; https://www.ncbi.nlm.nih.gov/pmc/articles/PMC4159698/pdf/nihms588573.pdf.

2. National Archives. Crimean Conference—Prime Minister Winston Churchill, President Franklin D. Roosevelt, and Marshal Joseph Stalin at the palace in Yalta, where the Big Three met, February 1945. http://loc.gov/pictures/resource/cph.3a10098/.

3. SS Mahmood et al.

4. *Ibid.*

5. K Tuthill and R Van Wyck (illustrator). John Snow and the Broad Street Pump: On the Trail of an Epidemic. *Cricket* Nov 2003; 31:23–31, https://www.ph.ucla.edu/epi/snow/snowcricketarticle.html.

6. Framingham Heart Study, https://en.wikipedia.org/wiki/Framingham_Heart_Study.

7. WB Kannel, TR Dawber, A Kagan, N Revotskie, J Stokes. Factors of risk in the development of coronary heart disease—six-year follow-up experience. The Framingham Heart Study. *Ann Intern Med* 1961; 55:33–50.

8. Framingham, Massachusetts, https://en.wikipedia.org/wiki/Framingham,_Massachusetts#Geography.

9. SM Grundy, RB d'Agostino, L Mosca, GL Burke, PWF Wilson, DJ Rader, EJ Rocella, JA Cutler, LM Friedman. Cardiovascular risk assessment based on U.S. cohort studies: Findings from a National Heart, Lung, and Blood Institute Workshop. *Circulation* 2001; 104:491–496. P Sorlie, G Wei. Population-based cohort studies: Still relevant? *J Am Coll Cardiol* 2011; 58:2010–13, http://www.onlinejacc.org/content/accj/58/19/2010.full.pdf.

10. AHA/ACC Heart Risk Calculator, http://www.cvriskcalculator.com/.

Chapter 3

1. JA Van Helmont. *Oriatrike*. London: Lodowick-Loyd, 1662, p. 526.

2. I Milne, I Chalmers. A controlled clinical trial in 1809? *J Epidemiol Community Health* 2002; 56:1a.

3. The Mysterious Death of George Washington, Constitution Daily, December 14, 2019, https://constitutioncenter.org/blog/the-mysterious-death-of-george-washington.

4. M Bliss. *William Osler: A Life in Medicine*. Oxford: Oxford University Press, 1999, p. 188.

5. LM Friedman, CD Furberg, DL DeMets, DM Reboussin, CB Granger. *Fundamentals of Clinical Trials*. New York: Springer Science & Business Media, 5th edition, 2015.

6. ClinicalTrials.gov. The Women's Health Study (WHS). https://clinicaltrials.gov/ct2/show/NCT00000479.

7. ClinicalTrials.gov. Action to Control Cardiovascular Risk in Diabetes (ACCORD). https://clinicaltrials.gov/ct2/show/NCT00000620?term=accord&draw=2&rank=1.

8. ClinicalTrials.gov. The Cardiac Arrhythmia Suppression Trial (CAST). https://clinicaltrials.gov/ct2/show/record/NCT00000526?term=flecanide&draw=5&rank=33&view=record.

9. Cardiac Arrhythmia Suppression Trial (CAST) Investigators. Preliminary report: effect of encainide and flecainide on mortality in a randomized trial of arrhythmia suppression after myocardial infarction. *N Engl J Med* 1989; 32:406–12.

10. HL Greene, DM Roden, RJ Katz, DM Slerno, RW Henthorn. The Cardiac Arrhythmia Suppression Trial: first CAST-I ... then CAST-II. *J Am Coll Cardiol* 1992; 19:894–98, https://clinicaltrials.gov/ct2/show/record/NCT00000526?term=flecanide&draw=5&rank=33&view=record.

11. Multiple Risk Factor Intervention Trial Research Group. Multiple Risk Factor Intervention Trial. Risk factor changes and mortality results. *JAMA* 1982; 248:1465–77.

12. ClinicalTrials.gov. Lipid Research Clinics Coronary Primary Prevention Trial (LRC-CPPT). https://clinicaltrials.gov/ct2/show/NCT00000488?term=Lipid+Research+Clinics&draw=2&rank=2.

13. ClinicalTrials.gov. Efficacy of pioglitazone on macrovascular outcome in

patients with type 2 diabetes (PROactive). https://clinicaltrials.gov/ct2/show/NCT0 0174993?term=PROactive+pioglitazone& draw=2&rank=1.

14. Editorial. The statin wars: why AstraZeneca must retreat. *Lancet* 2003; 362:1341.

15. DJ Gordon. Cholesterol and Mortality: What Can Meta-Analysis Tell Us? *Cardiovascular Disease 2: Cellular and Molecular Mechanisms, Prevention, and Treatment*, LL Gallo (ed.). New York: Plenum Press, 1995, pp. 333–340. DJ Gordon. Cholesterol Lowering Reduces Mortality. *Cholesterol Lowering Therapies 1999.* SM Grundy (ed.). New York: Marcel Dekker, Inc., 1999, pp. 299–311.

16. Cholesterol Treatment Trialists (CTC) Collaboration. Protocol for a prospective collaborative overview of all current and planned randomized trials of cholesterol treatment regimens. *Am J Cardiol* 1995; 75:1130–1134.

Chapter 4

1. Wikipedia. History of Hypertension. https://en.wikipedia.org/wiki/History_ of_hypertension. MG Sakayan, NV Deshpanda. Timeline of history of hypertension treatment. *Front Cardiovasc Med* 2016; 33:1–14, doi: 10.3389/fcvm.2016.00003, https://www.ncbi.nlm.nih.gov/pmc/ articles/PMC4763852.

2. TA Kotchen. Historical trends and milestones in hypertension research. A model of the process of translational research. *Hypertension* 2011; 58:522–538.

3. PD White. *Heart Disease.* New York: Macmillan, 2nd edition, 1937, p. 326.

4. J Hay. A British Medical Association Lecture on the Significance of a Raised Blood Pressure. *British Medical J* July 11, 1931; 2 (3679): 43–47.

5. Morbidity and Mortality. 2012 Chartbook on Cardiovascular, Lung and Blood Diseases, NIH-NHLBI. Chart 3–24. https://www.nhlbi.nih.gov/files/docs/ research/2012_ChartBook_508.pdf.

Centers for Disease Control. Age-adjusted death rates for 69 selected causes by race and sex using year 2000 standard population: United States, 1950–59. https:// www.cdc.gov/nchs/data/dvs/hist293_ 1950_59.pdf, 1960–67. https://www.cdc. gov/nchs/data/mortab/aadr6067.pdf, 1968–78. https://www.cdc.gov/nchs/data/ mortab/aadr6878.pdf.

Centers for Disease Control and Prevention (CDC), National Center of Health Statistics. Mortality Data Finder. Table 5: Age-adjusted death rates for selected causes of death by sex, race and Hispanic origin: United States, selected years 1950–2017, https://www.cdc.gov/nchs/hus/ contents2018.htm#Table_005 (Excel spreadsheet link).

6. M Moser. Historical perspective on management of hypertension. *J Clin Hypertens* 2006; 8:15–20. https://online library.wiley.com/doi/full/10.1111/ j.1524-6175.2006.05836.x.

7. W Goldring, H Chasis. Antihypertensive drug therapy: an appraisal. *Arch Intern Med* 1965; 115:523–25.

8. U.S. National Library of Medicine. The VA Cooperative Study and the Beginning of Routine Hypertension Screening, 1864–1980. The Edward D. Freis Papers. https://profiles.nlm.nih.gov/spotlight/xf/ feature/study.

9. J Cutler, SW MacMahon, CD Furberg. Controlled clinical trials of drug treatment for hypertension: A review. *Hypertension* 1989; 13(suppl I):I36-I44.

10. Veterans Administration Cooperative Study Group on Anti-Hypertensive Agents. Effects of treatment on morbidity in hypertension. Results in patients with diastolic blood pressures averaging 115–129 mm Hg. *JAMA* 1967; 202:1028–34.

11. Veterans Administration Cooperative Study Group on Anti-Hypertensive Agents. Effects of treatment on morbidity in hypertension. II Results in patients with diastolic blood pressure averaging 90–114 mm Hg. *JAMA* 1970; 213:1143–52.

12. VL Burt, JA Cutler, M Higgins, MJ Horan, D Labarth, P Whelton, C Brown, EJ Rocella. Trends in the prevalence, awareness, treatment, and control of hypertension in the adults U.S. population. Data from the Health Examination Surveys, 1960 to 1991. *Hypertension* 1995; 26:1–60, https://www.

ahajournals.org/doi/epub/10.1161/01.
HYP.26.1.60.

13. ClinicalTrials.gov. The Hypertension Detection and Follow-Up Study (HDFP). https://clinicaltrials.gov/ct2/show/NCT00000485?term=HDFP&draw=2&rank=1.

14. Hypertension Detection and Follow-Up Program Cooperative Group. Five Year Findings of the Hypertension Detection and Follow-Up Program. I. Reduction in mortality of persons with high blood pressure, including mild hypertension. *JAMA* 1979; 242:2562–71.

15. Hypertension Detection and Follow-Up Program Cooperative Group. Five Year Findings of the Hypertension Detection and Follow-Up Program. II. Mortality by age, race, and sex. JAMA 1979; 242:2572–77.

16. Hypertension Detection and Follow-Up Program Cooperative Group. Five Year Findings of the Hypertension Detection and Follow-Up Program. III. Reduction in stroke incidence among persons with high blood pressure. *JAMA* 1982; 247:633–638.

17. NO Borhani, WB Applegate, JA Cutler, BR Davis, CD Furberg, E Lakatos, L Page, M Perry, WM Smith, JL Probstfield. Part 1: Rationale and Design. *Hypertension* 1991; 17(suppl II):1–15. ClinicalTrials.gov. Systolic Hypertension in the Elderly Program (SHEP). https://clinicaltrials.gov/ct2/show/record/NCT0000514?term=SHEP&draw=2&rank=4.

18. SHEP Cooperative Research Group. Prevention of stroke by antihypertensive drug treatment in older persons with isolated systolic hypertension. Final results of the Systolic Hypertension in the Elderly Program (SHEP). *JAMA* 1991; 265:3255–64.

19. The Antihypertensive and Lipid Heart Attack Trial (ALLHAT) ClinicalTrials.gov. https://clinicaltrials.gov/ct2/show/NCT00000542?term=ALLHAT&draw=2&rank=3.

20. RH Grimm, KL Margolis, V Papademetriou, WC Cushman, CE Ford, J Bettencourt, MH Alderman, JN Basile, HR Black, V DeQuattro, J Eckfeldt, CM Hawkins, HM Perry, M Proschan. Baseline characteristics of participants in the Antihypertensive and Lipid Heart Attack Trial (ALLHAT). *Hypertension* 2001; 37:19–27.

21. The sixth report of the Joint National Committee on prevention, detection, evaluation, and treatment of high blood pressure. *Arch Intern Med* 1997; 157:2413–2446.

22. The Antihypertensive and Lipid Lowering Treatment to Prevent Heart Attack Trial (ALLHAT). *JAMA* 2000; 283:1967–1975. The Antihypertensive and Lipid Heart Attack Trial (ALLHAT) Research Group. Major outcomes in high-risk hypertensive patients randomized to angiotensin-converting enzyme inhibitor or calcium channel blocker vs diuretic. *JAMA* 2002; 288:2981–2997.

23. The ALLHAT Officers and Coordinators for the ALLHAT Collaborative Research Group. Major cardiovascular events in hypertensive patients randomized to doxazosin vs chlorthalidone: the Antihypertensive and Lipid-Lowering Treatment to Prevent Heart Attack Trial (ALLHAT). *JAMA* 2000; 283:1967–1975.

24. ClinicalTrials.gov. Action to Control Cardiovascular Risk in Diabetes (ACCORD). https://clinicaltrials.gov/ct2/show/NCT00000620?term=accord&draw=2&rank=1.

25. ClinicalTrials.gov. Systolic Blood Pressure Intervention Trial (SPRINT). https://clinicaltrials.gov/ct2/show/record/NCT01206062?term=sprint&cond=High+Blood+Pressure&draw=2&rank=4.

26. The SPRINT Research Group. A randomized trial of intensive versus standard blood pressure control. *N Engl J Med* 2015; 373:2103–2116.

27. The ACCORD Study Group. Effects of intensive blood-pressure control in type 2 diabetes mellitus. *N Engl J Med* 2010; 362:1575–1585.

28. S Beddhu, GM Chertow, T Greene, PK Whelton, WT Ambrosius, AK Cheung, J Cutler, L Fine, R Boucher, G Wei, C Zhang, H Kramer, AP Bress, PL Kimmel, S Oparil, CE Lewis, M Rahman, WC Cushman. Effects of intensive systolic blood pressure lowering on cardiovascular events and mortality in patients with type 2 diabetes mellitus on standard glycemic control and

in those without diabetes mellitus: Reconciling results from ACCORD BP and SPRINT. *J Am Heart Assoc* 2018; 7(18):1–14. doi: 10.1161/JAHA.118.009326.

29. JD Curb, SL Pressel, JA Cutler, PJ Savage, WB Applegate, H Black, G Carmel, BR Davis, PH Frost, N Gonzalez, G Guthrie, A Oberman, GH Rutan, J Stamler, for the Systolic Hypertension in the Elderly Program Cooperative Research Group. Effect of diuretic-based antihypertensive treatment on cardiovascular disease risk in older diabetic patients with isolated systolic hypertension. *JAMA* 1996; 276:1896–1892.

30. PK Whelton, RM Carey, WS Aronow, DE Casey, KJ Collins, CD Himmelfarb, SM DePalma, S Goldring, KA Jamerson, DW Jones, EJ MasLaughlin, P Munter, B Ovbiagele, SC Smith, CC Spencer, RS Stafford, SJ Taler, RJ Thomas, KA Williams, JD Williamson, JT Wright. 2017 ACC/AHA/AAPA/ABC/ACPM/AGS/APhA/ASH/ASPC/NMA/PCNA Guideline for the Prevention, Detection, Evaluation, and Management of High Blood Pressure in Adults: A Report of the American College of Cardiology/American Heart Association Task Force on Clinical Practice Guidelines. *Circulation* 2018; 138:e484-e594. DOI: 10.1161/CIR.0000000000000596. https://www.ahajournals.org/doi/pdf/10.1161/CIR.0000000000000596.

31. MA Pfeffer, JJV McMurray. Lessons in uncertainty and humility—clinical trials involving hypertension. *N Engl J Med* 2016; 375:1756–1766. DOI: 10:1056/NEJMra1510067.

32. D Ettehad, CA Emdin, A Kiran, SG Anderson, T Callender, J Emberson, J Chalmers, A Rodgers, K Rahimi. Blood pressure lowering for prevention of cardiovascular disease and death: a systematic review and meta-analysis. *Lancet* 2016; 387:957–967.

33. AHA/ACC Heart Risk Calculator, http://www.cvriskcalculator.com/.

34. ClinCalc DrugStats Database. The top 200 drugs of 2020. https://clincalc.com/DrugStats/Top200Drugs.aspx.

35. P Muntner, ST Hardy, LJ Fine, BC Jaeger, G Wozniak, EB Levitan, LD Colantonio. Trends in blood pressure control among U.S. adults with hypertension, 1999–2000 to 2017–2018. *JAMA* 2020; doi:10.1001/jama.2020.14545.

36. PA James, S Oparil, BL Carter, WC Cushman, D Dennison-Himmelfarb, J Handler, DT Lackland, ML LeFevre, TD MacKenzie, O Ogedegbe, SC Smith, LP Svetky, SJ Taler, RR Townsend, JT Wright, AS Narva, E Ortiz. Evidence-based guideline for the management of high blood pressure in adults: report from the panel members appointed to the Eighth Joint National Committee (JNC 8). *JAMA* 2014; 311(5):507–520. doi:10.1001/jama.2013.284427.

37. PK Whelton, et al.

38. ES Ford, UA Ajani, JB Croft, JA Critchley, DR Labarth, TE Kottke, WH Giles, S Capewell. Explaining the Decrease in U.S. Deaths from Coronary Disease, 1980–2000. *N Engl J Med* 2007; 356:2388–2398. DOI: 10.1056/NEJMsa053935.

39. VL Burt, et al., Munter, et al.

Chapter 5

1. DS Fredrickson, RI Levy, RS Lees. Fat Transport in Lipoproteins—An integrated approach to mechanisms and disorders. *N Engl J Med* 1967; 276:273–281, DOI: .1056/NEJM196702022760507.

2. AM Gotto, Jeremiah Metzger Lecture: Cholesterol, Inflammation and Atherosclerotic Cardiovascular Disease: Is it all LDL? JL Goldstein, MS Brown. A century of cholesterol and coronaries. From plaques to genes to statins. *Cell* 2015; 161:161–172. doi: 10.1016/j.cell.2015.01.036.

3. NN Anichkov, S Chalatow. Ueber experimentelle Cholesterinsteatose und ihre Bedeuting fur die Entstehung einer pathologischer Prozesse. *Zentralbl Allg Pathol* 1913; 24:1–9.

4. A Keys, JT Anderson, F Grande. Serum cholesterol response to changes in the diet. *Metabolism* 1965; 14:747–787.

5. University of Minnesota Driven to Discover. Heart Attack Prevention: A History of Cardiovascular Epidemiology—Mortality Statistics. http://www.epi.umn.edu/cvdepi/history-gallery/mortality-statistics/.

6. RM Worth, H Kato, GG Rhoads, A Kagan, SL Syme. Epidemiologic studies of coronary heart disease and stroke in Japanese men living in Japan, Hawaii and California: mortality. *Am J Epidemiol* 1975; 102:481–490.

7. A Keys, C Aravanis, H Blackburn, R Buzina, BS Djordjevic, AS Dontas, F Fidanza, MJ Karvonen, N Kimura, A Menotti , I Mohacek, S Nedeljkovic, V Puddu, S Punsar, HL Taylor, FSP Van Buchem. *Seven countries. A Multivariate Analysis of Death and Coronary Heart Disease.* Cambridge: Harvard University Press, 1980.

8. University of Minnesota Driven to Discover. Heart Attack Prevention: A History of Cardiovascular Epidemiology—Study Synopses. October 15, 2012. http://www.epi.umn.edu/cvdepi/the-research/study-synopses/?search_keyword=&search_title=yes&search_synopsis=yes&search_people=&search_study_topic=&search_study_category=527&filter_search=yes#-results-title.

9. ClinicalTrials.gov. Coronary Drug Project. https://clinicaltrials.gov/ct2/show/NCT00000482?term=coronary+drug+project&draw=2&rank=2.

10. The Coronary Drug Project. Clofibrate and niacin in coronary heart disease. *JAMA* 1975, Jan 27; 231(4):360–81.

11. The Coronary Drug Project. Initial findings leading to modifications of its research protocol. *JAMA* 1970, Nov 16; 214(7):1303–1313.

The Coronary Drug Project. Findings leading to further modifications of its protocol with respect to dextrothyroxine. The coronary drug project research group. *JAMA* 1972, May 15; 220(7):996–1008.

12. M Oliver. The clofibrate saga: a retrospective commentary. *Br J Clin Pharmacol* 2012; 74:907–910. doi: 10.1111/j.1365-2125.2012.04282.x.

13. WHO cooperative trial on primary prevention of ischaemic heart disease with clofibrate to lower serum cholesterol: final mortality follow-up. *Lancet* 1984; 2(8403):600–604.

14. MH Frick, O Elo, K Haapa, OP Heinonen, P Heinsalmi, P Helo, JK Huttunen, P Kaitaniemi, P Koskinen, V Manninen, H Maenpaa, M Malkonen, et al. Helsinki Heart Study: primary-prevention trial with gemfibrozil in middle-aged men with dyslipidemia. Safety of treatment, changes in risk factors, and incidence of coronary heart disease. *N Engl J Med* 1987; 317:1237–1245. HB Rubins, SJ Robins, D Collins, CL Fye, JW Anderson, MB Elam, FH Faas, E Linares, EJ Schaefer, G Schectman, TJ Wilt, J Wittes. Gemfibrozil for the secondary prevention of coronary heart disease in men with low levels of high-density lipoprotein cholesterol. Veterans Affairs High-Density Lipoprotein Cholesterol Intervention Trial Study Group. *N Engl J Med* 1999; 341:410–418. The ACCORD Study Group. The effect of combination lipid therapy in type 2 diabetes mellitus. *N Engl J Med* 2010; 362:1563–1574. DOI: 10.1056/NEJMoa1001282.

15. ClinicalTrials.gov. Lipid Research Clinics Coronary Primary Prevention Trial (LRC-CPPT). https://clinicaltrials.gov/ct2/show/NCT00000488?term=Lipid+Research+Clinics&draw=2&rank=2.

16. The Lipid Research Clinics Program. The Lipid Research Clinics Coronary Primary Prevention Trial Results I. Reduction in incidence of coronary heart disease. *JAMA* 251: 351–364, 1984.

17. The Lipid Research Clinics Program. The Lipid Research Clinics Coronary Primary Prevention Trial Results II. The relationship of reduction in incidence of coronary heart disease to cholesterol reduction. *JAMA* 1984; 251 365–374.

18. JL Goldstein, MS Brown. History of Discovery: The LDL Receptor. *Arterioscler Thromb Vasc Biol* 2009; 29:431–438.

19. MS Brown, JL Goldstein. A receptor-mediated pathway for cholesterol homeostasis. *Science* 1986; 232:34–47.

20. MS Brown, JL Goldstein JL. A tribute to Akira Endo, discoverer of a "Penicillin" for cholesterol. *Atherosclerosis Suppl* 2004; 5:13–6. A Endo. A historical perspective on the study of statins. *Proc Jpn Acad Ser B* 2010; 86:484–493.

21. ClinCalc DrugStats Database. The top 200 drugs of 2020. https://clincalc.com/DrugStats/Top200Drugs.aspx.

22. H Buchwald, RL Varco, JP Matts, JM Long, LL Fitch, GS Campbell, MB

Pearce, AE Yellin, WA Edmiston, RD Smink, HS Sawin, CT Campos, BJ Hansen, N Tuna, JN Karnegis, ME Sanmarco, K Amplatz, WR Casteneda-Zuniga, DW Hunter, JK Bissett, FW Weber, JW Stevenson, AS Leon, TC Chalmers, and the POSCH Group. Effect of Partial Ileal Bypass Surgery on Mortality and Morbidity from Coronary Heart Disease in Patients with Hypercholesterolemia—Report of the Program on the Surgical Control of the Hyperlipidemias (POSCH). *N Engl J Med* 1990; 323:946–355, DOI: 10.1056/NEJM199010043231404.

23. Report of the National Cholesterol Education Program Expert Panel on Detection, Evaluation, and Treatment of High Blood Cholesterol in Adults. The Expert Panel. *Arch Intern Med* 1988; 148:36–69.

24. TJ More. The Cholesterol Myth. *Atlantic Monthly*, September 1989, pp. 37–70.

25. Scandinavian Simvastatin Survival Study Group. Randomised trial of cholesterol lowering in 4444 patients with coronary heart disease: the Scandinavian Simvastatin Survival Study (4S). *Lancet* 1994; 344:1383–1389.

26. J Shepherd, SM Cobbe, I Ford, CG Isles, AR Lorimer, PW MacFarlane, JH McKillop, CJ Packard, West of Scotland Coronary Prevention Study Group. Prevention of coronary heart disease with pravastatin in men with hypercholesterolemia. *N Engl J Med* 1995; 333:1301–07.

27. Cholesterol Treatment Trialists Collaboration. Efficacy and safety of cholesterol-lowering treatment: prospective meta-analysis of data from 90,056 participants in 14 randomized trials of statins. *Lancet* 2005; 366:1267–1278. DOI:10.1016/S0140–6736(05)67394–1.

28. Cholesterol Treatment Trialists Collaboration. Efficacy and safety of more intensive lowering of LDL cholesterol: a meta-analysis of data from 170,000 participants in 26 randomised trials. *Lancet* 2010; 376:1670–1681.

29. Cholesterol Treatment Trialists Collaboration. Efficacy of cholesterol-lowering therapy in 18 686 people with diabetes in 14 randomised trials of statins: a meta-analysis. *Lancet* 2008; 371:117–125.

30. AS Peterson, LG Fong, SG Young. PCSK9 function and physiology. *J Lipid Res* 2008; 49:1152–1156. doi: 10.1194/jlr.E800008-JLR200.

31. Third Report of the National Cholesterol Education Program (NCEP) Expert Panel on Detection, Evaluation, and Treatment of High Blood Cholesterol in Adults (Adult Treatment Panel III). Executive Summary. National Cholesterol Education Program, National Heart, Lung, and Blood Institute, National Institutes of Health. NIH Publication No. 01–3670, May 2001.

32. MD Carroll, AK Kit, DA Lacher, ST Shero, ME Mussolino. Trends in lipids and lipoproteins of U.S. adults, 1988–2010. *JAMA* 2012; 308:1545–1554.

33. EM Sarpong, SH Zuvekas. Changes in statin therapy among adults (age 18+) by selected characteristics, United States, 2000–2001 to 2010–2011. Medical Expenditure Panel Survey (MEPS). Statistical Brief #459. November 2014. https://www.ncbi.nlm.nih.gov/books/NBK470833/.

34. Q Gu, R Paulose-Ram, VL Burt, BK Kit. Prescription cholesterol-lowering medication use in adults aged 40 and over: United States, 2003–2012. NCHS Data Brief No. 177, December 2014. https://www.cdc.gov/nchs/data/databriefs/db177.pdf.

35. SM Grundy, NJ Stone, AL Bailey, C Beam, KK Birtcher, RS Blumenthal, LT Braun, S de Ferranti, J Faiella-Tommasino, DE Forman, R Goldberg, PA Heidenreich, MA Hlatky, DW Jones, D Lloyd-Jones, N Lopez-Pajares, CE Ndumele, CE Orringer, CA Peralta, JJ Saseen, SC Smith, L Sperling, SS Virani, J Yeboah. 2018 AHA/ACC/AACVPR/AAPA/ABC/ACPM/ADA/AGS/APhA/ASPC/NLA/PCNA Guideline on the Management of Blood Cholesterol: A Report of the American College of Cardiology/American Heart Association Task Force on Clinical Practice Guidelines. *Circulation* 2019; 139:e1082-e1143. https://www.ahajournals.org/doi/10.1161/CIR.0000000000000625.

36. JA Salami, H Warralch, J Velardo-Elizondo, ES Spatz, NR Desai, JS Rana, SS Virani, R Blankstein, A Khera, MJ Blaha, RS Blumenthal, D Lloyd-Jones, K Nasir. National trends in statin use and

expenditures, in the U.S. adult population from 2002 to 2013: Insights from the Medical Expenditure Panel survey. *JAMA Cardiology* 2017; 2:56–65. doi.10.1001/jamacardio.2016.4700. file:///C:/Users/gordo/AppData/Local/Temp/jamacardiology_salami_2016_oi_160082.pdf.

37. NS Shah, MD Huffman, H Ning, DM Lloyd-Jones. Trends in myocardial infarction secondary prevention: The National Health and Nutrition Examination Surveys (NHANES), 1999–2012. *J Am Heart Assoc* 2015; 4:1–12. doi:10.1161/JAHA.114.001709. https://www.ahajournals.org/doi/pdf/10.1161/JAHA.114.001709.

38. ES Ford, UA Ajani, JB Croft, JA Critchley, DR Labarth, TE Kottke, WH Giles, S Capewell. Explaining the Decrease in U.S. Deaths from Coronary Disease, 1980–2000. *N Engl J Med* 2007; 356:2388–2398. DOI: 10.1056/NEJMsa053935. Cholesterol Treatment Trialists Collaboration (2010).

Chapter 6

1. JM Samet, FE Speizer. Sir Richard Doll, 1912–2005 (obituary). *Am J Epidiol* 2006; 164:95–100.

2. R Doll, AB Hill. A study of the aetiology of carcinoma of the lung. *Br Med J* 1952; 2:1271–1286.

3. R Doll R, AB Hill. The mortality of doctors in relation to their smoking habits. A preliminary report. *BMJ* 1954; 228(i):1451–55. EC Hammond, D Horn. The relationship between human smoking habits and death rates: A follow-up study of 187,766 men. *JAMA* 1954; 155:1316–1328. doi:10.1001/jama.1954.03690330020006.

4. L Terry, et al. Smoking and Health: Report of the Advisory Committee to the Surgeon General of the United States. U-23 Department of Health, Education, and Welfare. Public Health Service Publication No. 1103. 1964 https://profiles.nlm.nih.gov/spotlight/nn/catalog/nlm:nlmuid-101584932X202-doc.

5. Epidemiology of Tobacco Use: History and Current Trends. https://www.nap.edu/read/11795/chapter/4.

6. CDC MMMR Weekly. 1999 Tobacco Use—United States, 1900–1999. November 5, 1999; 48:986–993. https://www.cdc.gov/mmwr/preview/mmwrhtml/mm4843a2.htm.

7. American Lung Association. Overall Tobacco Trends. https://www.lung.org/research/trends-in-lung-disease/tobacco-trends-brief/overall-tobacco-trends. Accessed October 2020.

8. *Ibid.*

9. CA Ridge, AM McErlean, MS Ginsberg. Epidemiology of lung cancer. *Semin Intervent Radiol* 2013; 30:93–98.

10. Absurd Old Smoking Ads. https://www.google.com/search?q=absurd+old+smoking+ads&tbm=isch&client=firefox-b-1-d&hl=en&ved=2ahUKEwimp7H1l-vpAhWHON8KHRjeDHwQrNwCKAF6BQgBEOIB&biw=773&bih=560.

11. Epidemiology of Tobacco Use.

12. Centers for Disease Control and Prevention. Smoking & Tobacco Use: A Brief History. https://www.cdc.gov/tobacco/data_statistics/sgr/history/index.htm.

13. A Glass. Congress bans airing cigarette ads. April 1, 1970. https://www.politico.com/story/2018/04/01/congress-bans-airing-cigarette-ads-april-1-1970-489882.

14. A report of the Surgeon General. The Health Consequences of Involuntary Exposure to Tobacco Smoke. Centers for Disease Control and Prevention (U.S.), Atlanta, GA, 2006. https://www.ncbi.nlm.nih.gov/books/NBK44324/.

15. American Lung Association. Tobacco Control Milestones. https://www.lung.org/research/sotc/tobacco-timeline.

16. Centers for Disease Control. 1986 Surgeon General's Report: The Health Consequences of Involuntary Smoking. *MMWR Morb Mortal Wkly Rep* 1986; 35:769–70. PMID 3097495.

17. State Legislated Actions on Tobacco Issues (SLATI). https://www.lung.org/policy-advocacy/tobacco/slati.

18. EPA. Respiratory Health Effects of Passive Smoking: Lung Cancer and Other Disorders. Office of Health and Environmental Assessment, Office of Research and Development, U.S. Environmental Protection Agency, Washington, DC, December 1992.

19. C Crawford. Cigarette smoking among U.S. adults hits an all-time low. *AAFP News*. November 20, 2019. https://www.aafp.org/news/health-of-the-public/20191120mmwr-cigarettesmoking.html.

20. American Lung Association. Overall Tobacco Trends.

21. Epidemiology of Tobacco Use. Figure 1.4.

22. *Ibid.*

23. American Lung Association. Overall Tobacco Trends.

U.S. Food and Drug Administration. 2018 National Youth Tobacco Survey Finds Cause for Concern. https://www.fda.gov/tobacco-products/youth-and-tobacco/2018-nyts-data-startling-rise-youth-e-cigarette-use.

24. Centers for Disease Control and Prevention. Surgeon General's Advisory on E-cigarette Use Among Youth. February 2020. https://www.cdc.gov/tobacco/basic_information/e-cigarettes/surgeon-general-advisory/index.html.

25. TR Holford, R Meza, KE Warner, C Meernik, J Jeon, SH Moolgavkar, DT Levy. Tobacco Control and the Reduction in Smoking-Related Premature Deaths in the United States, 1964–2012. *JAMA* 2014; 311(2):164–171. doi:10.1001/jama.2013.285112.

26. ES Ford, UA Ajani, JB Croft, JA Critchley, DR Labarth, TE Kottke, WH Giles, S Capewell. Explaining the Decrease in U.S. Deaths from Coronary Disease, 1980–2000. *N Engl J Med* 2007; 356:2388–2398. DOI: 10.1056/NEJMsa053935.

27. JA Critchley, S Capewell. Mortality risk reduction associated with smoking cessation in patients with coronary heart disease: a systematic review. *JAMA* 2003; 290:86–97. Doi: 10.1001/jama.290.1.86.

28. AHA/ACC Heart Risk Calculator, http://www.cvriskcalculator.com/.

Chapter 7

1. National Institute of Diabetes and Digestive and Kidney Diseases (NIDDK) official website. Health Information/Diabetes. https://www.niddk.nih.gov/health-information/diabetes.

Centers for Disease Control and Prevention (CDC). National Diabetes Statistics Report 2020. Estimates of Diabetes and its Burden in the United States. https://www.cdc.gov/diabetes/pdfs/data/statistics/national-diabetes-statistics-report.Pdf.

2. AM Ahmed. History of Diabetes Mellitus. *Saudi Med J* 2002; 23:373–378.

3. National Institute of Diabetes and Digestive and Kidney Diseases (NIDDK) official website. Type 1 Diabetes. https://www.niddk.nih.gov/health-information/diabetes/overview/what-is-diabetes/type-1-diabetes.

4. M Bliss. *The Discovery of Insulin*. Toronto: McClelland & Steward, 1982.

5. NIDDK Type 1 Diabetes.

6. Jackie Robinson at age 53, shortly before his fatal heart attack on October 24, 1972. https://www.ebay.com/i/362305119438?chn=ps&norover=1&mkevt=1&mkrid=711-213727-13078-0&mkcid=2&itemid=362305119438&targetid=4580702888518295&device=c&mktype=&googleloc=&poi=&campaignid=395665092&mkgroupid=1233652256105976&rlsatarget=pla-4580702888518295&abcId=1129776&merchantid=51291&msclkid=8b01eecc521018263cc8b02a2adcb8a8.

7. CDC National Diabetes Statistics Report 2020.

8. National Institute of Diabetes and Digestive and Kidney Diseases (NIDDK) official website. Type 2 Diabetes. https://www.niddk.nih.gov/health-information/diabetes/overview/what-is-diabetes/type-2-diabetes.

9. A Cerami. The unexpected pathway to the creation of the HbA1c test and the discovery of AGE's. *J Intern Med* 2012; 271:218–226. Doi: 10.1111/j.1365-2796.2012.02514.x.

10. E Selvin, MW Steffes, H Zhu, K Matsushita, L Wagenknecht, J Panikow, J Coresh, FL Brancati. Glycated hemoglobin, diabetes, and cardiovascular risk in nondiabetic adults. *N Engl J Med* 2010; 800–811. doi: 10.1056/NEJMoa0908359.

11. Mayo Clinic. Type 2 Diabetes. https://www.mayoclinic.org/diseases-conditions/type-2-diabetes/diagnosis-treatment/drc-20351199.

12. American Diabetes Association.

Standards of Medical Care in Diabetes—2018. *Diabetes Care* 2018; 41 (supplement 1):S1-S159. http://diabetesed.net/wp-content/uploads/2017/12/2018-ADA-Standards-of-Care.pdf.

13. Mayo Clinic..

14. ADA Guidelines 2018, Figure 8.1.

15. ClinCalc DrugStats Database. The top 200 drugs of 2020. https://clincalc.com/DrugStats/Top200Drugs.aspx.

16. University of Minnesota Driven to Discover. Heart Attack Prevention. The University Group Diabetes Program (UGDP): A famous early randomized clinical trial (RCT). http://www.epi.umn.edu/cvdepi/essay/the-university-group-diabetes-program-ugdp-a-famousearly-randomized-clinical-trial-rct/.

17. TB Schwartz and CL Meinert. The UGDP controversy: Thirty-four years of contentious ambiguity laid to rest. *Perspect Biol Med* 2004; 47:564–574.

18. LA Conlay, JE Loewenstein. Phenformin and Lactic Acidosis. *JAMA* 1976; 235:1575–1578. doi:10.1001/jama.1976.03260410031019.

19. The Diabetes Control and Complications Trial Research Group. The effect of intensive treatment of diabetes on the development and progression of long-term complications in insulin-dependent diabetes mellitus. *N Engl J Med* 1993; 329:977–986.

20. P Reichard, BY Nilsson, U Rosenqvist. The effect of long-term intensified insulin treatment on the development of microvascular complications of diabetes mellitus. *N Engl J Med* 329: 304–309.

Y Ohkubo, H Kishikawa, E Araki, Y Kojima, N Furuyoshi, M Shichiri. Intensive insulin therapy prevents the progression of diabetic microvascular complications in Japanese patients with non-insulin dependent diabetes mellitus: a randomized prospective 6-year trial. *Diab Res Clin Pract* 1995; 28:103–117. https://www.diabetesresearchclinicalpractice.com/article/0168-8227(95)01064-K/pdf.

21. UK Prospective Diabetes Study (UKPDS) Group. Intensive blood-glucose control with sulphonylureas or insulin compared with conventional treatment and risk of complications in patients with type 2 diabetes (UKPDS 33). *Lancet* 1998; 352:837–853.

22. UK Prospective Diabetes Study (UKPDS) Group. Effect of intensive blood-glucose control with metformin on complications in overweight patients with type 2 diabetes (UKPDS 34). *Lancet* 1998; 352:854–865.

23. P King, I Peacock, R Donnelly. The UK Prospective Diabetes Study (UKPDS): clinical and therapeutic implications for type 2 diabetes. *J Clin Pharmacol* 1999; 48:643–649.

24. PD Home, SJ Pocock, H Beck-Nelson, R Gomis, M Hanefeld, NP Jones, M Komajada, JJV McMurray, for the RECORD Study Group. Rosiglitazone evaluated for cardiovascular outcomes—an interim analysis. *N Engl J Med* 2007; 357:28–38.

25. The BARI-2D Study Group. A randomized trial of therapies for type 2 diabetes and coronary artery disease. *N Engl J Med* 2009; 360:2503–2515.

26. JA Dormandy, B Charbonel, DJA Eckland, E Erdman, M Massi-Benedetti, IK Moules, MH Tan, PJ Lefebvre, GD Murray, E Standl, RG Wilcox, L Wilhelmsen, J Betteridge, K Birkeland, A Golay, RJ Heine, L Koranyi, M Laakso, M Mokan, A Norkus, V Pirags, T Podar, A Scheen, W Scherbaum, G Schernthaner, O Schmitz, J Skrha, U Smith, J Taton, on behalf of the PROActive Investigators. Secondary prevention of macrovascular events in patients with type 2 diabetes in the PROactive Study (PROspective pioglitzAzone Clinical Trial In macrovascular Events): a randomized controlled trial. *Lancet* 2005; 366:1279–1289. DOI: https://doi.org.10.1016/S0140-6736(05)67528-9.

27. S Singh, YK Loke, CD Furberg. Long-term risk of cardiovascular events with rosiglitazone: a meta-analysis. *JAMA* 2007; 298:1189–1195.

28. The Action to Control Cardiovascular Risk in Diabetes Study Group. Effects of intensive glucose lowering in type 2 diabetes. *N Engl J Med* 2008; 358:2545–2559.

29. The ADVANCE Collaborative Group. Intensive blood glucose control and vascular outcomes in patients with

type 2 diabetes. *N Engl J Med* 2008; 358: 2560–2572.

30. W Duckworth, C Abraira, T Moritz, D Reda, N Emanuele, PD Reaven, FJ Zieve, J Marks, SN Davis, R Hayward, SR Warren, S Goldman, M McCarren, ME Vitek, WG Henderson, GD Huang, for the VADT Investigators. Glucose control and vascular complications in veterans with type 2 diabetes. *N Engl J Med* 2009; 360:129–139.

31. The Look AHEAD Research Group. Cardiovascular effects of intensive lifestyle intervention in type 2 diabetes. *N Engl J Med* 2013; 369:145–154.

32. J Zhong, S Kankanala, S Rajagopalan. DPP4 inhibition: insights from the bench and recent clinical studies. *Curr Opin Lipidol* 2016; 27:484–492. doi: 10.1097/MOL.0000000000000340.

33. BM Scirica, DL Bhatt, E Braunwald, PG Steg, J Davidson, B Hirshberg, P Ohman, R Frederich, SD Wiviott, EB Hoffman, MA Cavender, JA Udell, NR Desai, O Mozenzon, DK McGuire, KK Ray, LA Leiter, I Raz, for the SAVOR-TIMI-53 Steering Committee and Investigators. Saxagliptin and cardiovascular outcomes in patients with type 2 diabetes mellitus. *N Eng J Med* 2013; 369:1317–1326. DOI: 10.1056/NEJMoa1307684.

WB White, CP Cannon, SR Heller, SE Nissen, RM Bergenstal, GL Bakris, AT Perez, PR Fleck, CR Mehta, S Kupfer, C Wilson, WC Cushman, F Zannad, for the Examine Investigators. Alogliptin after acute coronary syndrome in patients with type 2 diabetes. *N Engl J Med* 2013; 369:1327–1335. DOI: 10.1056/NEJMoa1305889.

JB Green, MA Bethel, PW Armstrong, JB Buse, SS Engel, J Garg, R Josse, KD Kaufman, J Koglin, S Korn, KM Lachin, DK McGuire, MJ Pencina, E Standl, PP Stein, S Suryawanshi, F Van de Werf, ED Peterson, RR Holman, for the TECOS Study Group. Effect of sitagliptin on cardiovascular outcomes in type 2 diabetes. *N Engl J Med* 2015; 373:232–242. DOI: 10.1056/NEJMoa1501352.

34. AJ Garber. Long-acting glucagon-like peptide 1 receptor agonists: a review of their efficacy and efficiency. *Diabetes Care* 2011; 34:S279-S284.

35. DS Hsia, O Grove, WT Cefalu. An update on SGLT2 inhibitors for the treatment of diabetes mellitus. *Curr Opin Diabetes Obes* 2017; 24:73–79.

36. JD Curb, SL Pressel, JA Cutler, PJ Savage, WB Applegate, H Black, G Carmel, BR Davis, PH Frost, N Gonzalez, G Guthrie, A Oberman, GH Rutan, J Stamler, for the Systolic Hypertension in the Elderly Program Cooperative Research Group. Effect of diuretic-based antihypertensive treatment on cardiovascular disease risk in older diabetic patients with isolated systolic hypertension. *JAMA* 1996; 276:1896–1892.

Cholesterol Treatment Trialists Collaboration. Efficacy of cholesterol-lowering therapy in 18,686 people with diabetes in 14 randomised trials of statins: a meta-analysis. *Lancet* 2008; 371:117–125.

37. CDC's Division of Diabetes Translation. United States Diabetes Surveillance System. Long-term Trends in Diabetes April 2017. https://www.cdc.gov/Diabetes/statistics/slides/long_term_trends.pdf.

CDC National Diabetes Statistical Report 2020. Estimates of Diabetes and its Burden in the United States. https://www.cdc.gov/diabetes/pdfs/data/statistics/national-diabetes-statistics-report.pdf.

38. A report from the American Heart Association. AHA Statistical Update Heart Disease and Stroke Statistics—2020 Update, Chapter 9: Diabetes Mellitus, Chart 9.6. *Circulation* 2020; 141:e139-e596. See p. e275. DOI: 10.1161/CIR.0000000000000757.

39. ES Ford, UA Ajani, JB Croft, JA Critchley, DR Labarth, TE Kottke, WH Giles, S Capewell. Explaining the Decrease in U.S. Deaths from Coronary Disease, 1980–2000. *N Engl J Med* 2007; 356:2388–2398. DOI: 10.1056/NEJMsa053935.

40. JA Salami, H Warralch, J Velardo-Elizondo, ES Spatz, NR Desai, JS Rana, SS Virani, R Blankstein, A Khera, MJ Blaha, RS Blumenthal, D Lloyd-Jones, K Nasir. National trends in statin use and expenditures, in the U.S. adult population from 2002 to 2013: Insights from the Medical Expenditure Panel survey. *JAMA Cardiology* 2017; 2:56–65. doi.10.1001/jamacardio.2016.4700. Cholesterol Treatment Trialists Collaboration.

Chapter 8

1. T Gordon, WP Castelli, MC Hjortland, WB Kannel, TR Dawber. High-density lipoprotein as a protective factor against coronary heart disease. The Framingham Study. *Am J Med* 1977; 62: 707–714.

2. M Krieger. The 'best' of cholesterols, the 'worst' of cholesterols: a tale of two receptors. *Proc Nat Acad Sci, USA* 1998; 95:4077–4080.

3. DJ Gordon, JL Probstfield, RJ Garrison, JD Neaton, WP Castelli, JD Knoke, DR Jacobs, S Bangdiwala, HA Tyroler. High-density lipoprotein and cardiovascular disease: Four American Studies. *Circulation* 1989; 79:8–15.

4. DJ Gordon, BM Rifkind. HDL—Clinical implications of recent studies. *N Engl J Med* 1989; 321:1311–1316.

DJ Gordon. Role of circulating HDL and triglycerides in coronary artery disease. *End Metab Clin N Amer* 1990; 19:299–310.

DJ Gordon. HDL and cardiovascular disease. *Cardiology Board Review* 1990; 7:29–40.

DJ Gordon. HDL and CHD—An epidemiologic perspective. *J Drug Devel* 1990, 3(suppl):11–17.

5. CE Kosmas, D Silverio, A Sourlas, F Garcia, PD Montan, E Guzman. Primary genetic disorders affecting high density lipoprotein (HDL). *Drugs in Context* 2018; 7: 212546. DOI: 10.7573/dic.212546.

6. MH Frick, O Elo, K Haapa, OP Heinonen, P Heinsalmi, P Helo, JK Huttunen, P Kaitaniemi, P Koskinen, V Manninen, H Maenpaa, M Malkonen, et al. Helsinki Heart Study: primary-prevention trial with gemfibrozil in middle-aged men with dyslipidemia. Safety of treatment, changes in risk factors, and incidence of coronary heart disease. *New England Journal of Medicine* 1987; 317: 1237–1245.

7. HB Rubins, SJ Robins, D Collins, CL Fye, JW Anderson, MB Elam, FH Faas, E Linares, EJ Schaefer, G Schectman, TJ Wilt, J Wittes. Gemfibrozil for the secondary prevention of coronary heart disease in men with low levels of high-density lipoprotein cholesterol. Veterans Affairs High-Density Lipoprotein Cholesterol Intervention Trial Study Group. *N Engl J Med* 1999; 341:410–418.

8. The ACCORD Study Group. The effect of combination lipid therapy in type 2 diabetes mellitus. *N Engl J Med* 2010; 362:1563–1574. DOI: 10.1056/NEJMoa1001282.

9. The AIM-HIGH Investigators. Niacin in patients with low HDL cholesterol levels receiving intensive statin therapy. *N Engl J Med* 2011; 365:2235–2267.

10. PJ Barter, HB Brewer, J Chapman, CH Hennekens, DJ Rader, AR Tall. Cholesteryl ester transfer protein. A novel target for raising HDL and inhibiting atherosclerosis. *Arteriosclerosis, Thrombosis, and Vascular Biology* 2003; 23:160–167.

11. AR Tall, DJ Rader. Trials and Tribulations of CETP inhibitors. *Circulation Research* 2018; 122:106–112. https://doi.org/10.1161/CIRCRESAHA.117.311978.

12. PJ Barter, M Caulfield, M Eriksson, SM Grundy, JJP Kastelein, M Kornajda, J Lopez-Sendon, L Mosca, JC Tardif, DD Waters, CL Shear, JH Revkin, KA Buhr, MR Fisher, AR Tall, HB Brewer, for the ILLUMINATE Investigators. Effects of torcetrapib in patients at high risk for coronary events. *N Engl J Med* 2007; 357:2109–2122. doi: 10.1056/NEJMoa0706628.

13. GG Schwartz, AG Olsson M Abt M, CM Ballantyne, PJ Barter, J Brumm, BR Chaitman, IM Holme, D Kallend, LA Leiter, E Leitersdorf, JJV McMurray, H Mundl, SJ Nicholls, PK Shah, JC Tardif, S Wright, dal-OUTCOMES Investigators. Effects of dalcetrapib in patients with a recent acute coronary syndrome. *N Engl J Med* 2012; 367:2089–2099. doi: 10.1056/NEJMoa1206797.

14. AM Lincoff, SJ Nicholls, JS Riesmeyer, PJ Barter, HB Brewer, KAA Fox, CM Gibson, C Granger, V Menon, G Montalescot, D Rader, AR Tall, E McErlean, K Wolski, G Ruatolo, B Vangerow, G Weerakkody, SG Goodman, D Conde, DK McGuire, JC Nicolau, JL Leiva-Pons, Y Pesant, W Li, D Kandath, S Kouz, N Takirkheli, D Mason, SE Nissen, for the ACCELERATE Investigators. Evacetrapib and cardiovascular outcomes in high-risk vascular disease. *N Engl J Med*

2017; 376:1933–1942. doi: 10.1056/NEJMoa1609581.

15. L Bowman, JC Hopewell, F Chen, K Wallendszus, W Stevens, R Collins, SD Wiviott, CP Cannon, E Braunwald, E Sammons, MJ Landray MJ. HPS3/TIMI55–REVEAL Collaborative Group. Effects of anacetrapib in patients with atherosclerotic vascular disease. *N Engl J Med* 2017; 377:1217–1227. doi: 10.1056/NEJMoa1706444.

Chapter 9

1. L Medina, S Sabo, J Vespa. Living Longer: Historical and Projected Life Expectancy in the United States, 1960–2060. Population Estimates and Projections. Current Population Reports. February 2020. https://www.census.gov/content/dam/Census/library/publications/2020/demo/p25-1145.pdf.

2. The Coronary Drug Project. Initial findings leading to modifications of its research protocol. *JAMA* 1970, Nov 16; 214(7):1303–1313.

3. TL Bush. Noncontraceptive estrogen use and risk of cardiovascular disease: an overview and critique of the literature. *The Menopause: Biological and Clinical Consequences of Ovarian Failure, Evolution and Management*. SG Korenman (ed.) Norwell, MA: Serono Symposia, USA, 1990, 211–2240.

D Grady, SM Rubin, DB Petiti, CS Fox, D Black, B Ettinger, VL Ernster, SR Cummings. Hormone therapy to prevent disease and prolog life in postmenopausal women. *Ann Intern Med* 1992; 117:1016–1037.

4. MJ Stampfer, GA Colditz. Estrogen replacement and coronary heart disease: a quantitative assessment of the epidemiologic evidence. *Prev Med* 1991; 20:47–63.

5. American Cancer Society. Menopausal hormone therapy and cancer risk. https://www.cancer.org/cancer/cancer-causes/medical-treatments/menopausal-hormone-replacement-therapy-and-cancer-risk.html.

6. HA Tyroler, CJ Glueck, B Christenson, PO Kwiterovich. Plasma high density lipoprotein cholesterol comparisons in black and white populations. The Lipid Research Clinics Prevalence Study. *Circulation* 1980; 62(suppl IV):99–107.

7. JC LaRosa, W Applegate, JR Crouse, D Hunninghake, R Grimm, R Knopp, J Eckfelt, CE Davis, DJ Gordon. Cholesterol lowering in the elderly: Results of the Cholesterol Reduction in Seniors Program (CRISP) pilot study. *Arch Int Med* 1994; 154:529–539.

8. The ALLHAT Officers and Coordinators for the ALLHAT Research Group. Major outcomes in moderately hypercholesterolemic, hypertensive patients randomized to pravastatin versus usual care: The Antihypertensive and Lipid Lowering Treatment to Prevent Heart Attack Trial. *JAMA* 2002; 288:2998–3007

9. The Writing Group for the PEPI Trial. Effects of Estrogen or Estrogen/Progestin Regimens on Heart Disease Risk Factors in Postmenopausal Women. The Postmenopausal Estrogen/Progestin Interventions (PEPI) Trial. *JAMA* 1995; 273:199–208.

10. JE Rossouw, LP Finnegan, WR Harlan, VW Pinn, C Clifford, JA McGowan. The evolution of the Women's Health Initiative: perspectives from the NIH. *J Am Med Women's Assoc* 1995; 50:50–55.

11. S Hulley, D Grady, T Bush, C Furberg, D Herrington, B Riggs, E Vittinghoff, for the Heart and Estrogen/Progestin Replacement Study (HERS) research group. Randomized trial of estrogen plus progestin for secondary prevention of coronary heart disease in postmenopausal women. *JAMA* 1998; 280:605–613.

12. The Women's Health Initiative Study Group. Design of the Women's Health Initiative Clinical Trial and Observational Study. *Controlled Clin Trials* 1998; 19:61–109.

13. DB Waters, EL Alderman, J Hsia, BV Howard, FR Cobb, WJ Rogers, P Ouyang, P Thompson, JC Tardif, L Higginson, V Bittner, M Steffes, DJ Gordon, M Proschan, N Younnes, J Verter. Effects of hormone replacement therapy and antioxidant vitamin supplements on coronary atherosclerosis in postmenopausal women. *JAMA* 2002; 288:2432–2440.

14. DM Herrington, DM Reboussin, B Brosnihan, PC Sharp, SA Schumaker, TE Snyder, CD Furberg, GJ Kowalchuk, TD

Stuckey, WJ Rogers, DH Givens, D Waters. Effects of estrogen replacement on the progression of coronary artery atherosclerosis. *N Engl J Med* 2000; 343:522–529.

HN Hodis, WJ Mack, SP Azen, RA Lobo, D Shoupe, PR Mahrer, DP Faxon, L Cashin-Hemphill, ME Sanmarco, WJ French, TL Shook, TD Gardner, AO Mehra, R Rabbani, A Sevanian, AB Shil, M Torres, KH Vogelbach, RH Selzer, for the Women's Estrogen/Progestin Lipid-Lowering Hormone Atherosclerosis Regression Trial.

15. DB Petiti. Hormone replacement therapy for prevention. More evidence, more pessimism. *JAMA* 2002; 288:99–101.

16. Writing Group for the Women's Health Study. Risks and benefits of estrogen plus progestin in healthy postmenopausal women. Principal results from the Women's Health Initiative randomized controlled trial. *JAMA* 2002; 288:321–333.

17. D Grady, D Herrington, V Bittner, R Blumenthal, M Davidson, M Hlatky, J Hsia, S Hulley, A Herd, S Khan, IK Newby, D Waters, E Vittinghoff, N Wenger, for the HERS Research Group. Cardiovascular disease outcomes during 6.8 years of hormone therapy. Heart and Estrogen/Progestin Replacement Study follow-up (HERS II). *JAMA* 2002; 288:49–57.

18. The Women's Health Initiative Steering Committee. Effects of conjugated equine estrogen in postmenopausal women with hysterectomy. The Women's Health Initiative randomized controlled trial. *JAMA* 2004; 291:1701–1712.

19. E Nabel. The Women's Health Initiative—a victory for women and their health. *JAMA* 2013; 310:1349–1350.

20. DS Buist, KM Newton, DL Miglioretti, K Beverly, MT Connelly, S Andrade, CL Hartsfield, F Wei, A Chan, L Kessler. Hormone therapy prescribing patterns in the United States. *Osbtet Gynecol* 2004; 104:1042–1050.

21. SA Tsai, ML Stefanik, RS Stafford. Trends in menopausal hormone therapy use of U.S. office-based physicians, 2000–2009. *Menopause* 2011; 18:285–392.

22. JA Roth, R Etzioni, TM Waters, M Pettinger, JE Rossouw, GL Anderson, RT Chlebowski, JE Manson, M Hlatky, KC Johnson, SD Ramsey. Economic return from the Women's Health Initiative estrogen plus progestin clinical trial: a modeling study. *Ann Intern Med* 2014, May 6; 160(9):594–602. doi: 10.7326/ M13–2348.

23. U.S. Department of Health and Human Services, National Institutes of Health, National Heart, Lung, and Blood Institute. Facts about Menopausal Hormone Therapy. NIH Publication No. 05–5200 (June 2005 Revision). https://www.nhlbi. nih.gov/files/docs/pht_facts.pdf.

24. JE Manson, RT Chebowski, ML Stefanick, AK Aragaki, JE Rossouw, RL Prentice, G Anderson, BV Howard, CA Thomson, AZ LaCroix, J Wactawski-Wende, RD Jackson, M Limacher, KL Margolis, S Wasserthal-Smoller, SA Beresford, JA Cauley, CB Eaton, M Gass, J Hsia, KC Johnson, C Kooperberg, LH Kuller, CE Lewis, S Liu, LW Martin, JK Ockene, MJ O'Sullivan, LH Powell, MS Simon, L Van Horn, MZ Vitolina, RB Wallace. Menopausal hormone therapy and health outcomes during the intervention and extended post-stopping phases of the Women's Health Initiative randomized trials. *JAMA* 2013; 310:1353–1368.

25. ClinicalTrials.gov. The Women's Health Initiative Memory Study (The WHIMS Study). https://clinicaltrials.gov/ ct2/show/NCT00685009?term=women% 27s+health+initiative&draw=2&rank=1.

ClinicalTrials.gov. The Women's Health Strong and Healthy Study (The WHISH Study). https://clinicaltrials.gov/ct2/ show/NCT02425345?term=women%27s +health+initiative&draw=1&rank=3.

26. ES Ford, UA Ajani, JB Croft, JA Critchley, DR Labarth, TE Kottke, WH Giles, S Capewell. Explaining the Decrease in U.S. Deaths from Coronary Disease, 1980–2000. *N Engl J Med* 2007; 356:2388–2398. DOI: 10.1056/NEJMsa053935.

Chapter 10

1. M Alkhouli, F Alqahtini, A Kalra, S Gafoor, M Alhajii, M Alreshidan, DR Holmes, A Leman. Trends in characteristics and outcomes of hospital inpatients

undergoing coronary revascularization in the United States, 2003–2016. *JAMA Network Open* 2020; 3(2):e1921326. doi:10.1001/jamanetworkopen.2019.21326. https://jamanetwork.com/journals/jamanetworkopen/fullarticle/2760898.

2. W Röntgen. Ueber eine neue Art von Strahlen. Vorläufige Mitteilung. *Aus den Sitzungsberichten der Würzburger Physik.-medic. Gesellschaft Würzburg*, pp. 137–147, 1895.

3. A Meyer. Werner Forssmann and the catheterization of the heart, 1929. *Ann Thorac Surg* 1990;49:497–499.

4. TJ Ryan. The coronary angiogram and its seminal contributions to cardiovascular medicine over five decades. Circulation 2002; 106:752-756.

5. RJ Morris. The history of cardiopulmonary bypass: medical advances. American College of Cardiology, June 19, 2019. https://www.acc.org/latest-in-cardiology/articles/2019/06/19/06/46/the-history-of-cardiopulmonary-bypass.

American College of Cardiology Expert Analysis. The history of cardiopulmonary bypass: medical advances. https://www.acc.org/latest-in-cardiology/articles/2019/06/19/06/46/the-history-of-cardiopulmonary-bypass.

6. L Melly, G Torregrossa, T Lee, JL Jansens, JD Puskas. Fifty years of coronary bypass grafting. *J Thoracic Dis* 2018; 1960–1967. Doi: 10.21037/jtd2018.02.43.

7. AL Hawkes, M Nowak, B Bidstrup, R Speare. Outcomes of coronary artery bypass graft surgery. *Vascular Health and Risk Management* 2006; 2:477–484.

8. ED Grech. Percutaneous coronary intervention. I. History and Development. *BMJ* 2003; 326:1080–1082.

9. M Barton, J Grüntzig, M Huisman, J Rüsch. Balloon angioplasty—the legacy of Andreas Grüntzig, M.D. (1939–1985). *Frontiers in Cardiovascular Medicine* 2014; 1(15):1–25. Doi: 10.3389/fcvm.2014.00015.

10. ED Grech.

11. A Roguin. Stent: The man and word behind the coronary metal prosthesis. *Circulation: Cardiovascular Interventions* 2011; 4:206–209. https://doi.org/10.1161/CIRCINTERVENTIONS.110.960872.

12. R Piccolo, KH Bonaa, O Efthimiou, O Varenne, A Baldo, P Urban, C Kaiser, W Remkes, L Raber, A de Belder, AWJ van't Hof, G Stankovic, PA Lemos, T Wilsgaard, J Reifart, AE Rodriguez, EE Ribeiro, PWJC Serruys, A Abizaid, M Sabate, RA Byrne, JMT Hernandez, W Wijns, P Juni, S Windecker, M Valgimigli, on behalf of the Coronary Stents Trialists' Collaboration. *Lancet* 2019; 393: 2503–2510. DOI: https://doi.org/10.1016/S0140-6736(19)30474-X.

LO Jansen and EH Christensen. Are drug-eluting stents safer than bare metal stents? *Lancet* 2019; 393:2472–2474. DOI: https://doi.org/10.1016/S0140-6736(19)31000-1.

13. European Coronary Surgery Study Group. Long-term results of prospective randomized study of coronary artery bypass surgery in stable angina patients. *Lancet* 1992; 320:1173–1180. DOI: https://doi.org/10.1016/S0140-6736(82)91200-4.

14. CASS Principal Investigators and Their Associates. Myocardial infarction and mortality in the Coronary Artery Surgery Study (CASS) randomized trial. *N Engl J Med* 1984; 310:750–758. DOI: 10.1056/NEJM198403223101204.

15. The VA Coronary Artery Bypass Surgery Cooperative Study Group. Eighteen-year follow-up in the Veterans Affairs Cooperative Study of Coronary Artery Bypass Surgery for Stable Angina. *Circulation* 1992; 86:121–130.

16. T Takaro, P Peduzzi, KM Detre, HN Hultgren, ML Murphy, J van der Bel-Kahn, J Thomsen, WR Meadows. Survival in subgroups of patients with left main coronary artery disease. Veterans Affairs Cooperative Study of Surgery for Coronary Arterial Occlusive Disease. *Circulation* 1982; 66:14–22.

17. ClinicalTrials.gov. Completed interventional trials of stents in coronary artery disease. Accessed July 5, 2020, https://clinicaltrials.gov/ct2/results?term=stents&cond=Coronary+Artery+Disease&recrs=e&age_v=&gndr=&type=Intr&rslt=&Search=Apply#.

18. RJ Gibbons, K Chatterjee, J Daley, JS Douglas, SD Fihn, JM Gardin, MA Grunwald, D Levy, BW Lytle, RA O'Rourke, WP Schafer, SV Williams, JL Ritchie,

MD Cheitlin, KA Eagle, TJ Gardner, A Garson, RO Russell, TJ Ryan, SC Smith. ACC/AHA/ACP—ASIM Guidelines for the Management of Patients with Chronic Stable Angina: Executive Summary and Recommendations. A report of the American College of Cardiology/American Heart Association task force on practice guidelines (Committee on Management of Patients with Chronic Stable Angina). *Circulation* 1999; 99:2829–2848. https://doi.org/10.1161/01.CIR.99.21.2829.

19. The Bypass Angioplasty Revascularization (BARI) Investigators. Comparison of coronary bypass surgery with angioplasty in patients with multivessel disease. *N Engl J Med* 1996; 335:217–225.

20. The BARI-2D Study Group. A randomized trial of therapies for type 2 diabetes and coronary artery disease. *N Engl J Med* 2009; 360:2503–2515.

21. WE Boden, RA O'Rourke, KK Teo, PM Hartigan, DJ Maron, WJ Kostuk, M Knudtson, M Dada, P Casperson, CL Harris, BR Chaitman, L Shaw, G Gosselin, S Nawaz, LM Title, G Gau, AS Blaustein, DC Booth, ER Bates, JA Spertus, DS Berman, J Mancini, WS Weintraub, for the COURAGE Trial Research Group. Optimal medical therapy with or without PCI for stable coronary disease. *N Engl J Med* 2007; 356:1503–1516.

22. CinicalTrials.gov. SYNTAX Study: TAXUS drug-eluting stent versus coronary artery bypass surgery for the treatment of narrowed arteries (SYNTAX). https://clinicaltrials.gov/ct2/show/NCT00114972?term=SYNTAX+Trial&draw=2&rank=2.

23. PW Serruys, MC Morice, AP Kappetein, A Columbo, DR Holmes, MJ Mack, E Stahle, TE Feldman, M van den Brand, EJ Bass, N Van Duck, K leadley, KD Dawkins, FW Mohr, for the SYNTAX Investigators. P ercutaneous coronary intervention versus coronary-artery bypass grafting for sever coronary artery disease. *N Engl J Med* 2009; 360:961–972.

24. SD Fihn, JM Gardin, J Abrams, K Berra, JC Blankenship, AP Dallas, PS Douglas, JM Foody, TC Gerber, AL Hinderliter, SB King, PD Kligfield, HM Krumholz, RYK Kwong, MJ Lim, JA Linderbaum, MJ Mack, MA Munger, RL Prager, JF Sabik, LJ Shaw, JD Sikkema, CR Smith, SC Smith, JA Spertus, SV Williams. 2012 ACCF/AHA/ACP/AATS/PCNA/SCAI/STS Guideline for the Diagnosis and Management of Patients with Stable Ischemic Heart Disease. A report of the American College of Cardiology Foundation/American Heart Association Task Force on Practice Guidelines, and the American College of Physicians, American Association for Thoracic Surgery, Preventive Cardiovascular Nurses Association, Society for Cardiovascular Angiography and Intervention, and Society of Thoracic Surgeons. *Circulation* 2012; 126:e354-e471. DOI: 10.1161/CIR.0b013e318277d6a0.

25. DJ Maron, JS Hochman, HR Reynolds, S Bangalore, SM O'Brien, WE Boden, BR Chaitman, R Senior, J López-Sendón, KP Alexander, RD Lopes, LJ Shaw, JS Berger, JD Newman, MS Sidhu, SG Goodman, W Ruzyllo, G Gosselin, AP Maggioni, HD White, B Bhargava, JK Min, GBJ Mancini, DS Berman, MH Picard, RY Kwong, ZA Ali, DB Mark, JA Spertus, MN Krishnan, A Elghamaz, N Moorthy, WA Hueb, M Demkow, K Mavromatis, O Bockeria, J Peteiro, TD Miller, H Szwed, R Doerr, M Keltai, JB Selvanayagam, PG Steg, C Held, S Kohsaka, S Mavromichalis, R Kirby, NO Jeffries, FE Harrell, FW Rockhold, S Broderick, TB Ferguson, DO Williams, RA Harrington, GW Stone, Y Rosenberg, ISCHEMIA Research Group. I nitial invasive or conservative strategy for stable coronary disease. *N Engl J Med* 2020; 382:1395–1407. doi: 10.1056/NEJMoa191592.

26. Maron, et al., Table 2.

27. N Sikri, A Bardia. A history of streptokinase use in acute myocardial infarction. *Texas Heart Inst J* 2007; 34:318–327.

28. JW Kennedy. Streptokinase for the treatment of acute myocardial infarction: a brief review of randomized trials. *J Am Coll Cardiol* 1987; 10:28B-32B.

29. GISSI. Effectiveness of intravenous thrombolytic treatment in acute myocardial infarction. *Lancet* 1986; 1:397-402.

30. F Rovelli, C De Vita, GA Feruglio, A Lotto, A Selvini, G Tognoni and GISSI Investigators. GISSI Trial: early results and

late follow-up. *J Am Coll Cardiol* 1987; 10:33B-39B.

31. E Braunwald, MS Sabatine. The Thrombolysis in Myocardial Infarction (TIMI) group experience. *J Thorac Cardiovasc Surg* 2012; 144:762–770.

The TIMI Study Group. The Thrombolysis in Myocardial Infarction Trial—Phase I Findings. *N Engl J Med* 1985; 312:932–936. DOI: 10.1056/NEJM19850404.

JH Chesebro, G Knatterud, R Roberts, J Borer, LS Cohen, J Dalen, HT Dodge, CK Francis, D Hillis, P Ludbrook, JE Markis, H Mueller, ER Passamani, ER Powers, AK Rao, T Robertson, A Ross, TJ Ryan, BE Sobel, J Willerson, DO Williams, BL Zaret, E Braunwald. Thrombolysis in Myocardial Infarction (TIMI) Trial, Phase I: a comparison between intravenous tissue plasminogen activator and intravenous streptokinase. Clinical findings through hospital discharge. *Circulation* 1987; 76:142–154.

Gruppo Italiano per la Sperimentazione della Streptchinasi nell'Infarto Miocardico. GISSI-2: a factorial randomized trial of altepase versus streptokinase and heparin versus no heparin among 12,490 patients with acute myocardial infarction. *Lancet* 1990; 8797:65–71.

ISIS-3 (Third International Study of Infarct Survival) Collaborative Group. ISIS-3: a randomized comparison of streptokinase vs tissue plasminogen activator vs anistreplase and of aspirin plus heparin versus aspirin alone among 41,299 cases of suspected acute myocardial infarction. *Lancet* 1992; 8976:753–770. DOI: https://doi.org/10.1016/0140-6736(92)91893-D.

32. The GUSTO Investigators. An international randomized trial comparing four thrombolytic strategies for acute myocardial infarction. *N Engl J Med* 1993; 329:673–672.

33. EJ Topol. Coronary angioplasty for acute myocardial infarction. *Ann Intern Med* 1988; 109:970–980.

34. KB Michels, S Yusuf. Does PTCA in acute myocardial infarction affect mortality and reinfarction rates? A quantitative overview (meta-analysis) of the randomized clinical trials. *Circulation* 1995; 91:476–485. https://doi.org/10.1161/01.CIR.91.2.476.

35. The Global Use of Strategies to Open Occluded Coronary Arteries in Acute Coronary Syndromes (GUSTO IIb) Angioplasty Substudy Investigators. A clinical trial comparing primary angioplasty with tissue plasminogen activator for acute myocardial infarction. *N Engl J Med* 1997; 336:1621–1628.

36. JS Hochman, LA Sleeper, JG Webb, TA Sanborn, HD White, JD Talley, CE Buller, AK Jacobs, JN Slater, J Col, SM McKinlay, TH LeMetel, for the SHOCK Investigators. *N Engl J Med* 1999; 341:625–634.

37. EC Keeley, JA Boura, CL Grines. Primary angioplasty versus intravenous thrombolytic therapy for acute myocardial infarction: a quantitative review of 23 randomized trials. *Lancet* 2003; 361:13–20.

38. JS Hochman, GA Lamas, CE Buller, V Dzavik, HR Reynolds, SJ Abramsky, S Forman, W Ruzyllo, AP Maggione, H White, Z Sadowski, AC Carvalho, JM Rankin, JP Renkin, PG Steg, AM Mascette, G Sopko, ME Pfisterer, J Leor, V Fridrich, DB Mark, GL Knatterud, for the Occluded Artery Trial Investigators. Coronary intervention for persistent occlusion after myocardial infarction. *N Engl J Med* 2006; 355:2395–2407.

39. ClinCalc DrugStats Database. The top 200 drugs of 2020. https://clincalc.com/DrugStats/Top200Drugs.aspx.

40. P O'Gara, FD Kushner, DD Ascheim, DE Casey, MK Chung, JA de Lemos, SM Ettinger, JC Fang, FM Fesmire, BA Franklin, CB Granger, HM Krumholz, JA Linderbaum, DA Morrow, LK Newby, JP Ornato, N Ou, MJ Radford, JE Tamis-Holland, CL Tommaso, CM Tracy, YJ Woo, DX Zhao. 2013 ACCF/AHA Guideline for the Management of ST-Elevation Myocardial Infarction. A report of the American College of Cardiology Foundation/American Heart Association Task Force on Practice Guidelines. *JACC* 2013; e78-e140.

EA Amsterdam, NK Wenger, RG Brindis, DE Casey, TG Ganiats, DR Holmes, AS Jaffe, H Jneid, RF Kelly, MC Kontos, GN Levine, PR Liebson, D Mukherjee, ED Peterson, MS Sabatine, RW Smalling, SJ Zieman. 2014 AHA/ACC Guidelines for the Management of Patients with Non-ST-Elevation Acute Coronary Syndromes. A report of the American College of Cardiology Foundation/American Heart Association Task Force on Practice Guidelines. *JACC* 2014; 64:e139-e228.

41. HM Krumholz, J Herrin, LE Miller, EE Drye, SM Ling, LF Han, MT Rapp, EH Bradley, BK Nallamothu, W Nsa, DW Bratzler, JP Curtis. Improvements in door-to-balloon time in the United States, 2005-2010. *Circulation* 2011; 124:1038-1045. doi:10.1161/CIRCULATIONAHA.111.044107.

42. ES Ford, UA Ajani, JB Croft, JA Critchley, DR Labarth, TE Kottke, WH Giles, S Capewell. Explaining the Decrease in U.S. Deaths from Coronary Disease, 1980-2000. *N Engl J Med* 2007; 356:2388-2398. DOI: 10.1056/NEJMsa053935.

43. L Chacko, JP Howard, C Rajkumar, AN Nowbar, C Kane, D Mahdi, M Foley, M Shun-Shin, G Cole, S Sen, A Al-Lamee, DP Francis, Y Ahmad. Effects of percutaneous coronary intervention on death and myocardial infarction stratified by stable and unstable coronary artery disease. A meta-analysis of randomized controlled trials. *Circ Cardiovasc Qual Outcomes* Feb. 2020; 13:e006363. DOI: 10.1161/CIRCOUTCOMES.119.006363. https://www.ahajournals.org/doi/pdf/10.1161/CIRCOUTCOMES.119.006363.

44. M Ragosta, S Dee, IJ Sarembock, LC Lipson, LW Gimple, ER Powers. Prevalence of unfavorable angiographic characteristics for percutaneous intervention in patients with unprotected left main coronary artery disease. *Catheter Cardiovasc Interv* 2007; 68:357-362. doi: 10.1002/ccd.20709.

45. D Maron, et al.

46. L Chacko, et al.

47. FA Masoudi, A Ponikaris, JA de Lemos, JG Jollis, M Kremers, JC Messinger, JWM Moore, I Moussa, WJ Oetgen, PD Varosy, RN Vincent, J Wei, JP Curtis, MT Roe, JA Spertus. Trends in U.S. cardiovascular Care. 2016 Reports from 4 ACC National Cardiovascular Registries. *J Am Col Cardiol* 2016; 69:1427-1450.

48. Morbidity and Mortality. 2012 Chartbook on Cardiovascular, Lung and Blood Diseases, NIH-NHLBI. Chart 3-22. https://www.nhlbi.nih.gov/files/docs/research/2012_ChartBook_508.pdf.

JE Dalen, JS Alpert, RJ Goldberg, RS Weinstein. The epidemic of the 20th century: Coronary Heart Disease. *The American Journal of Medicine* 2014; 127:807-812.

49. PA Kavsak, AR MacRae, V Lustig, R Bhargava, R Vandersluis, GE Polomaki, ML Yerna, AS Jaffe. The impact of the ESC/ACC redefinition of myocardial infarction and new sensitive troponin assays on the frequency of acute myocardial infarction. *Am Heart J* 2005; 152:118-125.

50. Morbidity and Mortality. 2012 Chartbook on Cardiovascular, Lung and Blood Diseases, NIH-NHLBI. Charts 3-22, 3-23, and 3-24. https://www.nhlbi.nih.gov/files/docs/research/2012_ChartBook_508.pdf.

Health, United States. 2012 Updates. https://www.cdc.gov/nchs/data/hus/2012/001.pdf.

51. RW Yeh, S Sydney, M Chandra, M Sorel, JV Selby, AS Go. Population trends in the incidence and outcomes of acute myocardial infarction. *N Engl J Med* 2010; 362:2155-2165.

Chapter 11

1. DR Ginsberg. Aspirin: turn-of-the-century miracle drug. *Distillations*, June 2, 2009. https://www.sciencehistory.org/distillations/aspirin-turn-of-the-century-miracle-drug.

2. PC Elwood, AL Cochrane, ML Burr, PM Sweetman, G Williams, E Welsby, SJ Hughes, R Renton. A randomized controlled trial of acetyl salicylic acid in the secondary prevention of mortality from myocardial infarction. *BMJ* 1974; 1:436-440.

3. Antiplatelet Trialists Collaboration. Collaborative overview of randomized trials of antiplatelet therapy—I. Prevention of death, myocardial infarction, and stroke by prolonged antiplatelet therapy in various categories of patients. *BMJ* 1994; 308:81-106.

4. The Aspirin Myocardial Infarction Study Research Group. A randomized

controlled trial of aspirin in persons recovered from a heart attack. *JAMA* 1980; 243:661–669.

5. Steering Committee of the Physicians' Health Study Research Group. *N Engl J Med* 1989; 321:129–135. DOI: 10.1056/NEJM198907203210301.

6. Antithrombotic Trialists (ATT) Collaboration. Aspirin in the primary and secondary prevention of vascular disease: collaborative meta-analysis of individual participant data from randomized trials. *Lancet* 2009; 373:1849–1860. Supplementary webappendix, https://researchonline.lshtm.ac.uk/id/eprint/19177/1/mmc1.pdf.

7. U.S. Preventive Services Task Force. Aspirin for the prevention of cardiovascular disease: U.S. Preventive Services Task Force recommendation statement. *Ann Intern Med* 2009; 150:396–404. https://doi.org/10.7326/0003-4819-150-6-200903170-00008.

8. The Norwegian Multicenter Study Group. Timolol-induced reduction in mortality and reinfarction in patients surviving acute myocardial infarction. *N Engl J Med* 1981; 304:801–807.

9. Beta-Blocker Heart Attack Trial Research Group. A randomized trial of propranolol in patients with acute myocardial infarction. I. Mortality results. *JAMA* 1982; 247:1707–1714.

10. First International Study of Infarct Survival Collaborative Group. Randomised trial of intravenous atenolol among 16,027 cases of suspected acute myocardial infarction: ISIS-1. *Lancet* 1986; 2:57–66.

11. N Freemantle, J Cleland, P Young, J Mason, J Harrison. Beta blockade after myocardial infarction: systematic review and meta regression analysis. *BMJ* 1999; 318:1730–1737.

12. The CAPRICORN Investigators. Effect of carvedilol on outcome after myocardial infarction in patients with left-ventricular dysfunction: the CAPRICORN randomized trial. *Lancet* 2001; 357:1385–1390.

13. J McMurray, L Kober, M Robertson, H Dargie, W Colucci, J Lopez-Sendon, W Remme, DN Sharpe, I Ford. Antiarrhythmic effect of carvedilol after acute myocardial infarction. Result of the Carvedilol Post-Infarct Survival Control in Left Ventricular Dysfunction (CAPRICORN) Trial. *JACC* 2005; 45:525–530.

CM Pratt. Three decades of clinical trials with beta-blockers. The Contribution of the CAPRICORN trial and the effect of carvedilol on serious arrhythmias. *JACC* 2005; 45:531–532.

14. P O'Gara, FD Kushner, DD Ascheim, DE Casey, MK Chung, JA de Lemos, SM Ettinger, JC Fang, FM Fesmire, BA Franklin, CB Granger, HM Krumholz, JA Linderbaum, DA Morrow, LK Newby, JP Ornato, N Ou, MJ Radford, JE Tamis-Holland, CL Tommaso, CM Tracy, YJ Woo, DX Zhao. 2013 ACCF/AHA Guideline for the Management of ST-Elevation Myocardial Infarction. A report of the American College of Cardiology Foundation/American Heart Association Task Force on Practice Guidelines. *JACC* 2013; e78-e140.

EA Amsterdam, NK Wenger, RG Brindis, DE Casey, TG Ganiats, DR Holmes, AS Jaffe, H Jneid, RF Kelly, MC Kontos, GN Levine, PR Liebson, D Mukherjee, ED Peterson, MS Sabatine, RW Smalling, SJ Zieman. 2014 AHA/ACC Guidelines for the Management of Patients with Non-ST-Elevation Acute Coronary Syndromes. A report of the American College of Cardiology Foundation/American Heart Association Task Force on Practice Guidelines. *JACC* 2014; 64:e139-e228.

15. ClinCalc DrugStats Database. The top 200 drugs of 2020. https://clincalc.com/DrugStats/Top200Drugs.aspx.

16. J Speller. The Renin-Angiotensin-Aldosterone System. Teach Me Physiology, April 20, 2020. https://teachmephysiology.com/urinary-system/regulation/the-renin-angiotensin-aldosterone-system/.

17. ClinCalc DrugStats Database.

18. J Bryan. How spironolactone became the next best thing for severe heart failure. *Pharmaceutical Journal*, January 18, 2012. https://www.pharmaceutical-journal.com/news-and-analysis/how-spironolactone-became-the-next-best-thing-for-severe-heart-failure/11093181.article?firstPass=false.

19. DW Cushman, MA Ondetti. History of the design of captopril and related

inhibitors of angiotensin converting enzyme. *Hypertension* 1991; 4:589–592.

20. The Consensus Trial Study Group. Effects of enalopril on mortality in severe congestive heart failure. *N Engl J Med* 1987; 316:1429–1435. DOI: 10.1056/NEJM198706043162301.

The SOLVD Investigators. Effect of enalopril on survival in patients with reduced left ventricular ejection fractions and congestive heart failure. *N Engl J Med* 1991; 325:293–302.

JN Cohn, G Johnson, S Ziesche, F Cobb, G Francis, F Tristani, R Smith, B Dunkman, H Loeb, M Wong, G Bhat, S Goldman, RD Fletcher, J Doherty, CV Hughes, P Carson, G Cintron, R Shabetai, C Haakenson. A comparison of enalopril with hydralazine-isosorbide dinitrate in the treatment of chronic congestive heart failure. *N Engl J Med* 1991; 325:303–310.

21. MA Pfeffer, E Braunwald, LA Moye, L Basta, EJ Brown, TF Cuddy, BR Davis, EM Geltman, S Goldman, GC Flaker, M Klein, GA Lamas, M Packer, J Rouleau, JL Rouleau, J Rutherford, JH Wertheimer, CM Hawkins, on behalf of the SAVE Investigators. Effect of captopril on mortality and morbidity in patients with left ventricular dysfunction after myocardial infarction. Results of the Survival and Ventricular Enlargement Trial. *N Engl J Med* 1992; 327:669–677.

22. L Kober, C Turp-Pedersen, JE Carlsen, H Bagger, P Eliasen, K Lyngborg, J Videbaek, DS Cole, L Auclert, NC Pauly, E Aliot, S Persson, AJ Camm, for the Trandolapril Cardiac Evaluation Study Group. A clinical trial of the angiotensin-converting enzyme inhibitor trandolapril in patients with left ventricular dysfunction after myocardial infarction. *N Engl J Med* 1995; 333:1670–1676.

23. JGF Cleland, L Erhardt, G Murray, AS Hall, SG Bell, on behalf of the AIRE Study Investigators. Effect of ramipril on morbidity and mode of death among survivors of acute myocardial infarction with clinical evidence of heart failure. A Report from the AIRE Study Investigators. *Eur Heart J* 1997; 18:41–51.

24. The Heart Outcomes Prevention Evaluation Study Investigators. Effects of an angiotensin-converting enzyme inhibitor, ramipril, on cardiovascular events in high risk patients. *N Engl J Med* 2000; 342:145–153.

25. S Bangalore, R Fakheri, B Toklu, G Ogedegbe, H Weintraub, FH Messerli. Angiotensin-Converting Enzyme Inhibitors or Angiotensin Receptor Blockers in Patients Without Heart Failure? Insights From 254,301 Patients From Randomized Trials. *Mayo Clin Proc* 2016; 91:51–60.

26. P O'Gara, et al., and EA Amsterdam. ACCF/AHA Guidelines.

27. ClinCalc DrugStats Database.

28. The Digitalis Investigators Group. The effect of digoxin on mortality and morbidity in patients with heart failure. *N Engl J Med* 1997; 336:525–533.

29. R Steckelberg, JS Newman. The fascinating foxglove. *ACP Hospitalist*, March 2010. https://acphospitalist.org/archives/2010/03/newman.htm.

30. FI Marcus. Editorial: Use of digitalis in acute myocardial infarction. *Circulation* 1980; 62:17–19.

31. SA Haji, A Mohaved. Update on digoxin therapy in congestive heart failure. *Am Fam Physician* 2000; 62:409–416.

32. Digoxin. Drug usage statistics, 2007–2017. https://clincalc.com/DrugStats/Drugs/Digoxin.

33. ES Ford, UA Ajani, JB Croft, JA Critchley, DR Labarth, TE Kottke, WH Giles, S Capewell. Explaining the Decrease in U.S. Deaths from Coronary Disease, 1980–2000. *N Engl J Med* 2007; 356:2388–2398. DOI: 10.1056/NEJMsa053935.

34. NS Shah, MD Huffman, H Ning, DM Lloyd-Jones. Trends in myocardial infarction secondary prevention: The National Health and Nutrition Examination Surveys (NHANES), 1999–2012. *J Am Heart Assoc* 2015; 4:1–12. doi:10.1161/JAHA.114.001709. https://www.ahajournals.org/doi/pdf/10.1161/JAHA.114.001709.

Chapter 12

1. A report from the American Heart Association. AHA Statistical Update: Heart Disease and Stroke Statistics—2020

Update, Chapters 14 and 17. *Circulation* 2020; 141:e139-e596. OI: 10.1161/ CIR.0000000000000757.

Cardiac Arrest Registry to Enhance Survival (CARES) website. https://mycares. net/.

2. RJ Myerburg, J Junttila. Sudden cardiac death caused by coronary heart disease. *Circulation* 2012; 125:1043–1052.

3. PCSB Protein Data Bank. Molecule of the Month. Sodium Potassium Pump. 2009–2010. https://cbm.msoe. edu/teacherWorkshops/ddtyResources/ documents/sodiumPotassiumPump.pdf.

4. CT January, LS Wann, JS Alpert, H Calkins, JE Cigarroa, JC Cleveland, JB Cont, PT Ellinor, MD Ezekowitz, ME Field, KT Murray. 2014 AHA/ACC/HRS Guideline for the Management of Patients with Atrial Fibrillation. A report of the American College of Cardiology/American Heart Association Task Force on Practice Guidelines and the Heart Rhythm Society. *JACC* 2014; 64:2246–2280. Developed in collaboration with the Society of Thoracic Surgeons. http://dx.doi.org/10.1016/j. jacc.2014.03.021.

5. LA Cobb, CE Fahrenbruch, M Olsufka, MK Copass. Changing incidence of out-of-hospital ventricular fibrillation, 1980–2000. *JAMA* 2002; 288:3008–3013.

6. AHA Statistical Update 2020, Chapters 14 and 17.

U.S. Population Age Profile 1960–97, Centers for Disease Control and Prevention (CDC), National Center of Health Statistics Mortality Data, Table 5: Age-adjusted death rates for selected causes of death by sex, race and Hispanic origin, United States, selected years 1950–2017. https:// www.cdc.gov/nchs/hus/contents2018. htm#Table_005.

7. SM Al-Khatib, WG Stevenson, MJ Ackerman, WJ Bryant, DJ Callans, AB Curtis, BJ Deal, T Dickfeld, ME Field, GC Fonarow, AM Gillis, CB Granger, SC Hammill, MA Hlatky, JA Joglar, GN Kay, DD Matlock, RJ Myerburg, RL Page. 2017 AHA/ACC/HRS Guideline for Management of Patients with Ventricular Arrhythmias and the Prevention of Sudden Cardiac Death. A report of the American College of Cardiology/American Heart Association Task Force on Clinical Practice Guidelines and the Heart Rhythm Society. *Circulation* 2018; 138:e272-e391. doi: 10.1161/ CIR.0000000000000549.

8. Cardiac Arrhythmia Suppression Trial (CAST) Investigators. Preliminary report: effect of encainide and flecainide on mortality in a randomized trial of arrhythmia suppression after myocardial infarction. *N Engl J Med* 1989; 32:406–12. https://www.ncbi.nlm.nih.gov/pub med/2473403?dopt=Abstract.

9. SJ Connolly. Meta-analysis of anti-arrhythmic drug trials. *Am J Cardiol* 2004; 84(supplement 1):90–93. DOI: https://doi.org/10.1016/S0002-9149(99)00708-0.

10. SJ Connolly, P Dorian, RS Roberts, M Gent, S Bailin, ES Fain, K Thorpe, J Champagne, M Talajic, B Coutu, GC Cronefield, SH Hohnloser, for the Optimal Pharmacological Therapy in Cardioverter Defibrillator Patients (OPTIC) Investigators. Comparison of beta-blockers, amiodarone plus beta-blockers, or sotalol for prevention of shocks from implantable cardioverter defibrillators. The OPTIC Study: a randomized trial. *JAMA* 2006; 295:165–171.

11. GH Bardy, KL Lee, DB Mark, JE Poole, DL Packer, R Boineau, M Domanski, C Troutman, J Anderson, SE McNulty, N Clapp-Channing, LD Davidson-Ray, ES Fraulo, DP Fishbein, RM Luceri, JH Ip, for the Sudden Cardiac Death in Heart Failure Trial (SCD-HeFT) Investigators. Amiodarone or an implantable cardioverter-defibrillator for congestive heart failure. *N Engl J Med* 2005; 352:225–237.

12. RN Fogoros. Amiodarone lung toxicity. verywellhealth. https://www. verywellhealth.com/amiodarone-lung-toxicity-1745988.

ClinCalc DrugStats Database. Amiodarone Hydrochloride. https:// clincalc.com/DrugStats/Drugs/ AmiodaroneHydrochloride.

13. AHA Statistical Update: Heart Disease and Stroke Statistics—2020 Update, Table 25.2 (2014 data). *Circulation* 2020; 141:e139-e596. OI: 10.1161/ CIR.0000000000000757.

14. The Antiarrhythmics Versus

Implantable Defibrillator (AVID) Investigators. A comparison of antiarrhythmic drug therapy with implantable defibrillators in patients resuscitated from near-fatal ventricular arrhythmias. *N Engl J Med* 1997; 337:1576–1583.

SJ Connolly, M Gent, RS Roberts, P Doran, D Roy, RS Sheldon, LB Mitchell, MS Green, GJ Klein, B O'Brien, for the CIDS Investigators. Canadian Implantable Defibrillator Study (CIDS): A randomized controlled trial of the implantable cardioverter defibrillator against amiodarone. *Circulation* 2000; 101:1297–1302.

KH Kuck, R Cappato, J Siebels, R Ruppel, for the CASH Investigators. Randomized comparison of antiarrhythmic drug therapy with implantable defibrillators in patients resuscitated from cardiac arrest. *Circulation* 2000; 102:748–754.

15. RT Borne, D Katz, J Betz, PN Peterson, FA Masouli. Cardioverter-defibrillators for secondary prevention of sudden cardiac death: a review. *J Am Heart Assoc* 2017; 6:e005515. DOI: 10.1161/JAHA.117.005515.

16. AJ Moss, WJ Hall, DS Cannom, JP Daubert, SL Higgins, H Klein, JH Levine, S Saksena, AL Waldo, D Wilber, MW Brown, M Heo, for the Multicenter Automatic Defibrillator Implantation Trial Investigators. Improved survival with an implanted defibrillator in patients with coronary disease at high risk for ventricular arrhythmia. *N Engl J Med* 1996; 335:1933–1940.

17. AJ Moss, W Zareba, WJ Hall, H Klein, DJ Wilber, DS Cannom, JP Daubert, SL Higgins, MW Brown, ML Andrews, for the Multicenter Automatic Defibrillator Implantation Trial II Investigators. Prophylactic implantation of a defibrillator in patients with myocardial infarction and reduced ejection fraction. *N Engl J Med* 2002; 346:877–883.

18. GH Bardy, et al., SCD-HeFT.

19. AHA Statistical Update 2020, Chapters 14 and 17, *ibid.*

20. The Public Access Defibrillation Trial Investigators. Public-access defibrillation and survival after out-of-hospital cardiac arrest. *N Engl J Med* 2004; 351:637–646.

21. GH Bardy, KL Lee, DB Mark, JE Poole, WD Toff, AM Tonkin, W Smith, P Dorian, DL Packer, RD White, WT Longstreth, J Anderson, G Johnson, E Bischoff, JJ Yallop, S McNulty, L Davidson, NE Clapp-Channing, Y Rosenberg, EB Schron, for the HAT Investigators. Home use of automated external defibrillators for sudden cardiac arrest. *N Engl J Med* 2008; 358:1790–1804. DII 10.1056/NEJMoa0801651.

22. RJ Franscone, KG Lurie, JM Goodloe. Resuscitation Outcomes Consortium (ROC) studies dig deep into the science of resuscitation. *Journal of Emergency Medical Services* 2016, 31 Dec; 42(1). https://www.jems.com/2016/12/31/resuscitation-outcomes-consortium-roc-studies-dig-deep-into-the-science-of-resuscitation/.

23. ES Ford, UA Ajani, JB Croft, JA Critchley, DR Labarth, TE Kottke, WH Giles, S Capewell. Explaining the Decrease in U.S. Deaths from Coronary Disease, 1980–2000. *N Engl J Med* 2007; 356:2388–2398. DOI: 10.1056/NEJMsa053935.

24. GH Bardy, et al., SCD-HeFT.

Chapter 13

1. P Libby. History of discovery: inflammation in atherosclerosis. *Arterioscler. Thromb. Vasc. Biol* 2012; 32:2045–2051. https://doi.org/10.1161/ATVBAHA.108.179705.

2. R Virchow. *Cellular Pathology.* London: John Churchill, 1858.

3. P Libby, PM Ridker. Novel inflammatory markers of coronary risk. Theory versus practice. *Circulation* 1999; 100:1148–1150.

P Libby, PM Ridker. Inflammation and atherothrombosis. From population biology and bench research to clinical practice. *J Am Coll Cardiol* 2006; 48:A33-A46. Doi:10.1016/j.jacc.2006.08.011.

Moriya, J. Critical roles of inflammation in atherosclerosis. *J Cardiol* 2018; 73:22–27. https://reader.elsevier.com/reader/sd/pii/S091450871830145X?token=3665FDB1173C3253AB6E8CF2CF06274E5CFE8783B7BE9D80D2A8C15EF779D7A2FACA4EAB32058F498A171AEBF6B8950B.

GR Giovanini, P Libby. Atherosclerosis

and inflammation: overview and updates. *Clinical Science* 2018; 132:1243–1252.

4. MB Pepys, GM Hirschfield. C-reactive protein: a critical update. *J Clin Invest* 2003; 111:1805–1812. doi:10.1172/JCI200318921.

5. WK Lagrand, CA Visser, WT Hermens, HWM Niessen, FWA Verheugt, GJ Wolbink, CE Hack. C-reactive protein as a cardiovascular risk factor: More than an epiphenomenon? *Circulation* 1999; 100:96–102.

6. J Danesh, JG Wheeler, GM Hirschfield, S Eda, G Eiriksdottir, A Rumley, GDO Lowe, MB Pepys, V Gudnason. C-reactive protein and other circulating markers of inflammation in the prediction of coronary heart disease. *N Engl J Med* 2004; 350:1387–1397.

7. M Helfand, DL Buckley, M Freeman, R Fu, K Rogers, C Fleming, LL Humphrey. Emerging risk factors for coronary heart disease: a summary of systematic reviews conducted for the U.S. Preventive Services Task Force. *Ann Intern Med* 2009; 151:496–507.

8. PM Ridker, E Danielson, FAH Fonseca, J Genest, AM Gotto, JJP Kastelein, W Koenig, P Libby, AJ Lorenzen, JG MacFayden, BG Nordestgaard, J Shephers, JT Willerson, RJ Glynn, for the JUPITER Study Group. Rosuvastatin to prevent vascular events in men and women with elevated C-reactive protein. *N Engl J Med* 2008; 359:2195–2207. DOI: 10.1056/NEJMoa0807646.

9. P Ridker. The JUPITER Trial: results, controversies, and implications for prevention. *Circ Cardiovasc Qual Outcomes* 2009; 279–285.

10. S Kaul, RP Morrissey, GA Diamond. By Jove! What is a clinician to make of JUPITER? *Arch Intern Med* 2010;170:1073–1077.

11. SM Grundy, NJ Stone, AL Bailey, C Beam, KK Birtcher, RS Blumenthal, LT Braun, S de Ferranti, J Faiella-Tommasino, DE Forman, R Goldberg, PA Heidenreich, MA Hlatky, DW Jones, D Lloyd-Jones, N Lopez-Pajares, CE Ndumele, CE Orringer, CA Peralta, JJ Saseen, SC Smith, L Sperling, SS Virani, J Yeboah. 2018 AHA/ACC/AACVPR/AAPA/ABC/ACPM/ADA/AGS/APhA/ASPC/NLA/PCNA Guideline on the Management of Blood Cholesterol: A Report of the American College of Cardiology/American Heart Association Task Force on Clinical Practice Guidelines. *Circulation* 2019; 139:e1082-e1143. https://www.ahajournals.org/doi/10.1161/CIR.0000000000000625

12. PM Ridker, BM Everett, T Thuren, JG MacFayden, WH Chang, C Ballantyne, F Fonseca, J Nicolau, W Koenig, SD Anker, JJP Kastelein, JH Cornel, P Pais, D Pella, J Genest, R Cifkova, A Lorenzatti, T Forster, Z Kobalava, L Vida-Smith, M Flather, H Shimokawa, H Ogawa, M Dellborg, PRF Ross, RPT Troquay, P Libby, RJ Glynn, for the CANTOS Trial Group. Antiinflammatory therapy with canakinumab for atherosclerotic disease. *N Engl J Med* 2017; 377:1119–1131. DOI: 10.1056/NEJMoa170791.

13. RA Herrington. Targeting inflammation in cardiovascular disease. *N Engl J Med* 2017; 377:1197–1198. DOI: 10.1056/NEJMe1709904.

14. PM Ridker, BM Everett, A Pradhan, JG MacFayden, DH Solomon, E Zaharris, V Mam, A Hasan, Y Rosenberg, E Iturriaga, M Gupta, M Tsigoulis, S Verma, M Clearfield, P Libby, SZ Goldhaber, R Seagle, C Ofori, M Saklayen, S Butman, J Johnston, NP Paynter, RJ Glynn, for the CIRT Investigators. Low-dose methotrexate for the prevention of atherosclerotic events. *N Engl J Med* 2019; 380:752–762. DOI: 10.1056/NEJMoa1809.

Chapter 14

1. W Osler. *Lectures on Angina Pectoris and Allied States.* New York: D. Appleton and Company, 1897, pp. 22–23.

2. BV Howard, L Van Horn, J Hsia, JE Manson, ML Stefanick, S Wassertheil-Smoller, LH Kuller, AZ LaCroix, RD Langer, NL Lasser, CE Lewis, MC Limacher, KL Margolis, J Mysiw, JK Ockene, LM Parker, MG Perri, L Phillips, RL Prentice, J Robbins, JE Rossouw, GE Sarto, IJ Schatz, LG Snetselaar, VJ Stevens, LF Tinker, M Trevisan, MZ Vitolins, GL Anderson, AR Assaf, T Bassford,

SAA Beresford, HR Black, RL Brunner, RG Brzyski, B Caan, RT Chebowski, M Gass, I Granek, P Greenland, J Hays, D Heber, G Heiss, SL Hendrix, FA Hubbell, KC Johnson, JM Kotchen. Low-fat dietary pattern and risk of cardiovascular disease. The Women's Health Initiative Randomized Dietary Modification Trial. *JAMA* 2006; 295:655–666.

3. The Look AHEAD Research Group. Cardiovascular effects of intensive lifestyle intervention in type 2 diabetes. *N Engl J Med* 2013; 369:145–154.

4. J Dorn, J Naughton, D Inamura, M Trevisian, for the NEHDP Project Staff. Results of a multicenter randomized clinical trial or exercise and long-term survival in myocardial infarction patients. The National Exercise and Heart Disease Project (NEHDP). *Circulation* 1999; 100:1764–1769.

5. GT O'Connor, JE Buring, S Yusuf, SZ Goldhaber, EM Olmstead, RS Paffenberger, CH Hennekens. An overview of randomized trials of rehabilitation with exercise after myocardial infarction. *Circulation* 1989; 80:234–244.

6. RH Eckel, JM Jacsic, JD Ard, JM de Jesus, NH Miller, VS Hubbard, IM Lee, AH Lichtenstein, CM Loria, BE Millen, CA Nonas, FM Sacks, SC Smith, LP Svetkey, TA Wadden, SZ Yanovski. 2013 AHA/ACC Guideline on Lifestyle Management to Reduce Cardiovascular Risk. A report of the American College of Cardiology/American Heart Association Task Force on Practice Guidelines. *Circulation* 2014; 129(suppl 2):S76-S99. DOI: 10.1161/01.cir.0000437740.48606.d1.

7. MD Jensen, DH Ryan, CM Apovian, JD Ard, AG Comuzzie, KA Donato, FB Hu, VS Hubbard, JM Jakicic, RF Kushner, CM Loria, BE Millen, CA Nonas, X Pi-Sunyer, J Stevens, VJ Stevens, TA Wadden, BM Wolfe, SZ Yanovski. 2013 AHA/ACC/TOS Guideline for the Management of Overweight and Obesity in Adults. A report the American College of Cardiology/American Heart Association Task Force on Practice Guidelines and the Obesity Society. *Circulation* 2014; 129(suppl 2):S102-S138. DOI: 10.1161/01.cir.0000437739.71477.ee.

8. A Keys, JT Anderson, F Grande. Serum cholesterol response to changes in the diet. I. Iodine value of dietary fat versus 2S-P; II The effect of cholesterol in the diet; II Differences among individuals; IV Particular fats in the diet. *Metabolism* 1965; 14:747–787.

DM Hegsted, RB McGandy, ML Myers, FJ Stare. Quantitative effects of dietary fat on serum cholesterol in men. *Am J Clin Nutr* 1965; 17:281–295.

9. DJ Gordon, KM Salz, KJ Roggenkamp, FA Franklin. Dietary determinants of plasma cholesterol change in the recruitment phase of the Lipid Research Clinics Coronary Primary Prevention Trial. *Arteriosclerosis* 1982; 2:537–548.

10. FM Sacks, E Obarzanek, MM Windhauser, LP Svetky, WM Vollmer, M McCollough, N Karanja, PH Lin, P Steele, MA Proschan, MA Evans, LJ Appel, GA Bray, TM Vogt, TJ Moore, DASH Investigators. Rationale and design of the Dietary Approaches to Stop Hypertension trial (DASH): a multicenter controlled-feeding study of dietary patterns to lower blood pressure. *Ann Epidemiol* 1995; 5:108–118.

11. LJ Appel, TJ Moore, E Obarzanek, WM Vollmer, LP Svetky, FM Sacks, GA Bray, TM Vogt, JA Cutler, MM Windhauser, PH Lin, N Karanja, for the DASH Collaborative Research Group. *N Engl J Med* 1997; 336:1117–1124.

12. E Obarzanek, FM Sacks, WM Vollmer, GA Bray, ER Miller, PH Lin, N Karanja, MM Windhauser, TJ Moore, JF Swain, CW Bales, MA Proschan, on behalf of the DASH Research Group. Effects on blood lipids of a blood pressure-lowering diet: the Dietary Approaches to Stop Hypertension (DASH) Trial. *Am J Clin Nutr* 2001; 74:80–89.

13. FM Sacks, LP Svetky, WM Vollmer, LJ Appel, GA Bray, D Harisha, E Obarzanek, PR Comlin, ER Miller, DG Simons-Morton, N Karanja, PH Lin, for the DASH-Sodium Collaborative Research Group. Effects on blood pressure of reduced dietary sodium and the Dietary Approaches to Stop Hypertension (DASH) diet. *N Engl J Med* 2001; 344:3–10.

14. Mayo Clinic Staff. Glycemic index diet: What's behind the claims. Mayo Clinic

Website. Healthy Lifestyle. Nutrition and Healthy Living. Accessed August 1, 2020, at https://www.mayoclinic.org/healthy-lifestyle/nutrition-and-healthy-eating/in-depth/glycemic-index-diet/art-20048478.

15. FM Sacks, VJ Carey, CAM Anderson, ER Miller, T Copeland, J Charleston, BJ Harshfield, N Laranjo, P McCarron, J Swain, K White, K Yee, LJ Appel. Effects of high vs low glycemic index of dietary carbohydrate on cardiovascular disease risk factors and insulin sensitivity. The Omni-Carb randomized clinical trial. *JAMA* 2014; 312:2531–2541. doi:10.1001/jama.2014.16658.

16. American Heart Association. What is the Mediterranean diet? https://www.heart.org/en/healthy-living/healthy-eating/eat-smart/nutrition-basics/mediterranean-diet.

17. R Estruch, E Ros, J Salas-Salvadó, MI Covas, D Corella, F Arós, E Gómez-Gracia, V Ruiz-Gutiérrez, M Fiol, J Lapetra, RM Lamuela-Raventos. Primary prevention of cardiovascular disease with a Mediterranean diet supplemented with extra-virgin olive oil or nuts. *N Engl J Med* 2018; 378;e34. DOI: 10.1056/NEJMoa1800389.

Harvard School of Public Health. The Nutrition Source. PREDIMED Study Retraction and Republication. What changed, what didn't, and the big picture. https://www.hsph.harvard.edu/nutritionsource/2018/06/22/predimed-retraction-republication/.

MA Martinez-Gonzalez, A Gea, M Ruiz-Canela. The Mediterranean diet and cardiovascular health. A Critical review. *Circ Res* 2019; 124:779–798.

18. LJ Appel, JM Clarke, HC Yeh, NY Wang, JW Coughlin, G Daumit, ER Miller, A Dalcin, GJ Jerome, S Geller, G Noronha, T Pozefsky, J Charleston, JB Reynolds, N Durkin, RR Rubin, TA Louis, FL Brancati. Comparative effectiveness of weight loss interventions in clinical practice. *N Engl J Med* 2011; 365:1959–1968.

19. SK Agarwal. Cardiovascular benefits of exercise. *Int J Gen Med* 2012; 5:541–545.

JN Morris, JA Heady, PA Raffle, CG Roberts, JW Parks. Coronary heart disease and physical activity of work. *Lancet* 1953;265(6795):1053–1057; contd.

JN Morris, JA Heady, PA Raffle, CG Roberts, JW Parks. Coronary heart disease and physical activity of work (part 2). *Lancet* 1953, Nov 28;265(6796):1111–1120; concl.

HL Taylor, E Klepetar, A Keys, W Parlin, H Blackburn, T Puchner. Death rates among physically active and sedentary employees in the railroad industry. *Am J Public Health Nations Health* 1962, Oct; 52:1697–1707.

20. J Myers. Exercise and cardiovascular health. *Circulation* 2003; 107:e2-e5.

21. N Pattyn, VA Cornelissen, SRT Eshgbi, L Vanhees. The effect of exercise on the cardiovascular risk factors constituting the metabolic syndrome. *Sports Med* 2013; 43:121–133.

22. CJ Lavie, RV Milani, HO Ventura. Obesity and cardiovascular disease. Risk factor, paradox, and impact of weight loss. *J Am Coll Cardiol* 2009; 53:1925–1932.

23. P Poirier, TD Giles, GA Bray, Y Hong, JS Stern, X Pi-Sunyer, RH Eckel. Obesity and cardiovascular disease: Pathophysiology, evaluation, and effect of weight loss. An update of the 1997 American Heart Association Scientific Statement on Obesity and Heart Disease from the Obesity Committee of the Council on Nutrition, Physical Activity, and Metabolism. *Circulation* 2006; 113:898–918.

24. CD Fryar, MD Carroll, CL Ogden. Prevalence of overweight, obesity, and severe obesity among adults aged 20 and over. United States, 1960–62 through 2015–2016. National Center for Health Statistics. Health E-Stats September 2018. https://stacks.cdc.gov/view/cdc/58670.

25. ZJ Ward, SN Bleich, AL Cradock, JL Barrett, CM Giles, C Flax, MW Long, CL Gortmaker. Projected U.S. state-level prevalence of adult obesity and severe obesity. *N Engl J Med* 2019; 381:2440–2450. DOI: 10.1056/NEJMsa1909301.

26. CL Beale. A century of population growth and change. *Food Review* 2000; 23:16–22. https://wayback.archive-it.org/5923/20110903152144/http://ers.usda.gov/publications/foodreview/jan2000/frjan2000c.pdf.

27. Achievements in Public Health, 1900–1999. Healthier Mothers and

Babies. *MMWR Weekly* 1999; 48:849–858. https://www.cdc.gov/mmwr/preview/ mmwrhtml/mm4838a2.htm.

28. Life Expectancy in the USA 1900–98, https://u.demog.berkeley. edu/~andrew/1918/figure2.html. Macrotrends, U.S. Life Expectancy 1950–2020, https://www.macrotrends.net/countries/ USA/united-states/life-expectancy.

29. LI Wilder. *Farmer Boy*, Chapter 8. New York: HarperCollins, 1933.

30. W Cather. *My Antonia*, Chapter 9. Boston: Houghton-Mifflin, 1918.

31. Food Timeline FAQs. Popular 20th Century American Foods. http:// www.foodtimeline.org/fooddecades. html#1900s.

32. HAB Hiza, L Bente. Nutrient Content of the U.S. Food Supply, 1909–2004: A Summary Report. (Home Economics Research Report No. 57). 2007. https:// fns-prod.azureedge.net/sites/default/ files/nutrient_content_of_the_us_food_ supply/FoodSupply1909-2004Report.pdf.

33. USDA Economic Research Service. Major trends in U.S. Food Supply, 1909–99. January-April 2000. https://webs. wofford.edu/boppkl/coursefiles/Interim/ CookingInterim/Readings.Exercises/ MajorTrendsinUSFoodSupply09_99.pdf.

34. Hiza, Bente.

35. National Health and Nutrition Examination Survey website. National Center for Health Statistics, Centers for Disease Control and Prevention. https://www.cdc. gov/nchs/about_nhanes.htm.

36. ES Ford, UA Ajani, JB Croft, JA Critchley, DR Labarth, TE Kottke, WH Giles, S Capewell. Explaining the Decrease in U.S. Deaths from Coronary Disease, 1980–2000. *N Engl J Med* 2007; 356:2388–2398. DOI: 10.1056/NEJMsa053935.

37. ES Ford, et al.

38. *Ibid.*

Chapter 15

1. Centers for Disease Control and Prevention. U.S. Public Health Service Syphilis Study at Tuskegee. Timeline. Accessed August 2020, at https://www.cdc.gov/ tuskegee/timeline.htm.

E Nix. Tuskegee Experiment: the infamous syphilis study. History.com. Updated July 29, 2019. https://www.history.com/ news/the-infamous-40-year-tuskegee-study/.

2. SO Sodeke, LR Powell. Paying Tribute to Henrietta Lacks at Tuskegee University and at The Virginia Henrietta Lacks Commission, Richmond, Virginia. *J Health Care Poor Underserved* 2019; 30(4s):1–11.

3. Morbidity and Mortality. 2012 Chartbook on Cardiovascular, Lung and Blood Diseases, NIH-NHLBI. Chart 3–24. https://www.nhlbi.nih.gov/files/docs/ research/2012_ChartBook_508.pdf.

Centers for Disease Control. Age-adjusted death rates for 69 selected causes by race and sex using year 2000 standard population: United States, 1950–59. https://www.cdc.gov/nchs/data/ dvs/hist293_1950_59.pdf, 1960–67. https://www.cdc.gov/nchs/data/mortab/ aadr6067.pdf, 1968–78. https://www.cdc. gov/nchs/data/mortab/aadr6878.pdf.

Centers for Disease Control and Prevention (CDC), National Center of Health Statistics. Mortality Data Finder. Table 5: Age-adjusted death rates for selected causes of death by sex, race and Hispanic origin: United States, selected years 1950–2017, https://www.cdc.gov/nchs/hus/ contents2018.htm#Table_005 (Excel spreadsheet link).

4. Proceedings of the Conference on the Decline in Coronary Heart Disease Mortality: National Heart, Lung, and Blood Institute, National Institute of Health, Bethesda, Maryland. NIH publication no. 79–1610, 1978. Bethesda, MD: National Heart, Lung, and Blood Institute, NIH, 1979. Oct 24–25. *Chartbook for the Conference on the Decline in Coronary Heart Disease Mortality.* Hyattsville, MD: NCHS, 1978. National Center for Health Statistics. Factors Obscuring the Downturn in IHD Mortality (p. 17) and Comparability of Mortality Statistics for Diseases of the Heart (Appendix II).

5. Centers for Disease Control and Prevention. Heart disease death rates among blacks and whites, aged > 35 years—United States, 1968–2015. *Morbidity*

and Mortality Weekly Report. Surveillance Summaries 2018, 30 March; 67(5):1–11. https://www.cdc.gov/mmwr/volumes/67/ss/ss6705a1.htm.

6. Morbidity and Mortality. 2012 Chartbook on Cardiovascular, Lung and Blood Diseases, NIH-NHLBI. Chart 3–26. https://www.nhlbi.nih.gov/files/docs/research/2012_ChartBook_508.pdf.

7. MW Lewis, Y Khodneva, N Redmond, RW Durant, LL Wilkinson, VJ Howard, MM Safford. The impact of the combination of income and education on the incidence of coronary heart disease in the prospective Reasons for Geographic and Racial Differences in Stroke (REGARDS) cohort study. *BMC Public Health* 2015; 15:1312–1321. DOI 10.1186/s12889–015–2630–4.

8. S Pruitt. What part of Africa did most slaves come from? History.com. Updated June 19, 2019. https://www.history.com/news/what-part-of-africa-did-most-slaves-come-from?.

9. DT Lackland. Racial differences in hypertension: implications for high blood pressure management. *Am J Med Sci* 2014; 348:135–138. doi:10.1097/MAJ.0000000000000308.

J Lindhorst, N Alexander, J Blignaut, B Rayner. Differences in hypertension between blacks and whites: an overview. *Cardiovasc J Afr* 2007; 18:241–247.

10. PD Curtin. The slavery hypothesis for hypertension among African Americans: The historical evidence. *Am J Publ Health* 1992; 82:1681–1686.

11. G Howard, M Cushman, CS Moy, S Oparil, P Muntner, DT Lackland, JJ Manly, ML Flaherty, SE Judd, VG Wadley, DL Long, VJ Howard. Association of clinical and social factors with excess hypertension risk in black compared with white U.S. adults. *JAMA* 2018; 320:1338–1348. doi:10.1001/jama.2018.13467.

12. J Addo, L Smeeth, DA Leon. Hypertension in sub-Saharan Africa: a systematic review. *Hypertension* 2007; 50:1012–1018.

13. TM Sprull. Chronic psychosocial stress and hypertension. *Curr Hypertens Rep* 2010; 12:10–16. doi:10.1007/s11906–009–0084–8.

14. J Addo, et al.

15. S Rao, MW Segar, AP Bress, W Vongpatanasin, V Agusala, UR Essien, A Correa, AA Morris, JA de Lemos, A Pandey. Association of genetic West African ancestry, blood pressure response to therapy, and cardiovascular risk among self-reported black individuals in the Systolic Blood Pressure Reduction Intervention Trial (SPRINT). *JAMA Cardiology*, published online November 13, 2020. Doi.10.1001/jamacardio.2020.6566. https://jamanetwork.com/journals/jamacardiology/fullarticle/10.1001/jamacardio.2020.6566?guestAccessKey=bef18712-8884-479c-9d99-024845d9c461&utm_source=silverchair&utm_medium=email&utm_campaign=article_alert-jamacardiology&utm_content=olf&utm_term=111320.

16. AR Omran. The epidemiologic transition: a theory of the epidemiology of population change. 1971. *Milbank Q* 2005; 83(4):731–757. TA Gaziano, A Bitton, S Anand, S Abrahams-Gessel, A Murphy. Growing epidemic of coronary heart disease in low- and middle-income countries. *Curr Probl Cardiol* 2010; 35:72–115. World Health Organization 2009. Global Health Risks. Mortality and burden of disease attributable to selected major risks. ISBN 978 92 4 56387 1. https://www.who.int/healthinfo/global_burden_disease/GlobalHealthRisks_report_full.pdf.

17. V Smil. China's great famine: 40 years later. *BMJ* 1999; 319:1619–1621.

18. Z Chen, R Peto, R Collins, S MacMahon, J Lu, W Li. Serum cholesterol concentration and coronary heart disease In population with low cholesterol concentrations. *BMJ* 1991; 303:276–282.

MJ Martin, SB Hulley, WS Browner, LH Kuller, D Wentworth. Serum cholesterol, blood pressure, and mortality: implications from a cohort of 361,662 men. *Lancet* 1986, Oct; 933–936.

19. J He, D Gu, K Reynolds, X Wu, P Muntner, J Zhao, J Chen, D Liu, J Mo, PK Whelton, InterASIA Collaborative Group. Serum total and lipoprotein cholesterol levels and awareness, treatment, and control of hypercholesterolemia in China. *Circulation* 2004; 110: 405–411. DOI: 10.1161/01.CIR.0000136583.52681.0D.

MD Carroll, AK Kit, DA Lacher, ST Shero, ME Mussolino. Trends in lipids and lipoproteins of U.S. adults, 1988–2010. *JAMA* 2012; 308:1545–1554.

20. MA Gonzalez, FR Artalejo, J Calero. Relationship between socioeconomic status and ischaemic heart disease in cohort and case-control studies: 1960–1993. *Int J Epidemiol* 1998; 27:350–358.

21. World Health Rankings. Live Longer Live Better. https://www.world lifeexpectancy.com/cause-of-death/coro nary-heart-disease/by-country/.

22. Centers for Disease Control. Online Table 22. Hypertension among adults aged 20 and over by selected characteristics. United States, selected years 1988–1994 through 2013–2016. https://www.cdc.gov/nchs/data/hus/2018/022.pdf.

23. MD Carroll, BK Kit, DA Lacher, SS Yoon. Total and high-density lipoprotein cholesterol in adults: National Health and Nutrition Exam Survey 2011–12. Figures 3, 4. https://www.cdc.gov/nchs/data/databriefs/db132.pdf.

24. American Lung Association. Tobacco Use in Racial and Ethnic Populations. https://www.lung.org/quit-smoking/smoking-facts/impact-of-tobacco-use/tobacco-use-racial-and-ethnic.

25. MR Carnethon, J Pu, G Howard, MA Albert, CAM Anderson, AG Bertoni, MS Mujahid, L Palaniappan, HA Taylor, M Willis, CW Yancy, on behalf of the American Heart Association Council on Epidemiology and Prevention; Council on Cardiovascular Disease in the Young, Council on Cardiovascular Nursing, Council on Clinical Cardiology, Council on Functional Genomics and Translational Biology, and Stroke Council. Cardiovascular Health in African Americans. A scientific statement from the American Heart Association. Endorsed by the American College of Cardiology. *Circulation* 2017; 136:e393-e403. DOI: 10.1161/CIR.0000000000000534.

26. Centers for Disease Control and Prevention. National Diabetes Statistical Report 2020. Figure 2. Estimates of Diabetes and its Burden in the United States. https://www.cdc.gov/diabetes/pdfs/data/statistics/national-diabetes-statistics-report.pdf.

27. Centers for Disease Control and Prevention. A Closer Look at African American Men and High Blood Pressure Control: A Review of Psychosocial Factors and Systems-Level Interventions. Atlanta: U.S. Department of Health and Human Services, 2010.

28. G Howard, R Prineas, C Moy, M Cushman, M Kellum, E Temple, A Graham, V Howard. Racial and geographic differences in awareness treatment, and control of hypertension. Reasons for Geographic and Racial Differences in Stroke study. *Stroke* 2006; 37:1171–1178.

29. J Crowe, C Lacy, Y Columbus. Barriers to food security and community stress in an urban food desert. *Urban Science* 2018; 2:45–61. doi:10.3390/urbansci2020046.

30. LR Dugas, TE Forrester, J Plange-Rhule, P Bovet, EV Lambert, RA Durazo-Arvizu, G Cao, RS Cooper, R Khatib, L Tonino, W Riesen, W Korte, S Kliethermes, A Luke. Cardiovascular risk status of Afro-origin populations across the spectrum of economic development: findings from the Modeling the Epidemiologic Transition Study. *BMC Public Health* 2017; 17(1):438.

31. S Arora, GA Stouffer, A Kucharska-Newton, M Vaduganathan, K Matsushita, D Kolte, HR Reynolds, S Bangilore, DL Bhatt, MC Caughey. Fifteen-year trends in management and outcomes of non-ST-segment elevation myocardial infarction among black and white patients: the ARIC Community Survey 2000–2014. *J Am Heart Assoc* 2018; 7:e010203. DOI: 10.1161/JAHA.118.010203.

32. KM Hoffman, S Trawalter, JR Axt, MN Oliver. Racial bias in pain assessment and treatment recommendations, and false beliefs about differences between blacks and whites. *Proc Nat Acad Sci* 2016; 113: 4296–4301. www.pnas.org/cgi/doi/10.1073/pnas.1516047113.

33. Health, United States. 2012 Updates. https://www.cdc.gov/nchs/data/hus/2012/001.pdf.

Appendix

1. ES Ford, UA Ajani, JB Croft, JA Critchley, DR Labarth, TE Kottke, WH Giles, S Capewell. Explaining the

Decrease in U.S. Deaths from Coronary Disease, 1980–2000. *N Engl J Med* 2007; 356:2388–2398. DOI: 10.1056/NEJMsa 053935.

2. Centers for Disease Control and Prevention (CDC), National Center of Health Statistics. Mortality Data Finder. Table 5: Age-adjusted death rates for selected causes of death by sex, race and Hispanic origin: United States, selected years 1950–2017 https://www.cdc.gov/nchs/hus/contents2018.htm#Table_005 (Excel spreadsheet link).

Morbidity and Mortality. 2012 Chartbook on Cardiovascular, Lung and Blood Diseases, NIH-NHLBI. Chart 3–24. https://www.nhlbi.nih.gov/files/docs/research/2012_ChartBook_508.pdf.

Age-adjusted death rates for 69 selected causes by race and sex using year 2000 standard population: United States, 1968–78 https://www.cdc.gov/nchs/data/mortab/aadr6878.pdf.

3. ES Ford et al.

4. EM Sarpong, SH Zuvekas. Changes in statin therapy among adults (age 18+) by selected characteristics, United States, 2000–2001 to 2010–2011. Medical Expenditure Panel Survey (MEPS). Statistical Brief #459. November 2014. https://www.ncbi.nlm.nih.gov/books/NBK470833/.

VL Burt, JA Cutler, M Higgins, MJ Horan, D Labarth, P Whelton, C Brown, EJ Rocella. Trends in the prevalence, awareness, treatment, and control of hypertension in the adults U.S. population. Data from the Health Examination Surveys, 1960 to 1991. *Hypertension* 1995; 26:1–60, https://www.ahajournals.org/doi/epub/10.1161/01.HYP.26.1.60.

P Muntner, ST Hardy, LJ Fine, BC Jaeger, G Wozniak, EB Levitan, LD Colantonio. Trends in blood pressure control among U.S. adults with hypertension, 1999–2000 to 2017–2018. *JAMA* 2020; doi:10.1001/jama.2020.14545.

American Lung Association. Overall Tobacco Trends. https://www.lung.org/research/trends-in-lung-disease/tobacco-trends-brief/overall-tobacco-trends. Accessed September 2020.

5. American Lung Association. Overall Tobacco Trends.

6. Centers for Disease Control and Prevention (CDC), National Center of Health Statistics Mortality Data, HIST293. Age-adjusted death rates for selected causes by race and sex using year 2000 standard population: death registration states, 1900-32 and United States, 1933-49, Diseases of the Heart. https://www.cdc.gov/nchs/data/dvs/hist293_1900_49.pdf. Morbidity and Mortality. 2012.

Centers for Disease Control and Prevention (CDC), National Center of Health Statistics. Mortality Data Finder. Table 5: Age-adjusted death rates for selected causes of death by sex, race and Hispanic origin: United States, selected years 1950–2017 https://www.cdc.gov/nchs/hus/contents2018.htm#Table_005 (Excel spreadsheet link).

7. JA Critchley, S Capewell. Mortality risk reduction associated with smoking cessation in patients with coronary heart disease: a systematic review. *JAMA* 2003; 290:86–97. Doi: 10.1001/jama.290.1.86.

8. ES Ford et al.

NS Shah, MD Huffman, H Ning, DM Lloyd-Jones. Trends in myocardial infarction secondary prevention: The National Health and Nutrition Examination Surveys (NHANES), 1999–2012. *J Am Heart Assoc* 2015; 4:1–12. doi:10.1161/JAHA.114.001709. https://www.ahajournals.org/doi/pdf/10.1161/JAHA.114.001709.

9. CDC National Diabetes Statistical Report 2020. Estimates of Diabetes and its Burden in the United States. https://www.cdc.gov/diabetes/pdfs/data/statistics/national-diabetes-statistics-report.pdf

AHA/ACC Heart Risk Calculator, http://www.cvriskcalculator.com/.

10. Morbidity and Mortality. 2012 Chartbook on Cardiovascular, Lung and Blood Diseases, NIH-NHLBI. Chart 3–22. https://www.nhlbi.nih.gov/files/docs/research/2012_ChartBook_508.pdf.

LM Howden, JA Meyer. 2010 Census Briefs: Age and Sex Composition 2010. U.S. Department of Commerce, Economics and Statistics Information, U.S. Census Bureau. May 2011. https://www.census.gov/prod/cen2010/briefs/c2010br-03.pdf.

11. PA Kavsak, AR MacRae, V Lustig,

R Bhargava, R Vandersluis, GE Polomaki, ML Yerna, AS Jaffe. The impact of the ESC/ACC redefinition of myocardial infarction and new sensitive troponin assays on the frequency of acute myocardial infarction. *Am Heart J* 2005; 152:118–125.

12. Morbidity and Mortality. 2012 Chartbook on Cardiovascular, Lung and Blood Diseases, NIH-NHLBI. Chart 3–23. https://www.nhlbi.nih.gov/files/docs/research/2012_ChartBook_508.pdf.

LM Howden, JA Meyer. 2010 Census Briefs.

Bibliography

The ACCORD Study Group. The effect of combination lipid therapy in type 2 diabetes mellitus. *N Engl J Med* 2010; 362:1563–1574. DOI: 10.1056/NEJMoa1001282.

Achievements in Public Health, 1900–1999. Healthier Mothers and Babies. *MMWR Weekly* 1999; 48:849–858. https://www.cdc.gov/mmwr/preview/mmwrhtml/mm4838a2.htm.

The Action to Control Cardiovascular Risk in Diabetes Study Group. Effects of intensive glucose lowering in type 2 diabetes. *N Engl J Med* 2008; 358:2545–2559.

J Addo, L Smeeth, DA Leon. Hypertension in sub-Saharan Africa: a systematic review. *Hypertension* 2007; 50:1012–1018.

The ADVANCE Collaborative Group. Intensive blood glucose control and vascular outcomes in patients with type 2 diabetes. *N Engl J Med* 2008; 358:2560–2572.

SK Agarwal. Cardiovascular benefits of exercise. *Int J Gen Med* 2012; 5:541–545.

AHA Statistical Update: Heart Disease and Stroke Statistics—2020 Update, Table 25.2 (2014 data). *Circulation* 2020; 141:e139-e596. OI: 10.1161/CIR.0000000000000757.

AHA/ACC Heart Risk Calculator, http://www.cvriskcalculator.com/.

AM Ahmed. History of Diabetes Mellitus. *Saudi Med J* 2002; 23:373–378.

The AIM-HIGH Investigators. Niacin in patients with low HDL cholesterol levels receiving intensive statin therapy. *N Engl J Med* 2011; 365:2235–2267.

SM Al-Khatib, WG Stevenson, MJ Ackerman, WJ Bryant, DJ Callans, AB Curtis, BJ Deal, T Dickfeld, ME Field, GC Fonarow, AM Gillis, CB Granger, SC Hammill, MA Hlatky, JA Joglar, GN Kay, DD Matlock, RJ Myerburg, RL Page. 2017 AHA/ACC/HRS Guideline for Management of Patients with Ventricular Arrhythmias and the Prevention of Sudden Cardiac Death. A report of the American College of Cardiology/American Heart Association Task Force on Clinical Practice Guidelines and the Heart Rhythm Society. *Circulation* 2018; 138:e272-e391. doi: 10.1161/CIR.0000000000000549.

M Alkhouli, F Alqahtini, A Kalra, S Gafoor, M Alhajii, M Alreshidan, DR Holmes, A Leman. Trends in characteristics and outcomes of hospital inpatients undergoing coronary revascularization in the United States, 2003–2016. *JAMA Network Open* 2020; 3(2):e1921326. doi:10.1001/jamanetworkopen.2019.21326. https://jamanetwork.com/journals/jamanetworkopen/fullarticle/2760898.

The ALLHAT Officers and Coordinators for the ALLHAT Collaborative Research Group. Major cardiovascular events in hypertensive patients randomized to doxazosin vs chlorthalidone: the Antihypertensive and Lipid-Lowering Treatment to Prevent Heart Attack Trial (ALLHAT). *JAMA* 2000; 283:1967–1975.

American Cancer Society. Menopausal hormone therapy and cancer risk. https://www.cancer.org/cancer/cancer-causes/medical-treatments/menopausal-hormone-replacement-therapy-and-cancer-risk.html.

American College of Cardiology Expert Analysis. The history of cardiopulmonary bypass: medical advances. https://www.acc.org/latest-in-cardiology/articles/2019/06/19/06/46/the-history-of-cardiopulmonary-bypass.

American Diabetes Association. Standards

of Medical Care in Diabetes—2018. Diabetes Care 2018; 41 (supplement 1):S1-S159. http://diabetesed.net/wp-content/uploads/2017/12/2018-ADA-Standards-of-Care.pdf.

American Heart Association. What is the Mediterranean diet? https://www.heart.org/en/healthy-living/healthy-eating/eat-smart/nutrition-basics/mediterranean-diet.

American Lung Association. Overall Tobacco Trends. https://www.lung.org/research/trends-in-lung-disease/tobacco-trends-brief/overall-tobacco-trends. Accessed October 2020.

American Lung Association. Tobacco Control Milestones. https://www.lung.org/research/sotc/tobacco-timeline.

American Lung Association. Tobacco Use in Racial and Ethnic Populations. https://www.lung.org/quit-smoking/smoking-facts/impact-of-tobacco-use/tobacco-use-racial-and-ethnic.

EA Amsterdam, NK Wenger, RG Brindis, DE Casey, TG Ganiats, DR Holmes, AS Jaffe, H Jneid, RF Kelly, MC Kontos, GN Levine, PR Liebson, D Mukherjee, ED Peterson, MS Sabatine, RW Smalling, SJ Zieman. 2014 AHA/ACC Guidelines for the Management of Patients with Non-ST-Elevation Acute Coronary Syndromes. A report of the American College of Cardiology Foundation/American Heart Association Task Force on Practice Guidelines. *JACC* 2014; 64:e139-e228.

NN Anichkov, S Chalatow. Ueber experimentelle Cholesterinsteatose und ihre Bedeutung fur die Entstehung einer pathologischer Prozesse. *Zentralbl Allg Pathol* 1913; 24:1–9.

The Antiarrhythmics Versus Implantable Defibrillator (AVID) Investigators. A comparison of antiarrhythmic drug therapy with implantable defibrillators in patients resuscitated from near-fatal ventricular arrhythmias. *N Engl J Med* 1997; 337:1576–1583.

The Antihypertensive and Lipid Lowering Treatment to Prevent Heart Attack Trial (ALLHAT). JAMA. 2000; 283:1967–1975. The Antihypertensive and Lipid Heart Attack Trial (ALLHAT) Research Group. Major outcomes in high-risk hypertensive patients randomized to angiotensin-converting enzyme inhibitor or calcium channel blocker vs diuretic. *JAMA* 2002; 288:2981–2997.

Antiplatelet Trialists Collaboration. Collaborative overview of randomized trials of antiplatelet therapy—I. Prevention of death, myocardial infarction, and stroke by prolonged antiplatelet therapy in various categories of patients. *BMJ* 1994; 308:81–106.

Antithrombotic Trialists (ATT) Collaboration. Aspirin in the primary and secondary prevention of vascular disease: collaborative meta-analysis of individual participant data from randomized trials. *Lancet* 2009; 373:1849–1860.

LJ Appel, JM Clarke, HC Yeh, NY Wang, JW Coughlin, G Daumit, ER Miller, A Dalcin, GJ Jerome, S Geller, G Noronha, T Pozefsky, J Charleston, JB Reynolds, N Durkin, RR Rubin, TA Louis, FL Brancati. Comparative effectiveness of weight loss interventions in clinical practice. *N Engl J Med* 2011; 365:1959–1968.

LJ Appel, TJ Moore, E Obarzanek, WM Vollmer, LP Svetky, FM Sacks, GA Bray, TM Vogt, JA Cutler, MM Windhauser, PH Lin, N Karanja, for the DASH Collaborative Research Group. *N Engl J Med* 1997; 336:1117–1124.

S Arora, GA Stouffer, A Kucharska-Newton, M Vaduganathan, K Matsuhita, D Kolte, HR Reynolds, S Bangilore, DL Bhatt, MC Caughey. Fifteen-year trends in management and outcomes of non-ST-segment elevation myocardial infarction among black and white patients: the ARIC Community Survey 2000-2014. *J Am Heart Assoc* 2018; 7:e010203. DOI: 10.1161/JAHA.118.010203.

The Aspirin Myocardial Infarction Study Research Group. A randomized controlled trial of aspirin in persons recovered from a heart attack. JAMA 1980; 243:661–669. Supplementary webappendix, https://researchonline.lshtm.ac.uk/id/eprint/19177/1/mmc1.pdf.

S Bangalore, R Fakheri, B Toklu, G Ogedegbe, H Weintraub, FH Messerli. Angiotensin-Converting Enzyme Inhibitors or Angiotensin Receptor Blockers in Patients Without Heart Failure? Insights From

254,301 Patients from Randomized Trials. *Mayo Clin Proc* 2016; 91:51–60.

GH Bardy, KL Lee, DB Mark, JE Poole, DL Packer, R Boineau, M Domanski, C Troutman, J Anderson, SE McNulty, N Clapp-Channing, LD Davidson-Ray, ES Fraulo, DP Fishbein, RM Luceri, JH Ip, for the Sudden Cardiac Death in Heart Failure Trial (SCD-HeFT) Investigators. Amiodarone or an implantable cardioverter-defibrillator for congestive heart failure. *N Engl J Med* 2005; 352: 225–237.

GH Bardy, KL Lee, DB Mark, JE Poole, WD Toff, AM Tonkin, W Smith, P Dorian, DL Packer, RD White, WT Longstreth, J Anderson, G Johnson, E Bischoff, JJ Yallop, S McNulty, L Davidson, NE Clapp-Channing, Y Rosenberg, EB Schron, for the HAT Investigators. Home use of automated external defibrillators for sudden cardiac arrest. *N Engl J Med* 2008; 358:1790–1804. DII 10.1056/NEJMoa0801651.

The BARI-2D Study Group. A randomized trial of therapies for type 2 diabetes and coronary artery disease. *N Engl J Med* 2009; 360:2503–2515.

JM Barry. *The Great Influenza: The Story of the Deadliest Pandemic in History*. New York: Penguin Random House, 2004, 2005, 2009, 2018.

PJ Barter, HB Brewer, J Chapman, CH Hennekens, DJ Rader, AR Tall. Cholesteryl ester transfer protein. A novel target for raising HDL and inhibiting atherosclerosis. *Arteriosclerosis, Thrombosis, and Vascular Biology* 2003; 23:160–167.

PJ Barter, M Caulfield, M Eriksson, SM Grundy, JJP Kastelein, M Kornajda, J Lopez-Sendon, L Mosca, JC Tardif, DD Waters, CL Shear, JH Revkin, KA Buhr, MR Fisher, AR Tall, HB Brewer, for the ILLUMINATE Investigators. Effects of torcetrapib in patients at high risk for coronary events. *N Engl J Med* 2007; 357:2109–2122. doi: 10.1056/NEJMoa0706628.

M Barton, J Grüntzig, M Huisman, J Rüsch. Balloon angioplasty—the legacy of Andreas Grüntzig, M.D. (1939–1985). *Frontiers in Cardiovascular Medicine* 2014; 1(15):1–25. Doi: 10.3389/fcvm.2014.00015.

CL Beale. A century of population growth and change. *Food Review* 2000; 23:16–22. https://wayback.archive-it.org/5923/20110903152144/http://ers.usda.gov/publications/foodreview/jan2000/frjan2000c.pdf.

S Beddhu, GM Chertow, T Greene, PK Whelton, WT Ambrosius, AK Cheung, J Cutler, L Fine, R Boucher, G Wei, C Zhang, H Kramer, AP Bress, PL Kimmel, S Oparil, CE Lewis, M Rahman, WC Cushman. Effects of intensive systolic blood pressure lowering on cardiovascular events and mortality in patients with type 2 diabetes mellitus on standard glycemic control and in those without diabetes mellitus: Reconciling results from ACCORD BP and SPRINT. *J Am Heart Assoc* 2018; 7(18):1–14. doi: 10.1161/JAHA.118.009326.

Beta-Blocker Heart Attack Trial Research Group. A randomized trial of propranolol in patients with acute myocardial infarction. I. Mortality results. *JAMA* 1982; 247:1707–1714.

M Bliss. *The Discovery of Insulin*. Toronto: McClelland & Steward, 1982.

M Bliss. *William Osler: A Life in Medicine*. Oxford: Oxford University Press, 1999.

WE Boden, RA O'Rourke, KK Teo, PM Hartigan, DJ Maron, WJ Kostuk, M Knudtson, M Dada, P Casperson, CL Harris, BR Chaitman, L Shaw, G Gosselin, S Nawaz, LM Title, G Gau, AS Blaustein, DC Booth, ER Bates, JA Spertus, DS Berman, J Mancini, WS Weintraub, for the COURAGE Trial Research Group. Optimal medical therapy with or without PCI for stable coronary disease. *N Engl J Med* 2007; 356:1503–1516.

NO Borhani, WB Applegate, JA Cutler, BR Davis, CD Furberg, E Lakatos, L Page, M Perry, WM Smith, JL Probstfield. Part 1: Rationale and Design. *Hypertension* 1991; 17(suppl II):1–15.

RT Borne, D Katz, J Betz, PN Peterson, FA Masouli. Cardioverter-defibrillators for secondary prevention of sudden cardiac death: a review. *J Am Heart Assoc* 2017; 6:e005515. DOI: 10.1161/JAHA.117.005515.

L Bowman, JC Hopewell, F Chen, K Wallendszus, W Stevens, R Collins, SD Wiviott, CP Cannon, E Braunwald, E Sammons,

Bibliography

MJ Landray MJ. HPS3/TIMI55–REVEAL Collaborative Group. Effects of anacetrapib in patients with atherosclerotic vascular disease. *N Engl J Med* 2017; 377:1217–1227. doi: 10.1056/NEJMoa1706444.

E Braunwald, MS Sabatine. The Thrombolysis in Myocardial Infarction (TIMI) group experience. *J Thorac Cardiovasc Surg* 2012; 144:762–770.

MS Brown, JL Goldstein. A receptor-mediated pathway for cholesterol homeostasis. *Science* 1986; 232:34–47.

MS Brown, JL Goldstein. A tribute to Akira Endo, discoverer of a "Penicillin" for cholesterol. *Atherosclerosis Suppl* 2004; 5:13–6.

J Bryan. How spironolactone became the next best thing for severe heart failure. *Pharmaceutical Journal*, January 18, 2012. https://www.pharmaceutical-journal.com/news-and-analysis/how-spironolactone-became-the-next-best-thing-for-severe-heart-failure/11093181.article?firstPass=false.

H Buchwald, RL Varco, JP Matts, JM Long, LL Fitch, GS Campbell, MB Pearce, AE Yellin, WA Edmiston, RD Smink, HS Sawin, CT Campos, BJ Hansen, N Tuna, JN Karnegis, ME Sanmarco, K Amplatz, WR Casteneda-Zuniga, DW Hunter, JK Bissett, FW Weber, JW Stevenson, AS Leon, TC Chalmers, and the POSCH Group. Effect of Partial Ileal Bypass Surgery on Mortality and Morbidity from Coronary Heart Disease in Patients with Hypercholesterolemia—Report of the Program on the Surgical Control of the Hyperlipidemias (POSCH). *N Engl J Med* 1990; 323:946–355, DOI: 10.1056/NEJM199010043231404.

DS Buist, KM Newton, DL Miglioretti, K Beverly, MT Connelly, S Andrade, CL Hartsfield, F Wei, A Chan, L Kessler. Hormone therapy prescribing patterns in the United States. *Osbtet Gynecol* 2004; 104:1042–1050.

VL Burt, JA Cutler, M Higgins, MJ Horan, D Labarth, P Whelton, C Brown, EJ Rocella. Trends in the prevalence, awareness, treatment, and control of hypertension in the adults US population. Data from the Health Examination Surveys, 1960 to 1991. *Hypertension* 1995; 26:1–60, https://www.ahajournals.org/doi/epub/10.1161/01.HYP.26.1.60.

TL Bush. Noncontraceptive estrogen use and risk of cardiovascular disease: an overview and critique of the literature. In: SG Korenman (ed.) *The Menopause: Biological and Clinical Consequences of Ovarian Failure; Evolution and Management.* Norwell, MA: Serono Symposia, USA, 1990.

The Bypass Angioplasty Revascularization (BARI) Investigators. Comparison of coronary bypass surgery with angioplasty in patients with multivessel disease. *N Engl J Med* 1996; 335:217–225.

The CAPRICORN Investigators. Effect of carvedilol on outcome after myocardial infarction in patients with left-ventricular dysfunction: the CAPRICORN randomized trial. *Lancet* 2001; 357:1385–1390.

Cardiac Arrest Registry to Enhance Survival (CARES) website. https://mycares.net/.

Cardiac Arrhythmia Suppression Trial (CAST) Investigators. Preliminary report: effect of encainide and flecainide on mortality in a randomized trial of arrhythmia suppression after myocardial infarction. *N Engl J Med* 1989; 32:406–12. https://www.ncbi.nlm.nih.gov/pubmed/2473403?dopt=Abstract.

MR Carnethon, J Pu, G Howard, MA Albert, CAM Anderson, AG Bertoni, MS Mujahid, L Palaniappan, HA Taylor, M Willis, CW Yancy, on behalf of the American Heart Association Council on Epidemiology and Prevention; Council on Cardiovascular Disease in the Young, Council on Cardiovascular Nursing, Council on Clinical Cardiology, Council on Functional Genomics and Translational Biology, and Stroke Council. Cardiovascular Health in African Americans. A scientific statement from the American Heart Association. Endorsed by the American College of Cardiology. *Circulation* 2017; 136:e393-e403. DOI: 10.1161/CIR.0000000000000534.

MD Carroll, AK Kit, DA Lacher, ST Shero, ME Mussolino. Trends in lipids and lipoproteins of US adults, 1988–2010. *JAMA* 2012; 308:1545–1554.

MD Carroll, BK Kit, DA Lacher, SS Yoon. Total and high-density lipoprotein cholesterol in adults: National Health and

Nutrition Exam Survey 2011–12. Figures 3, 4. https://www.cdc.gov/nchs/data/databriefs/db132.pdf.

CASS Principal Investigators and Their Associates. Myocardial infarction and mortality in the Coronary Artery Surgery Study (CASS) randomized trial. *N Engl J Med* 1984; 310:750–758. DOI: 10.1056/NEJM198403223101204.

CDC MMMR Weekly. 1999 Tobacco Use—United States, 1900–1999. November 5, 1999; 48:986–993. https://www.cdc.gov/mmwr/preview/mmwrhtml/mm4843a2.htm.

CDC National Diabetes Statistical Report 2020. Estimates of Diabetes and its Burden in the United States. https://www.cdc.gov/diabetes/pdfs/data/statistics/national-diabetes-statistics-report.pdf.

CDC's Division of Diabetes Translation. United States Diabetes Surveillance System. Long-term Trends in Diabetes April 2017. https://www.cdc.gov/Diabetes/statistics/slides/long_term_trends.pdf.

Centers for Disease Control. Age-adjusted death rates for 69 selected causes by race and sex using year 2000 standard population: United States, 1950–59 https://www.cdc.gov/nchs/data/dvs/hist293_1950_59.pdf, 1960–67 https://www.cdc.gov/nchs/data/mortab/aadr6067.pdf, 1968–78 https://www.cdc.gov/nchs/data/mortab/aadr6878.pdf.

Centers for Disease Control (CDC). Leading Causes of Death, 1990–1998. Data provided to NIH by the National Center for Health Statistics.

Centers for Disease Control. 1986 Surgeon General's Report: The Health Consequences of Involuntary Smoking. MMWR Morb Mortal Wkly Rep 1986; 35:769–70. PMID 3097495.

Centers for Disease Control. Online Table 22. Hypertension among adults aged 20 and over by selected characteristics. United States, selected years 1988–1994 through 2013–2016. https://www.cdc.gov/nchs/data/hus/2018/022.pdf.

Centers for Disease Control and Prevention. *A Closer Look at African American Men and High Blood Pressure Control: A Review of Psychosocial Factors and Systems-Level Interventions.* Atlanta: U.S. Department of Health and Human Services, 2010.

Centers for Disease Control and Prevention. Heart disease death rates among blacks and whites, aged > 35 years—United States, 1968–2015. Morbidity and Mortality Weekly Report. *Surveillance Summaries* 2018, 30 March; 67(5):1–11. https://www.cdc.gov/mmwr/volumes/67/ss/ss6705a1.htm.

Centers for Disease Control and Prevention. Heart Disease Facts, https://www.cdc.gov/heartdisease/facts.htm.

Centers for Disease Control and Prevention (CDC). National Diabetes Statistics Report 2020. Estimates of Diabetes and its Burden in the United States. https://www.cdc.gov/diabetes/pdfs/data/statistics/national-diabetes-statistics-report.Pdf.

Centers for Disease Control and Prevention. Smoking & Tobacco Use: A Brief History. https://www.cdc.gov/tobacco/data_statistics/sgr/history/index.htm.

Centers for Disease Control and Prevention. Surgeon General's Advisory on E-cigarette Use Among Youth. February 2020. https://www.cdc.gov/tobacco/basic_information/e-cigarettes/surgeon-general-advisory/index.html.

Centers for Disease Control and Prevention. US Public Health Service Syphilis Study at Tuskegee. Timeline. Accessed August 2020 at https://www.cdc.gov/tuskegee/timeline.htm.

Centers for Disease Control and Prevention (CDC), National Center of Health Statistics. Mortality Data Finder. Table 5: Age-adjusted death rates for selected causes of death by sex, race and Hispanic origin: United States, selected years 1950–2017 https://www.cdc.gov/nchs/hus/contents2018.htm#Table_005 (Excel spreadsheet link).

Centers for Disease Control and Prevention (CDC), National Center of Health Statistics. Mortality Data,HIST293. Age-adjusted death rates for selected causes by race and sex using year 2000 standard population: death registration states, 1900–32 and United States, 1933–49, Diseases of the Heart. https://www.cdc.gov/nchs/data/dvs/hist293_1900_49.pdf.

Bibliography

L Chacko, JP Howard, C Rajkumar, AN Nowbar, C Kane, D Mahdi, M Foley, M Shun-Shin, G Cole, S Sen, A Al-Lamee, DP Francis, Y Ahmad. Effects of percutaneous coronary intervention on death and myocardial infarction stratified by stable and unstable coronary artery disease. A meta-analysis of randomized controlled trials. *Circ Cardiovasc Qual Outcomes* 2020, Feb; 13:e006363. DOI: 10.1161/CIRCOUTCOMES.119.006363. https://www.ahajournals.org/doi/pdf/10.1161/CIRCOUTCOMES.119.006363.

Chartbook for the Conference on the Decline in Coronary Heart Disease Mortality. Hyattsville, MD: NCHS, 1978. National Center for Health Statistics, https://www.cdc.gov/nchs/data/misc/corltrtacc.pdf.

Z Chen, R Peto, R Collins, S MacMahon, J Lu, W Li. Serum cholesterol concentration and coronary heart disease In population with low cholesterol concentrations. *BMJ* 1991; 303:276–282.

JH Chesebro, G Knatterud, R Roberts, J Borer, LS Cohen, J Dalen, HT Dodge, CK Francis, D Hillis, P Ludbrook, JE Markis, H Mueller, ER Passamani, ER Powers, AK Rao, T Robertson, A Ross, TJ Ryan, BE Sobel, J Willerson, DO Williams, BL Zaret, E Braunwald. Thrombolysis in Myocardial Infarction (TIMI) Trial, Phase I: a comparison between intravenous tissue plasminogen activator and intravenous streptokinase. Clinical findings through hospital discharge. *Circulation* 1987; 76:142–154.

Cholesterol Treatment Trialists (CTC) Collaboration. Protocol for a prospective collaborative overview of all current and planned randomized trials of cholesterol treatment regimens. *Am J Cardiol* 1995; 75:1130–1134.

Cholesterol Treatment Trialists Collaboration. Efficacy and safety of cholesterol-lowering treatment: prospective meta-analysis of data from 90,056 participants in 14 randomized trials of statins. *Lancet* 2005; 366:1267–1278.DOI:10.1016/S0140–6736(05)67394–1.

Cholesterol Treatment Trialists Collaboration. Efficacy and safety of more intensive lowering of LDL cholesterol: a meta-analysis of data from 170,000 participants in 26 randomized trials. *Lancet* 2010; 376:1670–1681.

Cholesterol Treatment Trialists Collaboration. Efficacy of cholesterol-lowering therapy in 18 686 people with diabetes in 14 randomised trials of statins: a meta-analysis. *Lancet* 2008; 371:117–125.

JGF Cleland, L Erhardt, G Murray, AS Hall, SG Bell, on behalf of the AIRE Study Investigators. Effect of ramipril on morbidity and mode of death among survivors of acute myocardial infarction with clinical evidence of heart failure. A Report from the AIRE Study Investigators. *Eur Heart J* 1997; 18:41–51.

ClinCalc DrugStats Database. The top 200 drugs of 2020. https://clincalc.com/DrugStats/Top200Drugs.aspx.

ClinicalTrials.gov. https://clinicaltrials.gov.

LA Cobb, CE Fahrenbruch, M Olsufka, MK Copass. Changing incidence of out-of-hospital ventricular fibrillation, 1980–2000. *JAMA* 2002; 288:3008–3013.

JN Cohn, G Johnson, S Ziesche, F Cobb, G Francis, F Tristani, R Smith, B Dunkman, H Loeb, M Wong, G Bhat, S Goldman, RD Fletcher, J Doherty, CV Hughes, P Carson, G Cintron, R Shabetai, C Haakenson. A comparison of enalapril with hydralazine-isosorbide dinitrate in the treatment of chronic congestive heart failure. *N Engl J Med* 1991; 325:303–310.

LA Conlay, JE Loewenstein. Phenformin and Lactic Acidosis. *JAMA* 1976; 235:1575–1578. doi:10.1001/jama.1976.03260410031019.

SJ Connolly, P Dorian, RS Roberts, M Gent, S Bailin, ES Fain, K Thorpe, J Champagne, M Talajic, B Coutu, GC Cronefield, SH Hohnloser, for the Optimal Pharmacological Therapy in Cardioverter Defibrillator Patients (OPTIC) Investigators. Comparison of beta-blockers, amiodarone plus beta-blockers, or sotalol for prevention of shocks from implantable cardioverter defibrillators. The OPTIC Study: a randomized trial. JAMA 2006; 295:165–171.

SJ Connolly. Meta-analysis of anti-arrhythmic drug trials. Am J Cardiol 2004; 84(supplement 1):90–93. DOI: https://doi.org/10.1016/S0002-9149(99)00708-0.

SJ Connolly, M Gent, RS Roberts, P Doran,

D Roy, RS Sheldon, LB Mitchell, MS Green, GJ Klein, B O'Brien, for the CIDS Investigators. Canadian Implantable Defibrillator Study (CIDS): A randomized controlled trial of the implantable cardioverter defibrillator against amiodarone. *Circulation* 2000; 101:1297–1302.

The Consensus Trial Study Group. Effects of enalopril on mortality in severe congestive heart failure. *N Engl J Med* 1987; 316:1429–1435. DOI: 10.1056/NEJM198706043162301.

The Coronary Drug Project. Initial findings leading to modifications of its research protocol. *JAMA* 1970, Nov 16; 214(7):1303–1313.

The Coronary Drug Project research group. The Coronary Drug Project. Findings leading to further modifications of its protocol with respect to dextrothyroxine. *JAMA* 1972, May 15; 220(7):996–1008.

The Coronary Drug Project. Clofibrate and niacin in coronary heart disease. *JAMA* 1975, Jan 27; 231(4):360–81.

C Crawford. Cigarette smoking among US adults hits an all-time low. *AAFP News*. November 20, 2019. https://www.aafp.org/news/health-of-the-public/20191120mmwr-cigarettesmoking.html.

JA Critchley, S Capewell. Mortality risk reduction associated with smoking cessation in patients with coronary heart disease: a systematic review. *JAMA* 2003; 290:86–97. Doi: 10.1001/jama.290.1.86.

J Crowe, C Lacy, Y Columbus. Barriers to food security and community stress in an urban food desert. *Urban Science* 2018; 2:45–61. doi:10.3390/urbansci2020046.

JD Curb, SL Pressel, JA Cutler, PJ Savage, WB Applegate, H Black, G Carmel, BR Davis, PH Frost, N Gonzalez, G Guthrie, A Oberman, GH Rutan, J Stamler, for the Systolic Hypertension in the Elderly Program Cooperative Research Group. Effect of diuretic-based antihypertensive treatment on cardiovascular disease risk in older diabetic patients with isolated systolic hypertension. *JAMA* 1996; 276:1896–1892.

PD Curtin. The slavery hypothesis for hypertension among African Americans: The historical evidence. *Am J Publ Health* 1992; 82:1681–1686.

DW Cushman, MA Ondetti. History of the design of captopril and related inhibitors of angiotensin converting enzyme. *Hypertension* 1991; 4:589–592.

J Cutler, SW MacMahon, CD Furberg. Controlled clinical trials of drug treatment for hypertension: A review. *Hypertension* 1989; 13(suppl I):I36-I44.

JE Dalen, JS Alpert, RJ Goldberg, RS Weinstein. The epidemic of the 20th century: Coronary Heart Disease. *The American Journal of Medicine* 2014; 127:807–812.

C Dampier. At age 100, the father of preventive medicine is going strong—as living proof that he was right all along. *Chicago Tribune*, December 26, 2019. https://www.chicagotribune.com/lifestyles/ct-life-100-year-old-scientist-stamler-20191226-jeprzoeqazha7nuvs2prfcndwy-story.html.

J Danesh, JG Wheeler, GM Hirschfield, S Eda, G Eiriksdottir, A Rumley, GDO Lowe, MB Pepys, V Gudnason. C-reactive protein and other circulating markers of inflammation in the prediction of coronary heart disease. *N Engl J Med* 2004; 350:1387–1397.

The Diabetes Control and Complications Trial Research Group. The effect of intensive treatment of diabetes on the development and progression of long-term complications in insulin-dependent diabetes mellitus. *N Engl J Med* 1993; 329: 977–986.

The Digitalis Investigators Group. The effect of digoxin on mortality and morbidity in patients with heart failure. *N Engl J Med* 1997; 336:525–533.

R Doll R, AB Hill. The mortality of doctors in relation to their smoking habits. A preliminary report. *BMJ* 1954; 228 (i): 1451–55.

R Doll, AB Hill. A study of the aetiology of carcinoma of the lung. *Br Med J* 1952; 2:1271–1286.

JA Dormandy, B Charbonel, DJA Eckland, E Erdman, M Massi-Benedetti, IK Moules, MH Tan, PJ Lefebvre, GD Murray, E Standl, RG Wilcox, L Wilhelmsen, J Betteridge, K Birkeland, A Golay, RJ

Heine, L Koranyi, M Laakso, M Mokan, A Norkus, V Pirags, T Podar, A Scheen, W Scherbaum, G Schernthaner, O Schmitz, J Skrha, U Smith, J Taton, on behalf of the PROActive Investigators. Secondary prevention of macrovascular events in patients with type 2 diabetes in the PROactive Study (PROspective pioglitzAzone Clinical Trial In macrovascular Events): a randomized controlled trial. *Lancet* 2005; 366:1279–1289. DOI: https://doi.org.10.1016/S0140-6736(05)67528-9.

J Dorn, J Naughton, D Inamura, M Trevisian, for the NEHDP Project Staff. Results of a multicenter randomized clinical trial or exercise and long-term survival in myocardial infarction patients. The National Exercise and Heart Disease Project (NEHDP). *Circulation* 1999; 100: 1764–1769.

W Duckworth, C Abraira, T Moritz, D Reda, N Emanuele, PD Reaven, FJ Zieve, J Marks, SN Davis, R Hayward, SR Warren, S Goldman, M McCarren, ME Vitek, WG Henderson, GD Huang, for the VADT Investigators. Glucose control and vascular complications in veterans with type 2 diabetes. *N Engl J Med* 2009; 360:129–139.

LR Dugas, TE Forrester, J Plange-Rhule, P Bovet, EV Lambert, RA Durazo-Arvizu, G Cao, RS Cooper, R Khatib, L Tonino, W Riesen, W Korte, S Kliethermes, A Luke. Cardiovascular risk status of Afro-origin populations across the spectrum of economic development: findings from the Modeling the Epidemiologic Transition Study. *BMC public health* 2017; 17(1):438.

RH Eckel, JM Jacsic, JD Ard, JM de Jesus, NH Miller, VS Hubbard, IM Lee, AH Lichtenstein, CM Loria, BE Millen, CA Nonas, FM Sacks, SC Smith, LP Svetkey, TA Wadden, SZ Yanovski. 2013 AHA/ACC Guideline on Lifestyle Management to Reduce Cardiovascular Risk. A report of the American College of Cardiology/American Heart Association Task Force on Practice Guidelines. *Circulation* 2014; 129(suppl 2):S76-S99. DOI: 10.1161/01.cir.0000437740.48606.d1.

PC Elwood, AL Cochrane, ML Burr, PM Sweetman, G Williams, E Welsby, SJ Hughes, R Renton. A randomized controlled trial of acetyl salicylic acid in the secondary prevention of mortality from myocardial infarction. *BMJ* 1974; 1:436–440.

A Endo. A historical perspective on the study of statins. *Proc Jpn Acad Ser B* 2010; 86;484–493.

EPA. Respiratory Health Effects of Passive Smoking: Lung Cancer and Other Disorders. Office of Health and Environmental Assessment, Office of Research and Development, US Environmental Protection Agency, Washington, D.C., December 1992.

Epidemiology of Tobacco Use: History and Current Trends. https://www.nap.edu/read/11795/chapter/4.

R Estruch, E Ros, J Salas-Salvadó, MI Covas, D Corella, F Arós, E Gómez-Gracia, V Ruiz-Gutiérrez, M Fiol, J Lapetra, RM Lamuela-Raventos. Primary prevention of cardiovascular disease with a Mediterranean diet supplemented with extra-virgin olive oil or nuts. *N Engl J Med* 2018; 378;e34. DOI: 10.1056/NEJMoa1800389.

D Ettehad, CA Emdin, A Kiran, SG Anderson, T Callender, J Emberson, J Chalmers, A Rodgers, K Rahimi. Blood pressure lowering for prevention of cardiovascular disease and death: a systematic review and meta-analysis. Lancet 2016; 387;957–967.

European Coronary Surgery Study Group. Long-term results of prospective randomized study of coronary artery bypass surgery in stable angina patients. *Lancet* 1992; 320:1173–1180. DOI: https://doi.org/10.1016/S0140-6736(82)91200-4.

SD Fihn, JM Gardin, J Abrams, K Berra, JC Blankenship, AP Dallas, PS Douglas, JM Foody, TC Gerber, AL Hinderliter, SB King, PD Kligfield, HM Krumholz, RYK Kwong, MJ Lim, JA Linderbaum, MJ Mack, MA Munger, RL Prager, JF Sabik, LJ Shaw, JD Sikkema, CR Smith, SC Smith, JA Spertus, SV Williams. 2012 ACCF/AHA/ACP/AATS/PCNA/SCAI/STS Guideline for the Diagnosis and Management of Patients with Stable Ischemic Heart Disease. A report of the American College of Cardiology

Foundation/American Heart Association Task Force on Practice Guidelines, and the American College of Physicians, American Association for Thoracic Surgery, Preventive Cardiovascular Nurses Association, Society for Cardiovascular Angiography and Intervention, and Society of Thoracic Surgeons. *Circulation* 2012; 126:e354-e471. DOI: 10.1161/CIR.0b013e318277d6a0.

First International Study of Infarct Survival Collaborative Group. Randomised trial of intravenous atenolol among 16,027 cases of suspected acute myocardial infarction: ISIS-1. *Lancet* 1986; 2:57–66.

RN Fogoros. Amiodarone lung toxicity. verywellhealth. https://www.verywellhealth.com/amiodarone-lung-toxicity-1745988.

Food and Drug Administration. 2018 National Youth Tobacco Survey Finds Cause for Concern. https://www.fda.gov/tobacco-products/youth-and-tobacco/2018-nyts-data-startling-rise-youth-e-cigarette-use.

ES Ford, UA Ajani, JB Croft, JA Critchley, DR Labarth, TE Kottke, WH Giles, S Capewell. Explaining the Decrease in U.S. Deaths from Coronary Disease, 1980–2000. *N Engl J Med* 2007; 356:2388–2398. DOI: 10.1056/NEJMsa053935.

RJ Franscone, KG Lurie, JM Goodloe. Resuscitation Outcomes Consortium (ROC) studies dig deep into the science of resuscitation. *Journal of Emergency Medical Services* 2026, Dec 31; 42(1). https://www.jems.com/2016/12/31/resuscitation-outcomes-consortium-roc-studies-dig-deep-into-the-science-of-resuscitation/.

DS Fredrickson, RI Levy, RS Lees. Fat Transport in Lipoproteins—An integrated approach to mechanisms and disorders. *N Engl J Med* 1967; 276: 273–281, DOI: 1056/NEJM196702022760507.

N Freemantle, J Cleland, P Young, J Mason, J Harrison. Beta blockade after myocardial infarction: systematic review and meta regression analysis. *BMJ* 1999; 318:1730–1737.

MH Frick, O Elo, K Haapa, OP Heinonen, P Heinsalmi, P Helo, JK Huttunen, P Kaitaniemi, P Koskinen, V Manninen, H Maenpaa, M Malkonen, et al. Helsinki Heart Study: primary-prevention trial with gemfibrozil in middle-aged men with dyslipidemia. Safety of treatment, changes in risk factors, and incidence of coronary heart disease. *New England Journal of Medicine* 1987; 317: 1237–1245.

LM Friedman, CD Furberg, DL DeMets, DM Reboussin, CB Granger. *Fundamentals of Clinical Trials*. New York: Springer Science & Business Media, 5th edition, 2015.

Fryar CD, Carroll MD, Ogden CL. Prevalence of overweight, obesity, and severe obesity among adults aged 20 and over. United States, 1960–62 through 2015–2016. National Center for Health Statistics. Health E-Stats September 2018. https://stacks.cdc.gov/view/cdc/58670.

AJ Garber. Long-acting glucagon-like peptide 1 receptor agonists: a review of their efficacy and efficiency. *Diabetes Care* 2011; 34:S279-S284.

TA Gaziano, A Bitton, S Anand, S Abrahams-Gessel, A Murphy. Growing epidemic of coronary heart disease in low- and middle-income countries. *Curr Probl Cardiol* 2010; 35:72–115.

RJ Gibbons, K Chatterjee, J Daley, JS Douglas, SD Fihn, JM Gardin, MA Grunwald, D Levy, BW Lytle, RA O'Rourke, WP Schafer, SV Williams, JL Ritchie, MD Cheitlin, KA Eagle, TJ Gardner, A Garson, RO Russell, TJ Ryan, SC Smith. ACC/AHA/ACP—ASIM Guidelines for the Management of Patients with Chronic Stable Angina: Executive Summary and Recommendations. A report of the American College of Cardiology/American Heart Association task force on practice guidelines (Committee on Management of Patients with Chronic Stable Angina). *Circulation* 1999; 99:2829-2848. https://doi.org/10.1161/01.CIR.99.21.2829.

DR Ginsberg. Aspirin: turn-of-the-century miracle drug. *Distillations*, June 2, 2009. https://www.sciencehistory.org/distillations/aspirin-turn-of-the-century-miracle-drug.

GR Giovanini, P Libby. Atherosclerosis and inflammation: overview and updates. *Clinical Science* 2018; 132:1243–1252.

GISSI. Effectiveness of intravenous

thrombolytic treatment in acute myocardial infarction. *Lancet* 1986; 1:397-402.

A Glass. Congress bans airing cigarette ads, April 1, 1970. https://www.politico.com/story/2018/04/01/congress-bans-airing-cigarette-ads-april-1-1970-489882.

The Global Use of Strategies to Open Occluded Coronary Arteries in Acute Coronary Syndromes (GUSTO IIb) Angioplasty Substudy Investigators. A clinical trial comparing primary angioplasty with tissue plasminogen activator for acute myocardial infarction. *N Engl J Med* 1997; 336:1621–1628.

W Goldring, H Chasis. Antihypertensive drug therapy: an appraisal. *Arch Intern Med* 1965; 115:523–25.

JL Goldstein, MS Brown. History of Discovery: The LDL Receptor. *Arteriosclerosis, Thrombosis, and Vascular Biology* 2009; 29:431–438.

MA Gonzalez, FR Artalejo, J Calero. Relationship between socioeconomic status and ischaemic heart disease in cohort and case-control studies: 1960–1993. *Int J Epidemiol* 1998; 27:350–358.

DJ Gordon. Cholesterol and Mortality: What Can Meta-Analysis Tell Us? *Cardiovascular Disease 2: Cellular and Molecular Mechanisms, Prevention, and Treatment*. LL Gallo LL (ed.). New York: Plenum Press ,1995.

DJ Gordon. Cholesterol Lowering Reduces Mortality. *Cholesterol Lowering Therapies 1999*. SM Grundy (ed.). New York: Marcel Dekker, Inc., 1999.

DJ Gordon. HDL and cardiovascular disease. *Cardiology Board Review* 1990; 7:29–40.

DJ Gordon. HDL and CHD—An epidemiologic perspective. J Drug Devel 1990, 3 (suppl): 11–17.

DJ Gordon. Role of circulating HDL and triglycerides in coronary artery disease. End Metab Clin N Amer 1990; 19:299–310.

DJ Gordon, JL Probstfield, RJ Garrison, JD Neaton, WP Castelli, JD Knoke, DR Jacobs, S Bangdiwala, HA Tyroler. High-density lipoprotein and cardiovascular disease: Four American Studies, Circulation 1989; 79:8–15.

DJ Gordon, BM Rifkind. HDL—Clinical implications of recent studies. *N Engl J Med* 1989; 321:1311–1316.

DJ Gordon, KM Salz, KJ Roggenkamp, FA Franklin. Dietary determinants of plasma cholesterol change in the recruitment phase of the Lipid Research Clinics Coronary Primary Prevention Trial. *Arteriosclerosis* 1982; 2:537–548.

T Gordon, WP Castelli, MC Hjortland, WB Kannel, TR Dawber. High-density lipoprotein as a protective factor against coronary heart disease. The Framingham Study. *Am J Med* 1977; 62:707–714.

AM Gotto, Jeremiah Metzger Lecture: Cholesterol, Inflammation and Atherosclerotic Cardiovascular Disease: Is it all LDL? JL Goldstein, MS Brown. A century of cholesterol and coronaries. From plaques to genes to statins. *Cell* 2015; 161:161–172. doi: 10.1016/j.cell.2015.01.036.

D Grady, D Herrington, V Bittner, R Blumenthal, M Davidson, M Hlatky, J Hsia, S Hulley, A Herd, S Khan, IK Newby, D Waters, E Vittinghoff, N Wenger, for the HERS Research Group. Cardiovascular disease outcomes during 6.8 years of hormone therapy. Heart and Estrogen/Progestin Replacement Study follow-up (HERS II). *JAMA* 2002; 288:49–57.

D Grady, SM Rubin, DB Petiti, CS Fox, D Black, B Ettinger, VL Ernster, SR Cummings. Hormone therapy to prevent disease and prolog life in postmenopausal women. *Ann Intern Med* 1992; 117: 1016–1037.

ED Grech. Percutaneous coronary intervention. I. History and Development. *BMJ* 2003; 326:1080–1082.

JB Green, MA Bethel, PW Armstrong, JB Buse, SS Engel, J Garg, R Josse, KD Kaufman, J Koglin, S Korn, KM Lachin, DK McGuire, MJ Pencina, E Standl, PP Stein, S Suryawanshi, F Van de Werf, ED Peterson, RR Holman, for the TECOS Study Group. Effect of sitagliptin on cardiovascular outcomes in type 2 diabetes. *N Engl J Med* 2015; 373:232–242. DOI: 10.1056/NEJMoa1501352.

HL Greene, DM Roden, RJ Katz, DM Slerno, RW Henthorn. The Cardiac Arrhythmia Suppression Trial: first CAST-I ... then CAST-II. *J Am Coll Cardiol* 1992;

19:894–98, https://clinicaltrials.gov/ct2/show/record/NCT00000526?term=flecanide&draw=5&rank=33&view=record.

RH Grimm, KL Margolis, V Papademetriou, WC Cushman, CE Ford, J Bettencourt, MH Alderman, JN Basile, HR Black, V DeQuattro, J Eckfeldt, CM Hawkins, HM Perry, M Proschan. Baseline characteristics of participants in the Antihypertensive and Lipid Heart Attack Trial (ALLHAT). *Hypertension* 2001; 37:19–27.

SM Grundy, RB d'Agostino, L Mosca, GL Burke, PWF Wilson, DJ Rader, EJ Rocella, JA Cutler, LM Friedman. Cardiovascular risk assessment based on US cohort studies: Findings from a National Heart, Lung, and Blood Institute Workshop. Circulation 2001; 104:491–496. P Sorlie, G Wei. Population-based cohort studies: Still relevant? *J Am Coll Cardiol* 2011; 58:2010–13, http://www.onlinejacc.org/content/accj/58/19/2010.full.pdf.

SM Grundy, NJ Stone, AL Bailey, C Beam, KK Birtcher, RS Blumenthal, LT Braun, S de Ferranti, J Faiella-Tommasino, DE Forman, R Goldberg, PA Heidenreich, MA Hlatky, DW Jones, D Lloyd-Jones, N Lopez-Pajares, CE Ndumele, CE Orringer, CA Peralta, JJ Saseen, SC Smith, L Sperling, SS Virani, J Yeboah. 2018 AHA/ACC/AACVPR/AAPA/ABC/ACPM/ADA/AGS/APhA/ASPC/NLA/PCNA Guideline on the Management of Blood Cholesterol: A Report of the American College of Cardiology/American Heart Association Task Force on Clinical Practice Guidelines. *Circulation* 2019; 139:e1082-e1143. https://www.ahajournals.org/doi/10.1161/CIR.0000000000000625

Gruppo Italiano per la Sperimentazione della Streptchinasi nell'Infarto Miocardico. GISSI-2: a factorial randomized trial of altepase versus streptokinase and heparin versus no heparin among 12,490 patients with acute myocardial infarction. *Lancet* 1990; 8797:65–71.

Q Gu, R Paulose-Ram, VL Burt, BK Kit. Prescription cholesterol-lowering medication use in adults aged 40 and over: United States, 2003–2012. NCHS Data Brief No. 177, December 2014. https://www.cdc.gov/nchs/data/databriefs/db177.pdf.

The GUSTO Investigators. An international randomized trial comparing four thrombolytic strategies for acute myocardial infarction. *N Engl J Med* 1993; 329:673–672.

SA Haji, A Mohaved. Update on digoxin therapy in congestive heart failure. *Am Fam Physician* 2000; 62:409–416.

EC Hammond, D Horn. The relationship between human smoking habits and death rates: A follow-up study of 187,766 men. *JAMA* 1954; 155:1316–1328. doi:10.1001/jama.1954.03690330020006.

Harvard School of Public Health. The Nutrition Source. PREDIMED Study Retraction and Republication. What changed, what didn't, and the big picture. https://www.hsph.harvard.edu/nutritionsource/2018/06/22/predimed-retraction-republication/.

AL Hawkes, M Nowak, B Bidstrup, R Speare. Outcomes of coronary artery bypass graft surgery. *Vascular Health and Risk Management* 2006; 2:477–484.

J Hay, A British Medical Association, Lecture on the Significance of a Raised Blood Pressure, British Medical J July 11, 1931; 2 (3679): 43–47.

J He, D Gu, K Reynolds, X Wu, P Muntner, J Zhao, J Chen, D Liu, J Mo, PK Whelton, InterASIA Collaborative Group. Serum total and lipoprotein cholesterol levels and awareness, treatment, and control of hypercholesterolemia in China. *Circulation* 2004; 110: 405–411. DOI: 10.1161/01.CIR.0000136583.52681.0D.

Health, United States. 2012 Updates. https://www.cdc.gov/nchs/data/hus/2012/001.pdf.

The Heart Outcomes Prevention Evaluation Study Investigators. Effects of an angiotensin-converting enzyme inhibitor, ramipril, on cardiovascular events in high risk patients. *N Engl J Med* 2000; 342:145–153.

DM Hegsted, RB McGandy, ML Myers, FJ Stare, Quantitative effects of dietary fat on serum cholesterol in men. *Am J Clin Nutr* 1965; 17:281–295.

Bibliography

M Helfand, DL Buckley, M Freeman, R Fu, K Rogers, C Fleming, LL Humphrey. Emerging risk factors for coronary heart disease: a summary of systematic reviews conducted for the US Preventive Services Task Force. *Ann Intern Med* 2009; 151:496–507.

DM Herrington, DM Reboussin, B Brosnihan, PC Sharp, SA Schumaker, TE Snyder, CD Furberg, GJ Kowalchuk, TD Stuckey, WJ Rogers, DH Givens, D Waters. Effects of estrogen replacement on the progression of coronary artery atherosclerosis. *N Engl J Med* 2000; 343:522–529.

RA Herrington. Targeting inflammation in cardiovascular disease. *N Engl J Med* 2017; 377:1197–1198. DOI: 10.1056/NEJMe1709904.

HAB Hiza, L Bente. (2007). Nutrient Content of the U.S. Food Supply, 1909–2004: A Summary Report. (Home Economics Research Report No. 57). U.S. https://fns-prod.azureedge.net/sites/default/files/nutrient_content_of_the_us_food_supply/FoodSupply1909-2004Report.pdf.

JS Hochman, GA Lamas, CE Buller, V Dzavik, HR Reynolds, SJ Abramsky, S Forman, W Ruzyllo, AP Maggione, H White, Z Sadowski, AC Carvalho, JM Rankin, JP Renkin, PG Steg, AM Mascette, G Sopko, ME Pfisterer, J Leor, V Fridrich, DB Mark, GL Knatterud, for the Occluded Artery Trial Investigators. Coronary intervention for persistent occlusion after myocardial infarction. *N Engl J Med* 2006; 355:2395–2407.

JS Hochman, LA Sleeper, JG Webb, TA Sanborn, HD White, JD Talley, CE Buller, AK Jacobs, JN Slater, J Col, SM McKinlay, TH LeMetel, for the SHOCK Investigators. *N Engl J Med* 1999; 341:625–634.

HN Hodis, WJ Mack, SP Azen, RA Lobo, D Shoupe, PR Mahrer, DP Faxon, L Cashin-Hemphill, ME Sanmarco, WJ French, TL Shook, TD Gardner, AO Mehra, R Rabbani, A Sevanian, AB Shil, M Torres, KH Vogelbach, RH Selzer, for the Women's Estrogen/Progestin Lipid-Lowering Hormone Atherosclerosis Regression Trial.

KM Hoffman, S Trawalter, JR Axt, MN Oliver. Racial bias in pain assessment and treatment recommendations, and false beliefs about differences between blacks and whites. *Proc Nat Acad Sci* 2016; 113: 4296–4301. www.pnas.org/cgi/doi/10.1073/pnas.1516047113.

TR Holford, R Meza, KE Warner, C Meernik, J Jeon, SH Moolgavkar, DT Levy. Tobacco Control and the Reduction in Smoking-Related Premature Deaths in the United States, 1964–2012. *JAMA* 2014; 311(2):164–171. doi:10.1001/jama.2013.285112.

PD Home, SJ Pocock, H Beck-Nelson, R Gomis, M Hanefeld, NP Jones, M Komajada, JJV McMurray, for the RECORD Study Group. Rosiglitazone evaluated for cardiovascular outcomes—an interim analysis. *N Engl J Med* 2007; 357:28–38.

BV Howard, L Van Horn, J Hsia, JE Manson, ML Stefanick, S Wassertheil-Smoller, LH Kuller, AZ LaCroix, RD Langer, NL Lasser, CE Lewis, MC Limacher, KL Margolis, J Mysiw, JK Ockene, LM Parker, MG Perri, L Phillips, RL Prentice, J Robbins, JE Rossouw, GE Sarto, IJ Schatz, LG Snetselaar, VJ Stevens, LF Tinker, M Trevisan, MZ Vitolins, GL Anderson, AR Assaf, T Bassford, SAA Beresford, HR Black, RL Brunner, RG Brzyski, B Caan, RT Chebowski, M Gass, I Granek, P Greenland, J Hays, D Heber, G Heiss, SL Hendrix, FA Hubbell, KC Johnson, JM Kotchen. Low-fat dietary pattern and risk of cardiovascular disease. The Women's Health Initiative Randomized Dietary Modification Trial. *JAMA* 2006; 295:655–666.

G Howard, M Cushman, CS Moy, S Oparil, P Muntner, DT Lackland, JJ Manly, ML Flaherty, SE Judd, VG Wadley, DL Long, VJ Howard. Association of clinical and social factors with excess hypertension risk in black compared with white US adults. *JAMA* 2018; 320:1338–1348. doi:10.1001/jama.2018.13467.

G Howard, R Prineas, C Moy, M Cushman, M Kellum, E Temple, A Graham, V Howard. Racial and geographic differences in awareness treatment, and control of hypertension. Reasons for Geographic and Racial Differences in Stroke study. *Stroke* 2006; 37:1171–1178.

LM Howden, JA Meyer. 2010 Census

Briefs: Age and Sex Composition 2010. US Department of Commerce, Economics and Statistics Information, U.S. Census Bureau. May 2011. https://www.census.gov/prod/cen2010/briefs/c2010br-03.pdf.

DS Hsia, O Grove, WT Cefalu. An update on SGLT2 inhibitors for the treatment of diabetes mellitus. *Curr Opin Diabetes Obes* 2017: 24:73–79.

S Hulley, D Grady, T Bush, C Furberg, D Herrington, B Riggs, E Vittinghoff, for the Heart and Estrogen/Progestin Replacement Study (HERS) research group. Randomized trial of estrogen plus progestin for secondary prevention of coronary heart disease in postmenopausal women. *JAMA* 1998; 280:605–613.

Hypertension Detection and Follow-Up Program Cooperative Group. Five Year Findings of the Hypertension Detection and Follow-Up Program. I. Reduction in mortality of persons with high blood pressure, including mild hypertension. *JAMA* 1979; 242:2562–71.

Hypertension Detection and Follow-Up Program Cooperative Group. Five Year Findings of the Hypertension Detection and Follow-Up Program. II. Mortality by age, race, and sex. *JAMA* 1979; 242:2572–77.

Hypertension Detection and Follow-Up Program Cooperative Group. Five Year Findings of the Hypertension Detection and Follow-Up Program. III. Reduction in stroke incidence among persons with high blood pressure. *JAMA* 1982; 247:633–638.

ISIS-3 (Third International Study of Infarct Survival) Collaborative Group. ISIS-3: a randomized comparison of streptokinase vs tissue plasminogen activator vs anistreplase and of aspirin plus heparin versus aspirin alone among 41,299 cases of suspected acute myocardial infarction. *Lancet* 1992; 8976:753–770. DOI: https://doi.org/10.1016/0140-6736(92)91893-D.

PA James, S Oparil, BL Carter, WC Cushman, D Dennison-Himmelfarb, J Handler, DT Lackland, ML LeFevre, TD MacKenzie, O Ogedegbe, SC Smith, LP Svetky, SJ Taler, RR Townsend, JT Wright, AS Narva, E Ortiz. Evidence-based guideline for the management of high blood pressure in adults: report from the panel members appointed to the Eighth Joint National Committee (JNC 8). *JAMA* 2014; 311(5):507–520. doi:10.1001/jama.2013.284427.

LO Jansen and EH Christensen. Are drug-eluting stents safer than bare metal stents? *Lancet* 2019; 393:2472–2474. DOI: https://doi.org/10.1016/S0140-6736(19)31000-1.

CT January, LS Wann, JS Alpert, H Calkins, JE Cigarroa, JC Cleveland, JB Cont, PT Ellinor, MD Ezekowitz, ME Field, KT Murray. 2014 AHA/ACC/HRS Guideline for the Management of Patients with Atrial Fibrillation.

MD Jensen, DH Ryan, CM Apovian, JD Ard, AG Comuzzie, KA Donato, FB Hu, VS Hubbard, JM Jakicic, RF Kushner, CM Loria, BE Millen, CA Nonas, X Pi-Sunyer, J Stevens, VJ Stevens, TA Wadden, BM Wolfe, SZ Yanovski. 2013 AHA/ACC/TOS Guideline for the Management of Overweight and Obesity in Adults. A report the American College of Cardiology/American Heart Association Task Force on Practice Guidelines and the Obesity Society. *Circulation* 2014; 129(suppl 2):S102–S138. DOI: 10.1161/01.cir.0000437739.71477.ee.

WB Kannel, TR Dawber, A Kagan, Revotskie N, Stokes J. Factors of risk in the development of coronary heart disease—six-year follow-up experience. The Framingham Heart Study. *Ann Intern Med* 1961; 55:33–50.

S Kaul, RP Morrissey, GA Diamond. By Jove! What is a clinician to make of JUPITER? *Arch Intern Med* 2010; 170:1073–1077.

PA Kavsak, AR MacRae, V Lustig, R Bhargava, R Vandersluis, GE Polomaki, ML Yerna, AS Jaffe. The impact of the ESC/ACC redefinition of myocardial infarction and new sensitive troponin assays on the frequency of acute myocardial infarction. *Am Heart J* 2005; 152:118–125.

EC Keeley, JA Boura, CL Grines. Primary angioplasty versus intravenous thrombolytic therapy for acute myocardial infarction: a quantitative review of 23 randomized trials. *Lancet* 2003; 361:13-20.

JW Kennedy. Streptokinase for the treatment of acute myocardial infarction: a brief review of randomized trials. *J Am Coll Cardiol* 1987; 10:28B-32B.

A Keys, JT Anderson, F Grande. Serum cholesterol response to changes in the diet. I. Iodine value of dietary fat versus 2S-P; II The effect of cholesterol in the diet; II Differences among individuals; IV Particular fats in the diet. *Metabolism* 1965; 14:747-787.

A Keys, C Aravanis, H Blackburn, R Buzina, BS Djordjevic, AS Dontas, F Fidanza, MJ Karvonen, N Kimura, A Menotti, I Mohacek, S Nedeljkovic, V Puddu, S Punsar, HL Taylor, FSP Van Buchem. *Seven countries. A multivariate analysis of death and coronary heart disease.* Cambridge: Harvard University Press, 1980.

P King, I Peacock, R Donnelly. The UK Prospective Diabetes Study (UKPDS): clinical and therapeutic implications for type 2 diabetes. *J Clin Pharmacol* 1999; 48:643-649.

L Kober, C Turp-Pedersen, JE Carlsen, H Bagger, P Eliasen, K Lyngborg, J Videbaek, DS Cole, L Auclert, NC Pauly, E Aliot, S Persson, AJ Camm, for the Trandolapril Cardiac Evaluation Study Group. A clinical trial of the angiotensin-converting enzyme inhibitor trandolapril in patients with left ventricular dysfunction after myocardial infarction. *N Engl J Med* 1995; 333:1670-1676.

CE Kosmas, D Silverio, A Sourlas, F Garcia, PD Montan, E Guzman. Primary genetic disorders affecting high density lipoprotein (HDL). *Drugs in Context* 2018; 7: 212546. DOI: 10.7573/dic.212546.

TA Kotchen. Historical trends and milestones in hypertension research. A model of the process of translational research. *Hypertension* 2011; 58:522-538.

M Krieger. The "best of cholesterols, the "worst" of cholesterols: a tale of two receptors. *Proc Nat Acad Sci, USA* 1998; 95:4077-4080.

HM Krumholz, J Herrin, LE Miller, EE Drye, SM Ling, LF Han, MT Rapp, EH Bradley, BK Nallamothu, W Nsa, DW Bratzler, JP Curtis. Improvements in door-to-balloon time in the United States, 2005-2010. *Circulation* 2011; 124:1038-1045. doi:10.1161/CIRCULATIONAHA.111.044107.

KH Kuck, R Cappato, J Siebels, R Ruppel, for the CASH Investigators. Randomized comparison of antiarrhythmic drug therapy with implantable defibrillators in patients resuscitated from cardiac arrest. *Circulation* 2000; 102:748-754.

DT Lackland. Racial differences in hypertension: implications for high blood pressure management. *Am J Med Sci* 2014; 348:135-138. doi:10.1097/MAJ.0000000000000308.

WK Lagrand, CA Visser, WT Hermens, HWM Niessen, FWA Verheugt, GJ Wolbink, CE Hack. C-reactive protein as a cardiovascular risk factor: More than an epiphenomenon? *Circulation* 1999; 100:96-102.

JC LaRosa, W Applegate, JR Crouse, D Hunninghake, R Grimm, R Knopp, J Eckfelt, CE Davis, DJ Gordon. Cholesterol lowering in the elderly; Results of the Cholesterol Reduction in Seniors Program (CRISP) pilot study. *Arch Int Med* 1994; 154:529-539.

CJ Lavie, RV Milani, HO Ventura. Obesity and cardiovascular disease. Risk factor, paradox, and impact of weight loss. *J Am Coll Cardiol* 2009; 53:1925-1932.

MW Lewis, Y Khodneva, N Redmond, RW Durant, LL Wilkinson, VJ Howard, MM Safford. The impact of the combination of income and education on the incidence of coronary heart disease in the prospective Reasons for Geographic and Racial Differences in Stroke (REGARDS) cohort study. *BMC Public Health* 2015; 15:1312-1321. DOI 10.1186/s12889-015-2630-4.

P Libby. History of discovery: inflammation in atherosclerosis. *Arteriosclerosis, Thrombosis, and Vascular Biology* 2012; 32:2045-2051. https://doi.org/10.1161/ATVBAHA.108.179705.

P Libby, PM Ridker. Inflammation and atherothrombosis. From population biology and bench research to clinical practice. *J Am Coll Cardiol* 2006; 48:A33-A46. Doi:10.1016/j.jacc.2006.08.011.

P Libby, PM Ridker. Novel inflammatory markers of coronary risk. Theory versus practice. *Circulation* 1999; 100:1148–1150.

Life Expectancy in the USA 1900–98, https://u.demog.berkeley.edu/~andrew/1918/figure2.html.

AM Lincoff, SJ Nicholls, JS Riesmeyer, PJ Barter, HB Brewer, KAA Fox, CM Gibson, C Granger, V Menon, G Montalescot, D Rader, AR Tall, E McErlean, K Wolski, G Ruatolo, B Vangerow, G Weerakkody, SG Goodman, D Conde, DK McGuire, JC Nicolau, JL Leiva-Pons, Y Pesant, W Li, D Kandath, S Kouz, N Takirkheli, D Mason, SE Nissen, for the ACCELER-ATE Investigators. Evacetrapib and cardiovascular outcomes in high-risk vascular disease. *N Engl J Med* 2017; 376:1933–1942. doi: 10.1056/NEJMoa1609581.

J Lindhorst, N Alexander, J Blignaut, B Rayner. Differences in hypertension between blacks and whites: an overview. *Cardiovasc J Afr* 2007; 18:241–247.

The Lipid Research Clinics Program. The Lipid Research Clinics Coronary Primary Prevention Trial Results I. Reduction in incidence of coronary heart disease. *JAMA* 251: 351–364, 1984.

The Lipid Research Clinics Program. The Lipid Research Clinics Coronary Primary Prevention Trial Results II. The relationship of reduction in incidence of coronary heart disease to cholesterol reduction. *JAMA* 251: 365–374, 1984.

The Look AHEAD Research Group. Cardiovascular effects of intensive lifestyle intervention in type 2 diabetes. *N Engl J Med* 2013; 369:145–154.

Macrotrends, US Life Expectancy 1950–2020, https://www.macrotrends.net/countries/USA/united-states/life-expectancy.

SS Mahmood, D Levy, RS Vasan, TJ Wang. The Framingham Heart Study and the Epidemiology of Cardiovascular Diseases: A Historical Perspective. *Lancet* 2014 March 15; 383 (9921): 999–1008; doi 10.1016/S0140-6736(13)61752-3; https://www.ncbi.nlm.nih.gov/pmc/articles/PMC4159698/pdf/nihms588573.pdf.

JE Manson, RT Chebowski, ML Stefanick, AK Aragaki, JE Rossouw, RL Prentice, G Anderson, BV Howard, CA Thomson, AZ LaCroix, J Wactawski-Wende, RD Jackson, M Limacher, KL Margolis, S Wasserthal-Smoller, SA Beresford, JA Cauley, CB Eaton, M Gass, J Hsia, KC Johnson, C Kooperberg, LH Kuller, CE Lewis, S Liu, LW Martin, JK Ockene, MJ O'Sullivan, LH Powell, MS Simon, L Van Horn, MZ Vitolina, RB Wallace. Menopausal hormone therapy and health outcomes during the intervention and extended post-stopping phases of the Women's Health Initiative randomized trials. *JAMA* 2013; 310:1353–1368.

FI Marcus. Editorial: Use of digitalis in acute myocardial infarction. *Circulation* 1980; 62:17–19.

DJ Maron, JS Hochman, HR Reynolds, S Bangalore, SM O'Brien, WE Boden, BR Chaitman, R Senior, J López-Sendón, KP Alexander, RD Lopes, LJ Shaw, JS Berger, JD Newman, MS Sidhu, SG Goodman, W Ruzyllo, G Gosselin, AP Maggioni, HD White, B Bhargava, JK Min, GBJ Mancini, DS Berman, MH Picard, RY Kwong, ZA Ali, DB Mark, JA Spertus, MN Krishnan, A Elghamaz, N Moorthy, WA Hueb, M Demkow, K Mavromatis, O Bockeria, J Peteiro, TD Miller, H Szwed, R Doerr, M Keltai, JB Selvanayagam, PG Steg, C Held, S Kohsaka, S Mavromichalis, R Kirby, NO Jeffries, FE Harrell, FW Rockhold, S Broderick, TB Ferguson, DO Williams, RA Harrington, GW Stone, Y Rosenberg, ISCHEMIA Research Group. Initial invasive or conservative strategy for stable coronary disease. *N Engl J Med* 2020; 382:1395–1407. doi: 10.1056/NEJMoa191592.

MJ Martin, SB Hulley, WS Browner, LH Kuller, D Wentworth. Serum cholesterol, blood pressure, and mortality: implications from a cohort of 361,662 men. *Lancet* Oct 1986; 933–936.

MA Martinez-Gonzalez, A Gea, M Ruiz-Canela. The Mediterranean diet and cardiovascular health. A Critical review. *Circ Res* 2019; 124:779–798.

FA Masoudi, A Ponikaris, JA de Lemos, JG Jollis, M Kremers, JC Messinger, JWM Moore, I Moussa, WJ Oetgen, PD Varosy, RN Vincent, J Wei, JP Curtis, MT Roe,

Bibliography

JA Spertus. Trends in U.S. cardiovascular Care. 2016 Reports from 4 ACC National Cardiovascular Registries. *J Am Col Cardiol* 2016; 69:1427–1450.

Mayo Clinic. Type 2 Diabetes. https://www.mayoclinic.org/diseases-conditions/type-2-diabetes/diagnosis-treatment/drc-20351199.

Mayo Clinic Staff. Glycemic index diet: What's behind the claims. Mayo Clinic Website. Healthy Lifestyle. Nutrition and Haealthy Living. Accessed August 1, 2020, at https://www.mayoclinic.org/healthy-lifestyle/nutrition-and-healthy-eating/in-depth/glycemic-index-diet/art-20048478.

J McMurray, L Kober, M Robertson, H Dargie, W Colucci, J Lopez-Sendon, W Remme, DN Sharpe, I Ford. Antiarrhythmic effect of carvedilol after acute myocardial infarction. Result of the Carvedilol Post-Infarct Survival Control in Left Ventricular Dysfunction (CAPRICORN) Trial. *JACC* 2005; 45:525–530.

L Medina, S Sabo, J Vespa. Living Longer: Historical and Projected Life Expectancy in the United States, 1960–2060. Population Estimates and Projections. Current Population Reports. February 2020. https://www.census.gov/content/dam/Census/library/publications/2020/demo/p25-1145.pdf.

L Melly, G Torregrossa, T Lee, JL Jansens, JD Puskas. Fifty years of coronary bypass grafting. *J Thoracic Dis* 2018; 1960–1967. Doi: 10.21037/jtd2018.02.43.

GA Mensah, GS Wei, PD. Sorlie, LJ. Fine, Y Rosenberg, PG Kaufmann, ME. Mussolino, LL Hsu, E Addou, MM Engelgau, D Gordon. Decline in Cardiovascular Mortality: Possible Causes and Implications. *Circ Res* 2017; 366–380. doi:10.1161/CIRCRESAHA.116.309115.

A Meyer. Werner Forssmann and the catheterization of the heart, 1929. *Ann Thorac Surg* 1990; 49:497–499.

KB Michels, S Yusuf. Does PTCA in acute myocardial infarction affect mortality and reinfarction rates? A quantitative overview (meta-analysis) of the randomized clinical trials. *Circulation* 1995; 91:476–485. https://doi.org/10.1161/01.CIR.91.2.476.

I Milne, I Chalmers. *J Epidemiol Community Health* 2002;56:1a

Morbidity and Mortality. 2012 Chartbook on Cardiovascular, Lung and Blood Diseases, NIH-NHLBI. https://www.nhlbi.nih.gov/files/docs/research/2012_ChartBook_508.pdf.

TJ More. The Cholesterol Myth. *Atlantic Monthly*, September 1989, pp 37–70.

Moriya, J. Critical roles of inflammation in atherosclerosis. *J Cardiol* 2018; 73:22–27. https://reader.elsevier.com/reader/sd/pii/S091450871830145X?token=3665FDB1173C3253AB6E8CF2CF06274E5CFE8783B7BE9D80D2A8C15EF779D7A2FACA4EAB32058F498A171AEBF6B8950B.

JN Morris, JA Heady, PA Raffle, CG Roberts, JW Parks. Coronary heart disease and physical activity of work. *Lancet* 1953; 265(6795):1053–1057; contd.

JN Morris, JA Heady, PA Raffle, CG Roberts, JW Parks. Coronary heart disease and physical activity of work (part 2). *Lancet.* 1953, 28 Nov; 265(6796):1111–1120; concl.

RJ Morris. The history of cardiopulmonary bypass: medical advances. American College of Cardiology, June 19, 2019. https://www.acc.org/latest-in-cardiology/articles/2019/06/19/06/46/the-history-of-cardiopulmonary-bypass.

Mortality and Top 10 Causes of Death, USA, 1900 vs 2010, https://www.ncdemography.org/wp-content/uploads/2014/06/All-Cause-Mortality-and-Top-10_USA-e1402597040445.png.

M Moser. Historical perspective on management of hypertension. *J Clin Hypertens* 2006; 8:15–20. https://onlinelibrary.wiley.com/doi/full/10.1111/j.1524-6175.2006.05836.x.

AJ Moss, WJ Hall, DS Cannom, JP Daubert, SL Higgins, H Klein, JH Levine, S Saksena, AL Waldo, D Wilber, MW Brown, M Heo, for the Multicenter Automatic Defibrillator Implantation Trial Investigators. Improved survival with an implanted defibrillator in patients with coronary disease at high risk for ventricular arrhythmia. *N Engl J Med* 1996; 335:1933–1940.

AJ Moss, W Zareba, WJ Hall, H Klein, DJ Wilber, DS Cannom, JP Daubert, SL Higgins, MW Brown, ML Andrews, for the Multicenter Automatic Defibrillator Implantation Trial II Investigators. Prophylactic implantation of a defibrillator in patients with myocardial infarction and reduced ejection fraction. *N Engl J Med* 2002; 346:877–883.

Multiple Risk Factor Intervention Trial Research Group. Multiple Risk Factor Intervention Trial. Risk factor changes and mortality results. *JAMA* 1982; 248:1465–77.

P Muntner, ST Hardy, LJ Fine, BC Jaeger, G Wozniak, EB Levitan, LD Colantonio. Trends in blood pressure control among US adults with hypertension, 1999–2000 to 2017–2018. *JAMA* 2020; doi:10.1001/jama.2020.14545.

RJ Myerburg, J Junttila. Sudden cardiac death caused by coronary heart disease. *Circulation* 2012; 125:1043–1052.

J Myers. Exercise and cardiovascular health. *Circulation* 2003; 107:e2-e5.

The Mysterious Death of George Washington, Constitution Daily, December 14, 2019, https://constitutioncenter.org/blog/the-mysterious-death-of-george-washington.

E Nabel. The Women's Health Initiative—a victory for women and their health. *JAMA* 2013; 310:1349–1350.

National Archives, Vietnam War U.S. Military Fatal Casualty Statistics, Electronic Records Reference Report, https://www.archives.gov/research/military/vietnam-war/casualty-statistics.

National Health and Nutrition Examination Survey website. National Center for Health Statistics, Centers for Disease Control and Prevention. https://www.cdc.gov/nchs/nhanes/about_nhanes.htm.

National Institute of Diabetes and Digestive and Kidney Diseases (NIDDK) official website. Health Information/Diabetes. https://www.niddk.nih.gov/health-information/diabetes.

National Institute of Diabetes and Digestive and Kidney Diseases (NIDDK) official website. Type 1 Diabetes. https://www.niddk.nih.gov/health-information/diabetes/overview/what-is-diabetes/type-1-diabetes.

National Institute of Diabetes and Digestive and Kidney Diseases (NIDDK) official website. Type 2 Diabetes. https://www.niddk.nih.gov/health-information/diabetes/overview/what-is-diabetes/type-2-diabetes.

E Nix. Tuskegee Experiment: the infamous syphilis study. History.com. Updated July 29, 2019. https://www.history.com/news/the-infamous-40-year-tuskegee-study/.

The Norwegian Multicenter Study Group. Timolol-induced reduction in mortality and reinfarction in patients surviving acute myocardial infarction. *N Engl J Med* 1981; 304:801–807.

E Obarzanek, FM Sacks, WM Vollmer, GA Bray, ER Miller, PH Lin, N Karanja, MM Windhauser, TJ Moore, JF Swain, CW Bales, MA Proschan, on behalf of the DASH Research Group. Effects on blood lipids of a blood pressure-lowering diet: the Dietary Approaches to Stop Hypertension (DASH) Trial. *Am J Clin Nutr* 2001; 74:80–89.

GT O'Connor, JE Buring, S Yusuf, SZ Goldhaber, EM Olmstead, RS Paffenberger, CH Hennekens. An overview of randomized trials of rehabilitation with exercise after myocardial infarction. *Circulation* 1989; 80:234–244.

P O'Gara, FD Kushner, DD Ascheim, DE Casey, MK Chung, JA de Lemos, SM Ettinger, JC Fang, FM Fesmire, BA Franklin, CB Granger, HM Krumholz, JA Linderbaum, DA Morrow, LK Newby, JP Ornato, N Ou, MJ Radford, JE Tamis-Holland, CL Tommaso, CM Tracy, YJ Woo, DX Zhao. 2013 ACCF/AHA Guideline for the Management of ST-Elevation Myocardial Infarction. A report of the American College of Cardiology Foundation/American Heart Association Task Force on Practice Guidelines. *JACC* 2013; e78-e140.

Y Ohkubo, H Kishikawa, E Araki, Y Kojima, N Furuyoshi, M Shichiri. Intensive insulin therapy prevents the progression of diabetic microvascular complications in Japanese patients with non-insulin dependent diabetes mellitus: a randomized prospective 6-year trial. *Diab Res Clin Pract* 1995; 28:103–117. https://www.diabetesresearchclinicalpractice.com/article/0168-8227(95)01064-K/pdf.

M Oliver. The clofibrate saga: a retrospective commentary. *Br J Clin Pharmacol* 2012; 74:907–910. doi: 10.1111/j.1365-2125.2012.04282.x.

AR Omran. The epidemiologic transition: a theory of the epidemiology of population change. 1971. *Milbank Q* 2005; 83(4):731–757.

W Osler. *Lectures on Angina Pectoris and Allied States.* New York: D. Appleton and Company, 1897.

N Pattyn, VA Cornelissen, SRT Eshgbi, L Vanhees. The effect of exercise on the cardiovascular risk factors constituting the metabolic syndrome. *Sports Med* 2013; 43:121–133.

PCSB Protein Data Bank. Molecule of the Month. Sodium Potassium Pump. 2009–2010. https://cbm.msoe.edu/teacherWorkshops/ddtyResources/documents/sodiumPotassiumPump.pdf.

MB Pepys, GM Hirschfield. C-reactive protein: a critical update. *J Clin Invest* 2003; 111:1805–1812. doi:10.1172/JCI200318921.

AS Peterson, LG Fong, SG Young. PCSK9 function and physiology. *J Lipid Res* 2008; 49: 1152–1156. doi: 10.1194/jlr.E800008-JLR200.

DB Petiti. Hormone replacement therapy for prevention. More evidence, more pessimism. *JAMA* 2002; 288:99–101.

MA Pfeffer, E Braunwald, LA Moye, L Basta, EJ Brown, TF Cuddy, BR Davis, EM Geltman, S Goldman, GC Flaker, M Klein, GA Lamas, M Packer, J Rouleau, JL Rouleau, J Rutherford, JH Wertheimer, CM Hawkins, on behalf of the SAVE Investigators. Effect of captopril on mortality and morbidity in patients with left ventricular dysfunction after myocardial infarction. Results of the Survival and Ventricular Enlargement Trial. *N Engl J Med* 1992; 327:669–677.

MA Pfeffer, JJV McMurray. Lessons in uncertainty and humility—clinical trials involving hypertension. *N Engl J Med* 2016; 375:1756–1766. DOI: 10.1056/NEJMra1510067.

R Piccolo, KH Bonaa, O Efthimiou, O Varenne, A Baldo, P Urban, C Kaiser, W Remkes, L Raber, A de Belder, AWJ van't Hof, G Stankovic, PA Lemos, T Wilsgaard, J Reifart, AE Rodriguez, EE Ribeiro, PWJC Serruys, A Abizaid, M Sabate, RA Byrne, JMT Hernandez, W Wijns, P Juni, S Windecker, M Valgimigli, on behalf of the Coronary Stents Trialists' Collaboration. *Lancet* 2019; 393: 2503–2510. DOI: https://doi.org/10.1016/S0140-6736(19)30474-X.

P Poirier, TD Giles, GA Bray, Y Hong, JS Stern, X Pi-Sunyer, RH Eckel. Obesity and cardiovascular disease: Pathophysiology, evaluation, and effect of weight loss. An update of the 1997 American Heart Association Scientific Statement on Obesity and Heart Disease from the Obesity Committee of the Council on Nutrition, Physical Activity, and Metabolism. *Circulation* 2006; 113:898–918.

CM Pratt. Three decades of clinical trials with beta-blockers. The Contribution of the CAPRICORN trial and the effect of carvedilol on serious arrhythmias. *JACC* 2005; 45:531–532.

Proceedings of the Conference on the Decline in Coronary Heart Disease Mortality: National Heart, Lung, and Blood Institute, National Institute of Health, Bethesda, Maryland. NIH publication no. 79–1610, 1978. Bethesda, MD: National Heart, Lung, and Blood Institute, NIH, 1979. Oct 24–25.

S Pruitt. What part of Africa did most slaves come from? History.com. Updated June 19, 2019. https://www.history.com/news/what-part-of-africa-did-most-slaves-come-from?

The Public Access Defibrillation Trial Investigators. Public-access defibrillation and survival after out-of-hospital cardiac arrest. *N Engl J Med* 2004; 351:637–646.

M Ragosta, S Dee, IJ Sarembock, LC Lipson, LW Gimple, ER Powers. Prevalence of unfavorable angiographic characteristics for percutaneous intervention in patients with unprotected left main coronary artery disease. *Catheter Cardiovasc Interv* 2007; 68:357–362. doi: 10.1002/ccd.20709.

Bibliography

S Rao, MW Segar, AP Bress, W Vongpatanasin, V Agusala, UR Essien, A Correa, AA Morris, JA de Lemos, A Pandey. Association of genetic West African ancestry, blood pressure response to therapy, and cardiovascular risk among self-reported black individuals in the Systolic Blood Pressure Reduction Intervention Trial (SPRINT). *JAMA Cardiology*, published online November 13, 2020. Doi.10.1001/jamacardio.2020.6566. https://jamanetwork.com/journals/jamacardiology/fullarticle/10.1001/jamacardio.2020.6566?guestAccessKey=bef18712-8884-479c-9d99-024845d9c461&utm_source=silverchair&utm_medium=email&utm_campaign=article_alert-jamacardiology&utm_content=olf&utm_term=111320.

P Reichard, BY Nilsson, U Rosenqvist. The effect of long-term intensified insulin treatment on the development of microvascular complications of diabetes mellitus. *N Engl J Med* 329: 304–309.

A report of the American College of Cardiology/American Heart Association Task Force on Practice Guidelines and the Heart Rhythm Society. JACC 2014; 64:2246–2280. Developed in collaboration with the Society of Thoracic Surgeons. http://dx.doi.org/10.1016/j.jacc.2014.03.021 A report from the American Heart Association. AHA Statistical Update Heart Disease and Stroke Statistics—2020 Update. *Circulation* 2020; 141:e139-e596. DOI: 10.1161/CIR.0000000000000757.

Report of the National Cholesterol Education Program Expert Panel on Detection, Evaluation, and Treatment of High Blood Cholesterol in Adults. The Expert Panel. *Arch Intern Med* 1988; 148:36–69.

A report of the Surgeon General. The Health Consequences of Involuntary Exposure to Tobacco Smoke. Centers for Disease Control and Prevention (US), Atlanta, GA, 2006. https://www.ncbi.nlm.nih.gov/books/NBK44324/.

CA Ridge, AM McErlean, MS Ginsberg. Epidemiology of lung cancer. *Semin Intervent Radiol* 2013; 30:93–98.

P Ridker. The JUPITER Trial: results, controversies, and implications for prevention. *Circ Cardiovasc Qual Outcomes* 2009; 279–285.

PM Ridker, E Danielson, FAH Fonseca, J Genest, AM Gotto, JJP Kastelein, W Koenig, P Libby, AJ Lorenzen, JG MacFayden, BG Nordestgaard, J Shephers, JT Willerson, RJ Glynn, for the JUPITER Study Group. Rosuvastatin to prevent vascular events in men and women with elevated C-reactive protein. *N Engl J Med* 2008; 359:2195–2207. DOI: 10.1056/NEJMoa0807646.

PM Ridker, BM Everett, A Pradhan, JG MacFayden, DH Solomon, E Zaharris, V Mam, A Hasan, Y Rosenberg, E Iturriaga, M Gupta, M Tsigoulis, S Verma, M Clearfield, P Libby, SZ Goldhaber, R Seagle, C Ofori, M Saklayen, S Butman, J Johnston, NP Paynter, RJ Glynn, for the CIRT Investigators. Low-dose methotrexate for the prevention of atherosclerotic events. *N Engl J Med* 2019; 380:752–762. DOI: 10.1056/NEJMoa1809.

PM Ridker, BM Everett, T Thuren, JG MacFayden, WH Chang, C Ballantyne, F Fonseca, J Nicolau, W Koenig, SD Anker, JJP Kastelein, JH Cornel, P Pais, D Pella, J Genest, R Cifkova, A Lorenzatti, T Forster, Z Kobalava, L Vida-Smith, M Flather, H Shimokawa, H Ogawa, M Dellborg, PRF Ross, RPT Troquay, P Libby, RJ Glynn, for the CANTOS Trial Group. Antiinflammatory therapy with canakinumab for atherosclerotic disease. *N Engl J Med* 2017; 377:1119–1131. DOI: 10.1056/NEJMoa170791.

MD Ritchie, HK Wall, MG George, JS Wright. US trends in premature heart disease mortality over the past 5 years: Where do we go from here? *Trends in Cardiovascular Medicine* 2020, 30:364–374. Doi: org/10.1016/j.tcm.2019.09.005. https://reader.elsevier.com/reader/sd/pii/S1050173819301343?token=7F40CE58241E384675154F72DB6A47DA204635AA02005A37DE85A7A8ED4F1F679D9F00D9FDE3E1D64DC89666494E1ED0.

A Roguin. Stent: The man and word behind the coronary metal prosthesis. *Circulation: Cardiovascular Interventions* 2011; 4:206–209. https://doi.org/10.1161/CIRCINTERVENTIONS.110.960872.

Bibliography

W Röntgen. Ueber eine neue Art von Strahlen. Vorläufige Mitteilung. *Aus den Sitzungsberichten der Würzburger Physik.-medic.* Gesellschaft Würzburg, 1895.

JE Rossouw, LP Finnegan, WR Harlan, VW Pinn, C Clifford, JA McGowan. The evolution of the Women's Health Initiative: perspectives from the NIH. J *Am Med Women's Assoc* 1995; 50:50–55.

JA Roth, R Etzioni, TM Waters, M Pettinger, JE Rossouw, GL Anderson, RT Chlebowski, JE Manson, M Hlatky, KC Johnson, SD Ramsey. Economic return from the Women's Health Initiative estrogen plus progestin clinical trial: a modeling study. *Ann Intern Med* 2014 May 6;160(9):594–602. doi: 10.7326/M13-2348.

F Rovelli, C De Vita, GA Feruglio, A Lotto, A Selvini, G Tognoni and GISSI Investigators. GISSI Trial: early results and late follow-up. J Am Coll Cardiol 1987; 10:33B-39B.

HB Rubins, SJ Robins, D Collins, CL Fye, JW Anderson, MB Elam, FH Faas, E Linares, EJ Schaefer, G Schectman, TJ Wilt, J Wittes. Gemfibrozil for the secondary prevention of coronary heart disease in men with low levels of high-density lipoprotein cholesterol. Veterans Affairs High-Density Lipoprotein Cholesterol Intervention Trial Study Group. *N Engl J Med* 1999; 341:410–418.

TJ Ryan. The coronary angiogram and its seminal contributions to cardiovascular medicine over five decades.

FM Sacks, VJ Carey, CAM Anderson, ER Miller, T Copeland, J Charleston, BJ Harshfield, N Laranjo, P McCarron, J Swain, K White, K Yee, LJ Appel. Effects of high vs low glycemic index of dietary carbohydrate on cardiovascular disease risk factors and insulin sensitivity. The OmniCarb randomized clinical trial. *JAMA* 2014; 312:2531–2541. doi:10.1001/jama.2014.16658.

FM Sacks, E Obarzanek, MM Windhauser, LP Svetky, WM Vollmer, M McCollough, N Karanja, PH Lin, P Steele, MA Proschan, MA Evans, LJ Appel, GA Bray, TM Vogt, TJ Moore, DASH Investigators. Rationale and design of the Dietary Approaches to Stop Hypertension trial (DASH): a multicenter controlled-feeding study of dietary patterns to lower blood pressure. *Ann Epidemiol* 1995; 5:108–118.

FM Sacks, LP Svetky, WM Vollmer, LJ Appel, GA Bray, D Harisha, E Obarzanek, PR Comlin, ER Miller, DG Simons-Morton, N Karanja, PH Lin, for the DASH-Sodium Collaborative Research Group. Effects on blood pressure of reduced dietary sodium and the Dietary Approaches to Stop Hypertension (DASH) diet. *N Engl J Med* 2001; 344:3–10.

MG Sakayan, NV Deshpanda. Timeline of history of hypertension treatment. Front Cardiovasc Med 2016; 33:1–14, doi: 10.3389/fcvm.2016.00003, https://www.ncbi.nlm.nih.gov/pmc/articles/PMC4763852.

JA Salami, H Warralch, J Velardo-Elizondo, ES Spatz, NR Desai, JS Rana, SS Virani, R Blankstein, A Khera, MJ Blaha, RS Blumenthal, D Lloyd-Jones, K Nasir. National trends in statin use and expenditures, in the US adult population from 2002 to 2013: Insights from the Medical Expenditure Panel survey. *JAMA Cardiology* 2017; 2:56–65. doi.10.1001/jamacardio.2016.4700. file:///C:/Users/gordo/AppData/Local/Temp/jamacardiology_salami_2016_oi_160082.pdf.

JM Samet, FE Speizer. Sir Richard Doll, 1912–2005 (obituary). *Am J Epidiol* 2006; 164:95–100.

EM Sarpong, SH Zuvekas. Changes in statin therapy among adults (age 18+) by selected characteristics, United States, 2000–2001 to 2010–2011. Medical Expenditure Panel Survey (MEPS). Statistical Brief #459. November 2014. https://www.ncbi.nlm.nih.gov/books/NBK470833/.

Scandinavian Simvastatin Survival Study Group. Randomised trial of cholesterol lowering in 4444 patients with coronary heart disease: the Scandinavian Simvastatin Survival Study (4S). *Lancet* 1994; 344: 1383–1389.

GG Schwartz, AG Olsson M Abt M, CM Ballantyne, PJ Barter, J Brumm, BR Chaitman, IM Holme, D Kallend, LA Leiter, E Leitersdorf, JJV McMurray, H Mundl, SJ Nicholls, PK Shah, JC Tardif, S Wright, dal-OUTCOMES Investigators.

Effects of dalcetrapib in patients with a recent acute coronary syndrome. *N Engl J Med* 2012; 367:2089–2099. doi: 10.1056/NEJMoa1206797.

TB Schwartz, CL Meinert. The UGDP controversy: Thirty-four years of contentious ambiguity laid to rest. *Perspect Biol Med* 2004; 47:564–574.

BM Scirica, DL Bhatt, E Braunwald, PG Steg, J Davidson, B Hirshberg, P Ohman, R Frederich, SD Wiviott, EB Hoffman, MA Cavender, JA Udell, NR Desai, O Mozenzon, DK McGuire, KK Ray, LA Leiter, I Raz, for the SAVOR-TIMI-53 Steering Committee and Investigators. Saxagliptin and cardiovascular outcomes in patients with type 2 diabetes mellitus. *N Eng J Med* 2013; 369:1317–1326. DOI: 10.1056/NEJMoa1307684.

E Selvin, MW Steffes, H Zhu, K Matsushita, Lynne Wagenknecht, J Panikow, J Coresh, FL Brancati. Glycated hemoglobin, diabetes, and cardiovascular risk in nondiabetic adults. *N Engl J Med* 2010; 800–811. doi: 10.1056/NEJMoa0908359.

PW Serruys, MC Morice, AP Kappetein, A Columbo, DR Holmes, MJ Mack, E Stahle, TE Feldman, M van den Brand, EJ Bass, N Van Duck, K leadley, KD Dawkins, FW Mohr, for the SYNTAX Investigators. Percutaneous coronary intervention versus coronary-artery bypass grafting for sever coronary artery disease. *N Engl J Med* 2009; 360:961–972.

NS Shah, MD Huffman, H Ning, DM Lloyd-Jones. Trends in myocardial infarction secondary prevention: The National Health and Nutrition Examination Surveys (NHANES), 1999–2012. *J Am Heart Assoc* 2015; 4:1–12. doi:10.1161/JAHA.114.001709. https://www.ahajournals.org/doi/pdf/10.1161/JAHA.114.001709.

SHEP Cooperative Research Group. Prevention of stroke by antihypertensive drug treatment in older persons with isolated systolic hypertension. Final results of the Systolic Hypertension in the Elderly Program (SHEP). *JAMA* 1991; 265:3255–64.

J Shepherd, SM Cobbe, I Ford, CG Isles, AR Lorimer, PW MacFarlane, JH McKillop CJ Packard, West of Scotland Coronary Prevention Study Group. Prevention of coronary heart disease with pravastatin in men with hypercholesterolemia. *N Engl J Med* 1995; 333: 1301–07.

N Sikri, A Bardia. A history of streptokinase use in acute myocardial infarction. *Texas Heart Inst J* 2007; 34:318–327.

S Singh, YK Loke, CD Furberg. Long-term risk of cardiovascular events with rosiglitazone: a meta-analysis. *JAMA* 2007; 298:1189–1195.

The sixth report of the Joint National Committee on prevention, detection, evaluation, and treatment of high blood pressure. *Arch Intern Med* 1997; 157: 2413–2446.

V Smil. China's great famine: 40 years later. *BMJ* 1999; 319:1619–1621.

SO Sodeke, LR Powell. Paying Tribute to Henrietta Lacks at Tuskegee University and at The Virginia Henrietta Lacks Commission, Richmond, Virginia. *J Health Care Poor Underserved* 2019; 30(4s):1–11.

The SOLVD Investigators. Effect of enalapril on survival in patients with reduced left ventricular ejection fractions and congestive heart failure. *N Engl J Med* 1991; 325:293–302.

J Speller. The Renin-Angiotensin-Aldosterone System. Teach Me Physiology, April 20, 2020. https://teachmephysiology.com/urinary-system/regulation/the-renin-angiotensin-aldosterone-system/.

The SPRINT Research Group. A randomized trial of intensive versus standard blood pressure control. *N Engl J Med* 2015; 373:2103–2116.

TM Sprull. Chronic psychosocial stress and hypertension. *Curr Hypertens Rep* 2010; 12:10–16. doi:10.1007/s11906-009-0084-8.

MJ Stampfer, GA Colditz. Estrogen replacement and coronary heart disease: a quantitative assessment of the epidemiologic evidence. *Prev Med* 1991; 20:47–63.

State Legislated Actions on Tobacco Issues (SLATI). https://www.lung.org/policy-advocacy/tobacco/slati.

R Steckelberg, JS Newman. The fascinating foxglove. *ACP Hospitalist*, March 2010. https://acphospitalist.org/archives/2010/03/newman.htm.

Steering Committee of the Physicians'

Bibliography

Health Study Research Group. *N Engl J Med* 1989; 321:129–135. DOI: 10.1056/NEJM198907203210301.

S Sydney, CP Quesenberry, MG Jaffe, M Sorel, MN Nguyen-Huynh, LH Kushi, AS Go, JS Rana. Recent trends in cardiovascular mortality in the United States and public health goals. *JAMA Cardiology* 2016; 1:594–599. Doi:10.1001/jamacardio.2016.1326.

T Takaro, P Peduzzi, KM Detre, HN Hultgren, ML Murphy, J van der Bel-Kahn, J Thomsen, WR Meadows. Survival in subgroups of patients with left main coronary artery disease. Veterans Affairs Cooperative Study of Surgery for Coronary Arterial Occlusive Disease. *Circulation* 1982; 66:14–22.

AR Tall, DJ Rader. Trials and Tribulations of CETP inhibitors. *Circulation Research* 2018; 122:106–112. https://doi.org/10.1161/CIRCRESAHA.117.311978.

HL Taylor, E Klepetar, A Keys, W Parlin, H Blackburn, T Puchner. Death rates among physically active and sedentary employees in the railroad industry. *Am J Public Health Nations Health* 1962; 52:1697–1707.

L Terry, et al. Smoking and Health: Report of the Advisory Committee to the Surgeon General of the United States. U-23 Department of Health, Education, and Welfare. Public Health Service Publication No. 1103. 1964 https://profiles.nlm.nih.gov/spotlight/nn/catalog/nlm:nlmuid-101584932X202-doc.

Third Report of the National Cholesterol Education Program (NCEP) Expert Panel on Detection, Evaluation, and Treatment of High Blood Cholesterol in Adults (Adult Treatment Panel III). Executive Summary. National Cholesterol Education Program, National Heart, Lung, and Blood Institute, National Institutes of Health. NIH Publication No. 01–3670, May 2001.

The TIMI Study Group. The Thrombolysis in Myocardial Infarction Trial—Phase I Findings. *N Engl J Med* 1985; 312:932–936. DOI: 10.1056/NEJM19850404.

EJ Topol. Coronary angioplasty for acute myocardial infarction. *Ann Intern Med* 1988; 109:970–980.

SA Tsai, ML Stefanik, RS Stafford. Trends in menopausal hormone therapy use of U.S. office-based physicians, 2000–2009. *Menopause* 2011; 18:285–392.

K Tuthill, R Van Wyck (illustrator). John Snow and the Broad Street Pump: On the Trail of an Epidemic. Cricket Nov 2003; 31:23–31, https://www.ph.ucla.edu/epi/snow/snowcricketarticle.html.

HA Tyroler, CJ Glueck, B Christenson, PO Kwiterovich. Plasma high density lipoprotein cholesterol comparisons in black and white populations. The Lipid Research Clinics Prevalence Study. *Circulation* 1980; 62(suppl IV):99–107.

UK Prospective Diabetes Study (UKPDS) Group. Intensive blood-glucose control with sulphonylureas or insulin compared with conventional treatment and risk of complications in patients with type 2 diabetes (UKPDS 33) *Lancet* 1998; 352:837–853.

UK Prospective Diabetes Study (UKPDS) Group. Effect of intensive blood-glucose control with metformin on complications in overweight patients with type 2 diabetes (UKPDS 34). *Lancet* 1998; 352:854–865.

University of Minnesota Driven to Discover. Heart Attack Prevention: A History of Cardiovascular Epidemiology—Mortality. http://www.epi.umn.edu/cvdepi/.

US Department of Health and Human Services, National Institutes of Health, National Heart, Lung, and Blood Institute. Facts about Menopausal Hormone Therapy. NIH Publication No. 05–5200 (June 2005 Revision). https://www.nhlbi.nih.gov/files/docs/pht_facts.pdf.

USDA Economic Research Service. Major trends in U.S. Food Supply, 1909–99. January-April 2000. https://webs.wofford.edu/boppkl/coursefiles/Interim/CookingInterim/Readings.Exercises/MajorTrendsinUSFoodSupply09_99.pdf.

US National Library of Medicine. The VA Cooperative Study and the Beginning of Routine Hypertension Screening, 1864–1980. The Edward D. Freis Papers. https://profiles.nlm.nih.gov/spotlight/xf/feature/study.

US Population Age Profile 1960–97,

Centers for Disease Control and Prevention (CDC), National Center of Health Statistics Mortality Data, Table 5: Age-adjusted death rates for selected causes of death by sex, race and Hispanic origin, United States, selected years 1950–2017. https://www.cdc.gov/nchs/hus/contents2018.htm#Table_005.

U.S. Preventive Services Task Force. Aspirin for the prevention of cardiovascular disease: U.S. Preventive Services Task Force recommendation statement. *Ann Intern Med* 2009; 150:396–404. https://doi.org/10.7326/0003-4819-150-6-200903170-00008.

The VA Coronary Artery Bypass Surgery Cooperative Study Group. Eighteen-year follow-up in the Veterans Affairs Cooperative Study of Coronary Artery Bypass Surgery for Stable Angina. *Circulation* 1992; 86:121–130.

Veterans Administration Cooperative Study Group on Anti-Hypertensive Agents. Effects of treatment on morbidity in hypertension. Results in patients with diastolic blood pressures averaging 115–129 mm Hg. *JAMA* 1967; 202:1028–34.

Veterans Administration Cooperative Study Group on Anti-Hypertensive Agents. Effects of treatment on morbidity in hypertension. II Results in patients with diastolic blood pressure averaging 90–114 mm Hg. *JAMA* 1970; 213:1143–52.

Veterans Affairs High-Density Lipoprotein Cholesterol Intervention Trial Study Group. *N Engl J Med* 1999; 341:410–418.

R Virchow. *Cellular Pathology.* London: John Churchill, 1858.

ZJ Ward, SN Bleich, AL Cradock, JL Barrett, CM Giles, C Flax, MW Long, CL Gortmaker. Projected U.S. state-level prevalence of adult obesity and severe obesity. *N Engl J Med* 2019; 381:2440–2450. DOI: 10.1056/NEJMsa1909301.

DB Waters, EL Alderman, J Hsia, BV Howard, FR Cobb, WJ Rogers, P Ouyang, P Thompson, JC Tardif, L Higginson, V Bittner, M Steffes, DJ Gordon, M Proschan, N Younnes, J Verter. Effects of hormone replacement therapy and antioxidant vitamin supplements on coronary atherosclerosis in postmenopausal women. *JAMA* 2002; 288:2432–2440.

PK Whelton, RM Carey, WS Aronow, DE Casey, KJ Collins, CD Himmelfarb, SM DePalma, S Goldring, KA Jamerson, DW Jones, EJ MasLaughlin, P Munter, B Ovbiagele, SC Smith, CC Spencer, RS Stafford, SJ Taler, RJ Thomas, KA Williams, JD Williamson, JT Wright. 2017 ACC/AHA/AAPA/ABC/ACPM/AGS/APhA/ASH/ASPC/NMA/PCNA Guideline for the Prevention, Detection, Evaluation, and Management of High Blood Pressure in Adults: A Report of the American College of Cardiology/American Heart Association Task Force on Clinical Practice Guidelines. *Circulation* 2018; 138:e484-e594. DOI: 10.1161/CIR.0000000000000596. https://www.ahajournals.org/doi/pdf/10.1161/CIR.0000000000000596.

PD White. *Heart Disease.* New York: Macmillan, second edition, 1937.

WB White, CP Cannon, SR Heller, SE Nissen, RM Bergenstal, GL Bakris, AT Perez, PR Fleck, CR Mehta, S Kupfer, C Wilson, WC Cushman, F Zannad, for the Examine Investigators. Alogliptin after acute coronary syndrome in patients with type 2 diabetes. *N Engl J Med* 2013; 369:1327–1335. DOI: 10.1056/NEJMoa1305889.

WHO cooperative trial on primary prevention of ischaemic heart disease with clofibrate to lower serum cholesterol: final mortality follow-up. *Lancet* 1984; 2(8403):600–604.

The Women's Health Initiative Study Group. Design of the Women's Health Initiative Clinical Trial and Observational Study. *Controlled Clin Trials* 1998; 19:61–109.

The Women's Health Initiative Steering Committee. Effects of conjugated equine estrogen in postmenopausal women with hysterectomy. The Women's Health Initiative randomized controlled trial. *JAMA* 2004; 291:1701–1712.

World Health Organization 2009. Global Health Risks. Mortality and burden of disease attributable to selected major risks. ISBN 978 92 4 56387 1. https://www.who.int/healthinfo/global_burden_disease/GlobalHealthRisks_report_full.pdf.

Bibliography

World Health Rankings. Live Longer Live Better. https://www.world lifeexpectancy.com/cause-of-death/coronary-heart-disease/by-country/.

RM Worth, H Kato, GG Rhoads, A Kagan, SL Syme. Epidemiologic studies of coronary heart disease and stroke in Japanese men living in Japan, Hawaii and California: mortality. *Am J Epidemiol* 1975; 102:481–490.

The Writing Group for the PEPI Trial. Effects of Estrogen or Estrogen/Progestin Regimens on Heart Disease Risk Factors in Postmenopausal Women. The Postmenopausal Estrogen/Progestin Interventions (PEPI) Trial. *JAMA* 1995; 273:199–208.

Writing Group for the Women's Health Study. Risks and benefits of estrogen plus progestin in healthy postmenopausal women. Principal results from the Women's Health Initiative randomized controlled trial. *JAMA* 2002; 288:321–333.

RW Yeh, S Sydney, M Chandra, M Sorel, JV Selby, AS Go. Population trends in the incidence and outcomes of acute myocardial infarction. *N Engl J Med* 2010; 362:2155–2165.

J Zhong, S Kankanala, S Rajagopalan. DPP4 inhibition: insights from the bench and recent clinical studies. *Curr Opin Lipidol* 2016; 27:484–492. doi: 10.1097/MOL.0000000000000340.

INDEX

Index

Index

Index

Index